MW00651260

上海市重点图书

Full View of Yangtze River Pharmaceuticals Group (Taizhou,Jiangsu,China)

扬子江药业集团全景（中国·江苏·泰州）

A Newly Compiled
Practical English-Chinese Library
of Traditional Chinese Medicine
(英汉对照)新编实用中医文库

General Compiler-in-Chief Zuo Yanfu
总主编 左言富
Translators-in-Chief
Zhu Zhongbao Huang Yuezhong Tao Jinwen Li Zhaoguo
总编译 朱忠宝 黄月中 陶锦文 李照国(执行)

Compiled by Nanjing University of Traditional Chinese Medicine
Translated by Shanghai University of Traditional Chinese Medicine
南京中医药大学 主编
上海中医药大学 主译

SCIENCE OF CHINESE MATERIA MEDICA

中药学

Examiner-in-Chief	Chen Songyu
Compiler-in-Chief	Tang Decai
Compilers	Yao Yingzhi
	Yuan Ying
Translator-in-Chief	Xun Jianying
Translators	Zhang Wei
	Jing Zhen
	Yu Xin

主 审 陈松育
主 编 唐德才
编 者 姚映芷
袁 颖
主 译 寻建英
译 者 张 维
荆 蓁
于 新

PUBLISHING HOUSE OF SHANGHAI UNIVERSITY
OF TRADITIONAL CHINESE MEDICINE
上海中医药大学出版社

Publishing House of Shanghai University of Traditional Chinese Medicine
530 Lingling Road, Shanghai, 200032, China

Science of Chinese Materia Medica
Compiler-in-Chief Tang Decai Translator-in-Chief Xun Jianying
(A Newly Compiled Practical English-Chinese Library of Traditional Chinese Medicine General Compiler-in-Chief Zuo Yanfu)

All rights reserved. No part of this book may be reproduced, stored in a retrieval system, or transmitted in any form or by any means, electronic, mechanical, photocopying, recording or otherwise, without the prior written permission in writing of the Publisher.

ISBN 7-81010-658-9/R·624 paperback
ISBN 7-81010-682-1/R·647 hardback
Printed in Shanghai Xinhua Printing Works

图书在版编目(CIP)数据

中药学/唐德才主编;寻建英主译.—上海:上海中医药大学出版社,2003
(英汉对照新编实用中医文库/左言富总主编)
ISBN 7-81010-658-9

Ⅰ.中... Ⅱ.①唐...②寻... Ⅲ.中药学—英、汉 Ⅳ.R28

中国版本图书馆CIP数据核字(2003)第010455号

中药学 主编 唐德才 主译 寻建英

上海中医药大学出版社出版发行 (零陵路530号 邮政编码200032)
新华书店上海发行所经销 上海新华印刷厂印刷
开本 787 mm×1092 mm 1/18 印张 23.333 字数 557千字 印数 1—3 600册
版次 2003年2月第1版 印次 2003年2月第1次印刷

ISBN 7-81010-658-9/R·624 定价 56.10元

Compilation Board of the Library

Honorary Director Zhang Wenkang

General Advisor Chen Keji Xu Jingren

Advisors (Listed in the order of the number of strokes in the Chinese names)

Gan Zuwang You Songxin Liu Zaipeng Xu Zhiyin
Sun Tong Song Liren Zhang Minqing Jin Shi
Jin Miaowen Shan Zhaowei Zhou Fuyi Shi Zhen
Xu Jingfan Tang Shuhua Cao Shihong Fu Weimin

International Advisors M. S. Khan (Ireland) Alessandra Gulí (Italy) Secondo Scarsella (Italy) Raymond K. Carroll (Australia) Shulan Tang (Britain) Glovanni Maciocia (Britain) David Molony (America) Tzu Kuo Shih (America) Isigami Hiroshi (Japan) Helmut Ziegler (Germany)

Director Xiang Ping

Executive Director Zuo Yanfu

Executive Vice-Directors Ma Jian Du Wendong Li Zhaoguo

Vice-Directors Huang Chenghui Wu Kunping Liu Shenlin Wu Mianhua Chen Diping Cai Baochang

Members (Listed in the order of the number of strokes in the Chinese names)

Ding Anwei Ding Shuhua Yu Yong Wan Lisheng Wang Xu
Wang Xudong Wang Lingling Wang Lufen Lu Zijie Shen Junlong
Liu Yu Liu Yueguang Yan Daonan Yang Gongfu Min Zhongsheng
Wu Changguo Wu Yongjun Wu Jianlong He Wenbin
He Shuxun (specially invited) He Guixiang Wang Yue
Wang Shouchuan Shen Daqing Zhang Qing Chen Yonghui
Chen Tinghan (specially invited) Shao Jianmin Lin Xianzeng (specially invited)
Lin Duanmei (specially invited) Yue Peiping Jin Hongzhu
Zhou Ligao (specially invited) Zhao Xia Zhao Jingsheng Hu Lie
Hu Kui Zha Wei Yao Yingzhi Yuan Ying Xia Youbing
Xia Dengjie Ni Yun Xu Hengze Guo Haiying Tang Chuanjian
Tang Decai Ling Guizhen (specially invited) Tan Yong Huang Guicheng
Mei Xiaoyun Cao Guizhu Jiang Zhongqiu Zeng Qingqi Zhai Yachun
Fan Qiaoling

《(英汉对照)新编实用中医文库》编纂委员会

名誉主任 张文康

总 顾 问 陈可冀 徐镜人

顾　　问 (按姓氏笔画为序)

干祖望 尤松鑫 刘再朋 许芝银 孙 桐 宋立人 张民庆 金 实
金妙文 单兆伟 周福贻 施 震 徐景藩 唐蜀华 曹世宏 符为民

外籍顾问

萨利姆(爱尔兰) 亚历山大·古丽(意大利) 卡塞拉·塞肯多(意大利)
雷蒙特·凯·卡罗(澳大利亚) 汤淑兰(英国) 马万里(英国)
大卫·莫罗尼(美国) 施祖谷(美国) 石上博(日本) 赫尔木特(德国)

主　　任 项 平

执行主任 左言富

执行副主任 马 健 杜文东 李照国

副 主 任 黄成惠 吴坤平 刘沈林 吴勉华 陈涤平 蔡宝昌

编　　委 (按姓氏笔画为序)

丁安伟 丁淑华 于 勇 万力生 王 旭
王旭东 王玲玲 王鲁芬 卢子杰 申俊龙
刘 玉 刘跃光 严道南 杨公服 闵仲生
吴昌国 吴拥军 吴建龙 何文彬 何树勋(特邀)
何贵翔 汪 悦 汪受传 沈大庆 张 庆
陈永辉 陈廷汉(特邀) 邵健民 林显增(特邀)
林端美(特邀) 岳沛平 金宏柱 周礼杲(特邀)
赵 霞 赵京生 胡 烈 胡 葵 查 炜
姚映芷 袁 颖 夏有兵 夏登杰 倪 云
徐恒泽 郭海英 唐传俭 唐德才 凌桂珍(特邀)
谈 勇 黄桂成 梅晓芸 曹贵珠 蒋中秋
曾庆琪 翟亚春 樊巧玲

Translation Committee of the Library

Advisors Shao Xundao Ou Ming

Translators-in-Chief Zhu Zhongbao Huang Yuezhong Tao Jinwen

Executive Translator-in-Chief Li Zhaoguo

Vice-Translators-in-Chief (Listed in the order of the number of strokes in the Chinese names)

Xun Jianying Li Yong'an Zhang Qingrong Zhang Dengfeng Yang Hongying Huang Guoqi Xie Jinhua

Translators (Listed in the order of the number of strokes in the Chinese names)

Yu Xin	Wang Ruihui	Tian Kaiyu	Shen Guang
Lan Fengli	Cheng Peili	Zhu Wenxiao	Zhu Yuqin
Zhu Jinjiang	Zhu Guixiang	Le Yimin	Liu Shengpeng
Li Jingyun	Yang Ying	Yang Mingshan	He Yingchun
Zhang Jie	Zhang Haixia	Zhang Wei	Chen Renying
Zhou Yongming	Zhou Suzhen	Qu Yusheng	Zhao Junqing
Jing Zhen	Hu Kewu	Xu Qilong	Xu Yao
Guo Xiaomin	Huang Xixuan	Cao Lijuan	Kang Qin
Dong Jing	Qin Baichang	Zeng Haiping	Lou Jianhua
Lai Yuezhen	Bao Bai	Pei Huihua	Xue Junmei
Dai Wenjun	Wei Min		

Office of the Translation Committee

Director Yang Mingshan

Secretaries Xu Lindi Chen Li

《(英汉对照)新编实用中医文库》编译委员会

顾　　问　邵循道　欧　明

总 编 译　朱忠宝　黄月中　陶锦文

执行总编译　李照国

副 总 编 译　(按姓氏笔画为序)

寻建英　李永安　张庆荣　张登峰　杨洪英　黄国琪　谢金华

编 译 者　(按姓氏笔画为序)

于　新　王瑞辉　田开宇　申　光　兰凤利　成培莉　朱文晓
朱玉琴　朱金江　朱桂香　乐毅敏　刘升鹏　李经蕴　杨　莹
杨明山　何迎春　张　杰　张海峡　张　维　陈仁英　周永明
周素贞　屈榆生　赵俊卿　荆　蓁　胡克武　徐启龙　徐　瑶
郭小民　黄熙璇　曹丽娟　康　勤　董　晶　覃百长　曾海苹
楼建华　赖月珍　鲍　白　裴慧华　薛俊梅　戴文军　魏　敏

编译委员会办公室

主　任　杨明山

秘　书　徐林娣　陈　力

Approval Committee of the Library

Director Li Zhenji

Vice-Directors Shen Zhixiang Chen Xiaogu Zhou Zhongying Wang Canhui Gan Zuwang Jiang Yuren

Members (Listed in the order of the number of strokes in the Chinese names)

Ding Renqiang	Ding Xiaohong	Wang Xinhua	You Benlin
Shi Yanhua	Qiao Wenlei	Yi Sumei	Li Fei
Li Guoding	Yang Zhaomin	Lu Mianmian	Chen Songyu
Shao Mingxi	Shi Bingbing	Yao Xin	Xia Guicheng
Gu Yuehua	Xu Fusong	Gao Yuanhang	Zhu Fangshou
Tao Jinwen	Huang Yage	Fu Zhiwen	Cai Li

General Compiler-in-Chief Zuo Yanfu

Executive Vice-General-Compilers-in-Chief Ma Jian Du Wendong

Vice-General-Compilers-in-Chief (Listed in the order of the number of strokes in the Chinese names)

Ding Shuhua	Wang Xudong	Wang Lufen	Yan Daonan
Wu Changguo	Wang Shouchuan	Wang Yue	Chen Yonghui
Jin Hongzhu	Zhao Jingsheng	Tang Decai	Tan Yong
Huang Guicheng	Zhai Yachun	Fan Qiaoling	

Office of the Compilation Board Committee

Directors Ma Jian Du Wendong

Vice-Directors Wu Jianlong Zhu Changren

Publisher Zhu Bangxian

Chinese Editors (Listed in the order of the number of strokes in the Chinese names)

Ma Shengying	Wang Lingli	Wang Deliang	He Qianqian
Shen Chunhui	Zhang Xingjie	Zhou Dunhua	Shan Baozhi
Jiang Shuiyin	Qin Baoping	Qian Jingzhuang	Fan Yuqi
Pan Zhaoxi			

English Editors Shan Baozhi Jiang Shuiyin Xiao Yuanchun

Cover Designer Wang Lei

Layout Designer Xu Guomin

《(英汉对照)新编实用中医文库》审定委员会

主　　任　李振吉

副 主 任　沈志祥　陈啸谷　周仲瑛　王灿晖　干祖望　江育仁

委　　员　(按姓氏笔画为序)

丁仁强　丁晓红　王新华　尤本林　石燕华　乔文雷　衣素梅　李　飞

李国鼎　杨兆民　陆绵绵　陈松育　邵明熙　施冰冰　姚　欣　夏桂成

顾月华　徐福松　高远航　诸方受　陶锦文　黄雅各　傅志文　蔡　丽

总 主 编　左言富

执行副总主编　马　健　杜文东

副总主编　(按姓氏笔画为序)

丁淑华　王旭东　王鲁芬　严道南　吴昌国　汪　悦　汪受传　陈永辉

金宏柱　赵京生　唐德才　谈　勇　黄桂成　翟亚春　樊巧玲

编纂委员会办公室

主　　任　马　健　杜文东

副 主 任　吴建龙　朱长仁

出 版 人　朱邦贤

中文责任编辑　(按姓氏笔画为序)

马胜英　王玲琍　王德良　何倩倩　沈春晖　张杏洁　周敦华　单宝枝

姜水印　秦葆平　钱静庄　樊玉琦　潘朝曦

英文责任编辑　单宝枝　姜水印　肖元春

美术编辑　王　磊

技术编辑　徐国民

Foreword I

As we are walking into the 21st century, "health for all" is still an important task for the World Health Organization (WHO) to accomplish in the new century. The realization of "health for all" requires mutual cooperation and concerted efforts of various medical sciences, including traditional medicine. WHO has increasingly emphasized the development of traditional medicine and has made fruitful efforts to promote its development. Currently the spectrum of diseases is changing and an increasing number of diseases are difficult to cure. The side effects of chemical drugs have become more and more evident. Furthermore, both the governments and peoples in all countries are faced with the problem of high cost of medical treatment. Traditional Chinese medicine (TCM), the complete system of traditional medicine in the world with unique theory and excellent clinical curative effects, basically meets the need to solve such problems. Therefore, bringing TCM into full play in medical treatment and healthcare will certainly become one of the hot points in the world medical business in the 21st century.

Various aspects of work need to be done to promote the course of the internationalization of TCM, especially the compilation of works and textbooks suitable for international readers. The impending new century has witnessed the compilation of such a

序　一

人类即将迈入21世纪,"人人享有卫生保健"仍然是新世纪世界卫生工作面临的重要任务。实现"人人享有卫生保健"的宏伟目标,需要包括传统医药学在内的多种医学学科的相互协作与共同努力。世界卫生组织越来越重视传统医药学的发展,并为推动其发展做出了卓有成效的工作。目前,疾病谱正在发生变化,难治疾病不断增多,化学药品的毒副作用日益显现,日趋沉重的医疗费用困扰着各国政府和民众。中医药学是世界传统医学体系中最完整的传统医学,其独到的学科理论和突出的临床疗效,较符合当代社会和人们解决上述难题的需要。因此,科学有效地发挥中医药学的医疗保健作用,必将成为21世纪世界卫生工作的特点之一。

加快中医药走向世界的步伐,还有很多的工作要做,特别是适合国外读者学习的中医药著作、教材的编写是极其重要的方面。在新千年来临之际,由南京中医药大学

series of books known as *A Newly Compiled Practical English-Chinese Library of Traditional Chinese Medicine* published by the Publishing House of Shanghai University of TCM, compiled by Nanjing University of TCM and translated by Shanghai University of TCM. Professor Zuo Yanfu, the general compiler-in-chief of this Library, is a person who sets his mind on the international dissemination of TCM. He has compiled *General Survey on TCM Abroad*, a monograph on the development and state of TCM abroad. This Library is another important works written by the experts organized by him with the support of Nanjing University of TCM and Shanghai University of TCM. The compilation of this Library is done with consummate ingenuity and according to the development of TCM abroad. The compilers, based on the premise of preserving the genuineness and gist of TCM, have tried to make the contents concise, practical and easy to understand, making great efforts to introduce the abstruse ideas of TCM in a scientific and simple way as well as expounding the prevention and treatment of diseases which are commonly encountered abroad and can be effectively treated by TCM.

主编、上海中医药大学主译、上海中医药大学出版社出版的《(英汉对照)新编实用中医文库》的即将问世,正是新世纪中医药国际传播更快发展的预示。本套文库总主编左言富教授是中医药学国际传播事业的有心人,曾主编研究国外中医药发展状况的专著《国外中医药概览》。本套文库的编撰,是他在南京中医药大学和上海中医药大学支持下,组织许多著名专家共同完成的又一重要专著。本套文库的作者们深谙国外的中医药发展现状,编写颇具匠心,在注重真实,不失精华的前提下,突出内容的简明、实用,易于掌握,力求科学而又通俗地介绍中医药学的深奥内容,重点阐述国外常见而中医药颇具疗效的疾病的防治。

This Library encompasses a systematic summarization of the teaching experience accumulated in Nanjing University of TCM and Shanghai University of TCM that run the collaborating centers of traditional medicine and the international training centers on acupuncture and moxibustion set by WHO. I am sure that the publication of this Library will further promote the development of traditional Chinese med-

本套文库蕴含了南京中医药大学和上海中医药大学作为WHO传统医学合作中心、国际针灸培训中心多年留学生教学的实践经验和系统总结,更为全面、系统、准确地向世界传播中医药学。相信本书的出版将对中医更好地走向世界,让世界更好地了解中医产生更

icine abroad and enable the whole world to have a better understanding of traditional Chinese medicine.

为积极的影响。

Professor Zhu Qingsheng

Vice-Minister of Health Ministry of the People's Republic of China

Director of the State Administrative Bureau of TCM

December 14, 2000 Beijing

朱庆生教授

中华人民共和国卫生部副部长

国家中医药管理局局长

2000 年 12 月 14 日于北京

Foreword Ⅱ

Before the existence of the modern medicine, human beings depended solely on herbal medicines and other therapeutic methods to treat diseases and preserve health. Such a practice gave rise to the establishment of various kinds of traditional medicine with unique theory and practice, such as traditional Chinese medicine, Indian medicine and Arabian medicine, etc. Among these traditional systems of medicine, traditional Chinese medicine is a most extraordinary one based on which traditional Korean medicine and Japanese medicine have evolved.

Even in the 21st century, traditional medicine is still of great vitality. In spite of the fast development of modern medicine, traditional medicine is still disseminated far and wide. In many developing countries, most of the people in the rural areas still depend on traditional medicine and traditional medical practitioners to meet the need for primary healthcare. Even in the countries with advanced modern medicine, more and more people have begun to accept traditional medicine and other therapeutic methods, such as homeopathy, osteopathy and naturopathy, etc..

With the change of the economy, culture and living style in various regions as well as the aging in the world population, the disease spectrum has changed. And such a change has paved the way for the new application of traditional medicine. Besides,

序　二

在现代医学形成之前，人类一直依赖草药和其他一些疗法治病强身，从而发展出许多有理论、有实践的传统医学，例如中医学、印度医学、阿拉伯医学等。中医学是世界林林总总的传统医学中的一支奇葩，在它的基础上还衍生出朝鲜传统医学和日本汉方医学。在跨入 21 世纪的今天，古老的传统医学依然焕发着活力，非但没有因现代医学的发展而式微，其影响还有增无减，人们对传统医学的价值也有了更深刻的体会和认识。在许多贫穷国家，大多数农村人口仍然依赖传统医学疗法和传统医务工作者来满足他们对初级卫生保健的需求。在现代医学占主导地位的许多国家，传统医学及其他一些“另类疗法”，诸如顺势疗法、整骨疗法、自然疗法等，也越来越被人们所接受。

伴随着世界各地经济、文化和生活的变革以及世界人口的老龄化，世界疾病谱也发生了变化。传统医学有了新的应用，而新疾病所引起的新需求以及现代医学的成

the new requirements initiated by the new diseases and the achievements and limitations of modern medicine have also created challenges for traditional medicine.

就与局限又向传统医学提出了挑战,推动它进一步发展。

WHO sensed the importance of traditional medicine to human health early in the 1970s and have made great efforts to develop traditional medicine. At the 29th world health congress held in 1976, the item of traditional medicine was adopted in the working plan of WHO. In the following world health congresses, a series of resolutions were passed to demand the member countries to develop, utilize and study traditional medicine according to their specific conditions so as to reduce medical expenses for the realization of "health for all".

世界卫生组织早在20世纪70年代就意识到传统医学对人类健康的重要性,并为推动传统医学的发展做了努力。1976年举行的第二十九届世界卫生大会将传统医学项目纳入世界卫生组织的工作计划。其后的各届世界卫生大会又通过了一系列决议,要求各成员国根据本国的条件发展、使用和研究传统医学,以降低医疗费用,促进"人人享有初级卫生保健"这一目标的实现。

WHO has laid great stress on the scientific content, safe and effective application of traditional medicine. It has published and distributed a series of booklets on the scientific, safe and effective use of herbs and acupuncture and moxibustion. It has also made great contributions to the international standardization of traditional medical terms. The safe and effective application of traditional medicine has much to do with the skills of traditional medical practitioners. That is why WHO has made great efforts to train them. WHO has run 27 collaborating centers in the world which have made great contributions to the training of acupuncturists and traditional medical practitioners. Nanjing University of TCM and Shanghai University of TCM run the collaborating centers with WHO. In recent years it has, with the cooperation of WHO and other countries, trained about ten thousand international students from over

世界卫生组织历来重视传统医学的科学、安全和有效使用。它出版和发行了一系列有关科学、安全、有效使用草药和针灸的技术指南,并在专用术语的标准化方面做了许多工作。传统医学的使用是否做到安全和有效,是与使用传统疗法的医务工作者的水平密不可分的。因此,世界卫生组织也十分重视传统医学培训工作。它在全世界有27个传统医学合作中心,这些中心对培训合格的针灸师及使用传统疗法的其他医务工作者做出了积极的贡献。南京中医药大学、上海中医药大学是世界卫生组织传统医学合作中心之一,近年来与世界卫生组织和其他国家合作,培训了近万名来自90多个国

90 countries.

家和地区的留学生。

In order to further promote the dissemination of traditional Chinese medicine in the world, *A Newly Compiled Practical English-Chinese Library of Traditional Chinese Medicine*, compiled by Nanjing University of TCM with Professor Zuo Yanfu as the general compiler-in-chief and published by the Publishing House of Shanghai University of TCM, aims at systematic, accurate and concise expounding of traditional Chinese medical theory and introducing clinical therapeutic methods of traditional medicine according to modern medical nomenclature of diseases. Undoubtedly, this series of books will be the practical textbooks for the beginners with certain English level and the international enthusiasts with certain level of Chinese to study traditional Chinese medicine. Besides, this series of books can also serve as reference books for WHO to internationally standardize the nomenclature of acupuncture and moxibustion.

在南京中医药大学左言富教授主持下编纂的、由上海中医药大学出版社出版的《(英汉对照)新编实用中医文库》,旨在全面、系统、准确、简要地阐述中医基础理论,并结合西医病名介绍中医临床治疗方法。因此,这套文库可望成为具有一定英语水平的初学中医者和具有一定中文水平的外国中医爱好者学习基础中医学的系列教材。这套文库也可供世界卫生组织在编写国际针灸标准术语时参考。

The scientific, safe and effective use of traditional medicine will certainly further promote the development of traditional medicine and traditional medicine will undoubtedly make more and more contributions to human health in the 21st century.

传统医学的科学、安全、有效使用必将进一步推动传统医学的发展。传统医学一定会在 21 世纪为人类健康做出更大的贡献。

Zhang Xiaorui

WHO Coordination Officer

December, 2000

张小瑞

世界卫生组织传统医学协调官员

2000 年 12 月

Preface

The Publishing House of Shanghai University of TCM published *A Practical English-Chinese Library of Traditional Chinese Medicine* in 1990. The Library has been well-known in the world ever since and has made great contributions to the dissemination of traditional Chinese medicine in the world. In view of the fact that 10 years has passed since its publication and that there are certain errors in the explanation of traditional Chinese medicine in the Library, the Publishing House has invited Nanjing University of TCM and Shanghai University of TCM to organize experts to recompile and translate the Library.

Nanjing University of TCM and Shanghai University of TCM are well-known for their advantages in higher education of traditional Chinese medicine and compilation of traditional Chinese medical textbooks. The compilation of *A Newly Compiled Practical English-Chinese Library of Traditional Chinese Medicine* has absorbed the rich experience accumulated by Nanjing University of Traditional Chinese Medicine in training international students of traditional Chinese medicine. Compared with the previous Library, the Newly Compiled Library has made great improvements in many aspects, fully demonstrating the academic system of traditional Chinese medicine. The whole series of books has systematically introduced the basic theory and thera-

前　言

上海中医药大学出版社于1990年出版了一套《(英汉对照)实用中医文库》，发行10年来，在海内外产生了较大影响，对推动中医学走向世界起了积极作用。考虑到该套丛书发行已久，对中医学术体系的介绍还有一些欠妥之处，因此，上海中医药大学出版社特邀南京中医药大学主编、上海中医药大学主译，组织全国有关专家编译出版《(英汉对照)新编实用中医文库》。

《(英汉对照)新编实用中医文库》的编纂，充分发挥了南京中医药大学和上海中医药大学在高等中医药教育教学和教材编写方面的优势，吸收了作为WHO传统医学合作中心之一的两校，多年来从事中医药学国际培训和留学生学历教育的经验，对原《(英汉对照)实用中医文库》整体结构作了大幅度调整，以突出中医学术主体内容。全套丛书系统介绍了中医基础理论和中医辨证论治方法，讲解了中药学和方剂学的基本理论，详细介绍了236味中药、152首常用方剂和100种常用中成药；详述

peutic methods based on syndrome differentiation, expounding traditional Chinese pharmacy and prescriptions; explaining 236 herbs, 152 prescriptions and 100 commonly-used patent drugs; elucidating 264 methods for differentiating syndromes and treating commonly-encountered and frequently-encountered diseases in internal medicine, surgery, gynecology, pediatrics, traumatology and orthopedics, ophthalmology and otorhinolaryngology; introducing the basic methods and theory of acupuncture and moxibustion, massage (tuina), life cultivation and rehabilitation, including 70 kinds of diseases suitable for acupuncture and moxibustion, 38 kinds of diseases for massage, examples of life cultivation and over 20 kinds of commonly encountered diseases treated by rehabilitation therapies in traditional Chinese medicine. For better understanding of traditional Chinese medicine, the books are neatly illustrated. There are 296 line graphs and 30 colored pictures in the Library with necessary indexes, making it more comprehensive, accurate and systematic in disseminating traditional Chinese medicine in the countries and regions where English is the official language.

264 种临床内、外、妇、儿、骨伤、眼、耳鼻喉各科常见病与多发病的中医辨证论治方法;系统论述针灸、推拿、中医养生康复的基本理论和基本技能,介绍针灸治疗病种 70 种、推拿治疗病种 38 种、各类养生实例及 20 余种常见病证的中医康复实例。为了更加直观地介绍中医药学术,全书选用线图 296 幅、彩图 30 幅,并附有必要的索引,从而更加全面、系统、准确地向使用英语的国家和地区传播中医学术,推进中医学走向世界,造福全人类。

This Library is characterized by following features:

1. Scientific Based on the development of TCM in education and research in the past 10 years, efforts have been made in the compilation to highlight the gist of TCM through accurate theoretical exposition and clinical practice, aiming at introducing authentic theory and practice to the world.

2. Systematic This Library contains 14 sepa-

本丛书主要具有以下特色:

(1) 科学性:在充分吸收近 10 余年来中医教学和科学研究最新进展的基础上,坚持突出中医学术精华,理论阐述准确,临床切合实用,向世界各国介绍"原汁原味"的中医药学术。

(2) 系统性:本套丛书包括《中医基础理论》、《中医诊断学》、《中药

rate fascicles, i. e. *Basic Theory of Traditional Chinese Medicine*, *Diagnostics of Traditional Chinese Medicine*, *Science of Chinese Materia Medica*, *Science of Prescriptions*, *Internal Medicine of Traditional Chinese Medicine*, *Surgery of Traditional Chinese Medicine*, *Gynecology of Traditional Chinese Medicine*, *Pediatrics of Traditional Chinese Medicine*, *Traumatology and Orthopedics of Traditional Chinese Medicine*, *Ophthalmology of Traditional Chinese Medicine*, *Otorhinolaryngology of Traditional Chinese Medicine*, *Chinese Acupuncture and Moxibustion*, *Chinese Tuina (Massage)*, *and Life Cultivation and Rehabilitation of Traditional Chinese Medicine*.

3. Practical Compared with the previous Library, the Newly Compiled Library has made great improvements and supplements, systematically introducing therapeutic methods for treating over 200 kinds of commonly and frequently encountered diseases, focusing on training basic clinical skills in acupuncture and moxibustion, tuina therapy, life cultivation and rehabilitation with clinical case reports.

4. Standard This Library is reasonable in structure, distinct in categorization, standard in terminology and accurate in translation with full consideration of habitual expressions used in countries and regions with English language as the mother tongue.

学》、《方剂学》、《中医内科学》、《中医外科学》、《中医妇科学》、《中医儿科学》、《中医骨伤科学》、《中医眼科学》、《中医耳鼻喉科学》、《中国针灸》、《中国推拿》、《中医养生康复学》14 个分册，系统反映了中医各学科建设与发展的最新成果。

(3) 实用性：临床各科由原来的上下两册，根据学科的发展进行大幅度的调整和增补，比较详细地介绍了 200 多种各科常见病、多发病的中医治疗方法，重点突出了针灸、推拿、养生康复等临床基本技能训练，并附有部分临证实例。

(4) 规范性：全书结构合理，层次清晰，对中医各学科名词术语表述规范，对中医英语翻译执行了更为严格的标准化方案，同时又充分考虑到使用英语国家和地区人们的语言习惯和表达方式。

This series of books is not only practical for the beginners with certain competence of English to study TCM, but also can serve as authentic textbooks for international students in universities and colleges of TCM in China to study and practice TCM. For those from TCM field who are going to go

本丛书不仅能满足具有一定英语水平的初学中医者系统学习中医之用，而且也为中医院校外国留学生教育及国内外开展中医双语教学提供了目前最具权威的系列教材，同时也是中医出国人员进

abroad to do academic exchange, this series of books will provide them with unexpected convenience.

Professor Xiang Ping, President of Nanjing University of TCM, is the director of the Compilation Board. Professor Zuo Yanfu from Nanjing University of TCM, General Compiler-in-Chief, is in charge of the compilation. Zhang Wenkang, Minister of Health Ministry, is invited to be the honorary director of the Editorial Board. Li Zhenji, Vice-Director of the State Administrative Bureau of TCM, is invited to be the director of the Approval Committee. Chen Keji, academician of China Academy, is invited to be the General Advisor. International advisors invited are Mr. M. S. Khan, Chairman of Ireland Acupuncture and Moxibustion Fund; Miss Alessandra Gulí, Chairman of "Nanjing Association" in Rome, Italy; Doctor Secondo Scarsella, Chief Editor of YI DAO ZA ZHI; President Raymond K. Carroll from Australian Oriental Touching Therapy College; Ms. Shulan Tang, Academic Executive of ATCM in Britain; Mr. Glovanni Maciocia from Britain; Mr. David, Chairman of American Association of TCM; Mr. Tzu Kuo Shih, director of Chinese Medical Technique Center in Connecticut, America; Mr. Helmut Ziegler, director of TCM Center in Germany; and Mr. Isigami Hiroshi from Japan. Chen Ken, official of WHO responsible for the Western Pacific Region, has greatly encouraged the compilers in compiling this series of books. After the accomplishment of the compilation, Professor Zhu Qingsheng, Vice-Minister of Health Ministry and Director of the State Administrative Bureau of TCM, has set a high value on the books in his fore-

行中医药国际交流的重要工具书。

全书由南京中医药大学校长项平教授担任编委会主任、左言富教授任总主编，主持全书的编写。中华人民共和国卫生部张文康部长担任本丛书编委会名誉主任，国家中医药管理局李振吉副局长担任审定委员会主任，陈可冀院士欣然担任本丛书总顾问指导全书的编纂。爱尔兰针灸基金会主席萨利姆先生、意大利罗马"南京协会"主席亚历山大·古丽女士、意大利《医道》杂志主编卡塞拉·塞肯多博士、澳大利亚东方触觉疗法学院雷蒙特·凯·卡罗院长、英国中医药学会学术部长汤淑兰女士、英国马万里先生、美国中医师公会主席大卫先生、美国康州中华医疗技术中心主任施祖谷先生、德国中医中心主任赫尔木特先生、日本石上博先生担任本丛书特邀外籍顾问。世界卫生组织西太平洋地区官员陈恳先生对本丛书的编写给予了热情鼓励。全书完成后，卫生部副部长兼国家中医药管理局局长朱庆生教授给予了高度评价，并欣然为本书作序；WHO传统医学协调官员张小瑞对于本丛书的编写给予高度关注，百忙中也专为本书作序。我国驻外教育机构，特别是中国驻英国曼彻斯特领事张益群先生、中国驻美国休斯敦领事严美华

word for the Library. Zhang Xiaorui, an official from WHO's Traditional Medicine Program, has paid great attention to the compilation and written a foreword for the Library. The officials from the educational organizations of China in other countries have provided us with some useful materials in our compilation. They are Mr. Zhang Yiqun, China Consul to Manchester in Britain; Miss Yan Meihua, Consul to Houston in America; Mr. Wang Jiping, First Secretary in the Educational Department in the Embassy of China to France; and Mr. Gu Shengying, the Second Secretary in the Educational Department in the Embassy of China to Germany. We are grateful to them all.

The Compilers
December, 2000

女士、中国驻法国使馆教育处一秘王季平先生、中国驻德国使馆教育处二秘郭胜英先生在与我们工作联系中，间接提供了不少有益资料。在此一并致以衷心感谢！

编　者
2000年12月

Note for Compilation

编写说明

Chinese medicinal herbs are used in TCM (Traditional Chinese Medicine) as the main means to prevent and treat diseases and maintain health. As one of the basic subjects of Traditional Chinese Medicine, Chinese Materia Medica centers the elaboration and study on the theories and clinical practice of Chinese medicinal herbs. This book, under the guidance of the theories of Traditional Chinese Medicine and according to practical and effective principles, systematically introduces the basic theories concerning traditional Chinese Materia Medica, methods and principles in using Chinese medicinal herbs as well. The whole book consists of General Introduction, Specific Discussions and Appendix.

General Introduction mainly introduces common knowledge about Chinese medicinal herbs, including properties, processing, compatibility, contraindication, dosage and administration of Chinese medicinal herbs.

Specific Discussions, containing 236 kinds of Chinese medicinal herbs (including 10 kinds of added medicines), is divided into 16 chapters according to their specific efficacy. Each sort of Chinese medicinal herbs is illustrated in the order of formal name, source, applying parts, habitat, collecting and processing methods, properties, efficacy and application, usage and dosage as well as cautions, the efficacy and application of which are the focal points. The category of explanation particularly lays emphasis on

中药来自于天然药物，是中医用来防治疾病、保障健康的主要手段。中药学是阐述、研究中药的基础理论和临床应用的学科，是中医药各专业的基础学科之一。本书以中医药传统理论为指导，从实用、有效的原则出发，系统介绍传统中药学的基本理论和中药的使用原则与方法。全书包括总论、各论、附录三部分。

总论部分主要介绍中药的一般知识。内容包括中药的性能、炮制、配伍、用药禁忌、剂量、煎服法等。

各论共收载常用中药 236 味（含附药 10 味），按主要功效分为十六章。各药按正名、药物来源、药用部位、主要产地、采集和炮制方法、药性、功效和应用、用法用量、使用注意等项分别说明，其中功效与应用是介绍的重点。另设说明项，主要介绍功效类似药物间的比较、附药运用及其他需要说明的事项等。药物的正名、来源、临

the comparison between some Chinese medicinal herbs which have similar actions, application of added medicines, and other items in need of further explanation, etc.. All of names, sources and clinical dosage appeared in the book are quoted from *the Pharmacopoeia of the People's Republic of China* (1995 Edition) as standard.

床用量均以《中华人民共和国药典》1995年版一部为规范依据。

Appendix contains index of Chinese medicinal herb Latin names. For convenience, the index of Latin names is arranged in the order of alphabets.

附录包括中药拉丁名索引，拉丁名索引按拉丁字母顺序排列，以便检索。

Compilers
December, 2000

编　者
2000年12月

Contents

General Introduction ······ 1

1 Properties and Actions of Chinese Medicinal Herbs ······ 1

1.1 Four natures and five flavors ······ 2

1.2 Lifting, lowering, floating and sinking ······ 7

1.3 Meridian tropism of Chinese medicinal herbs ······ 10

1.4 Toxicity ······ 13

2 Processing of Chinese Medicinal Herbs ······ 16

2.1 Purposes of processing Chinese medicinal herbs ······ 16

2.2 Methods of processing medicinal materials ······ 18

3 Compatibility of Chinese Medicinal Herbs ······ 24

4 Contraindication of Chinese Medicinal Herbs ······ 28

5 Dosage and Administration ······ 33

5.1 Dosage ······ 33

5.2 Administration ······ 35

Specific Discussions ······ 40

1 Diaphoretics or Exterior Syndrome Relieving Chinese Medicinal Herbs ······ 40

1.1 Diaphoretics with pungent-warm property ······ 41

Mahuang *Herba Ephedrae* ······ 42

Guizhi *Ramulus Cinnamomi* ······ 43

Zisuye *Folium Perillae* ······ 45

Xiangru *Herba Elsholtziae* ······ 47

Jingjie *Herba Schizonepetae* ······ 48

Fangfeng *Radix Saposhnikoviae* ······ 50

Qianghuo *Rhizoma et Radix Notopterygii* ······ 52

Xixin *Herba Asari* ······ 53

Cang'erzi *Fructus Xanthii* ······ 55

Xinyi *Flos Magnoliae* ······ 56

目　录

总论 …… 1
第一章　中药的性能 …… 1
　第一节　四气五味 …… 2
　第二节　升降浮沉 …… 7
　第三节　归经 …… 10
　第四节　毒性 …… 13
第二章　中药的炮制 …… 16
　第一节　炮制的目的 …… 16
　第二节　炮制的方法 …… 18
第三章　中药的配伍 …… 24
第四章　用药禁忌 …… 28
第五章　剂量与煎服法 …… 33
　第一节　剂量 …… 33
　第二节　煎服法 …… 35
各论 …… 40
第一章　解表药 …… 40
　第一节　辛温解表药 …… 41
　　麻黄 …… 42
　　桂枝 …… 43
　　紫苏叶 …… 45
　　香薷 …… 47
　　荆芥 …… 48
　　防风 …… 50
　　羌活 …… 52
　　细辛 …… 53
　　苍耳子 …… 55
　　辛夷 …… 56

1.2 Diaphoretics with pungent-cool property ··· 57
Bohe *Herba Menthae* ··· 57
Juhua *Flos Chrysanthemi* ··· 58
Chantui *Periostracum Cicadae* ··· 60
Niubangzi *Fructus Arctii* ··· 61
Sangye *Folium Mori* ··· 62
Chaihu *Radix Bupleuri* ··· 63
Gegen *Radix Puerariae* ··· 65
Shengma *Rhizoma Cimicifugae* ··· 67
2 Heat Clearing Chinese Medicinal Herbs ··· 70
2.1 Heat clearing and fire purging Chinese medicinal herbs ··· 72
Shigao *Gypsum Fibrosum* ··· 72
Zhimu *Rhizoma Anemarrhenae* ··· 74
Zhizi *Fructus Gardeniae* ··· 75
Xiakucao *Spica Prunellae* ··· 76
Lugen *Rhizoma Phragmitis* ··· 77
Tianhuafen *Radix Trichosanthis* ··· 79
Danzhuye *Herba Lophatheri* ··· 80
Juemingzi *Semen Cassiae* ··· 81
2.2 Chinese medicinal herbs for eliminating heat and dampness ··· 82
Huangqin *Radix Scutellariae* ··· 83
Huanglian *Rhizoma Coptidis* ··· 85
Huangbai *Cortex Phellodendri* ··· 88
Longdan *Radix Gentianae* ··· 90
Kushen *Radix Sophorae Flavescentis* ··· 91
2.3 Heat clearing and blood cooling Chinese medicinal herbs ··· 92
Shengdihuang *Radix Rehmanniae* ··· 93
Xuanshen *Radix Scrophulariae* ··· 95
Mudanpi *Cortex Moutan Radicis* ··· 97
Chishaoyao *Radix Paeoniae Rubra* ··· 98
Shuiniujiao *Cornu Bubali* ··· 100
2.4 Chinese medicinal herbs for eliminating heat and toxin ··· 101
Jinyinhua *Flos Lonicerae* ··· 101
Lianqiao *Fructus Forsythiae* ··· 103

第二节　辛凉解表药 …… 57
薄荷 …… 57
菊花 …… 58
蝉蜕 …… 60
牛蒡子 …… 61
桑叶 …… 62
柴胡 …… 63
葛根 …… 65
升麻 …… 67
第二章　清热药 …… 70
第一节　清热泻火药 …… 72
石膏 …… 72
知母 …… 74
栀子 …… 75
夏枯草 …… 76
芦根 …… 77
天花粉 …… 79
淡竹叶 …… 80
决明子 …… 81
第二节　清热燥湿药 …… 82
黄芩 …… 83
黄连 …… 85
黄柏 …… 88
龙胆 …… 90
苦参 …… 91
第三节　清热凉血药 …… 92
生地黄 …… 93
玄参 …… 95
牡丹皮 …… 97
赤芍药 …… 98
水牛角 …… 100
第四节　清热解毒药 …… 101
金银花 …… 101
连翘 …… 103

Zihuadiding *Herba Violae* ······ 104
Banlangen *Radix Isatidis* ······ 105
Qingdai *Indigo Naturalis* ······ 106
Chuanxinlian *Herba Andrographitis* ······ 108
Banbianlian *Herba Lobeliae Chinensis* ······ 109
Guanzhong *Rhizoma Dryopteris Crassirhizomae* ······ 110
Baitouweng *Radix Pulsatillae* ······ 111
Yuxingcao *Herba Houttuyniae* ······ 112
Jinqiaomai *Rhizoma Fagopyri Cymosi* ······ 113
Hongteng *Caulis Sargentodoxae* ······ 114
Baijiangcao *Herba Patriniae* ······ 115
2.5 Asthenic-heat clearing Chinese medicinal herbs ······ 116
Qinghao *Herba Artemisiae Annuae* ······ 117
Digupi *Cortex Lycii Radicis* ······ 118
Baiwei *Radix Cynanchi Atrati* ······ 119
Huhuanglian *Rhizoma Picrorrhizae* ······ 120
Yinchaihu *Radix Stellariae* ······ 122
3 Cathartics ······ 123
3.1 Purgatives ······ 123
Dahuang *Radix et Rhizoma Rhei* ······ 124
Mangxiao *Natrii Sulfas* ······ 127
Luhui *Aloe* ······ 129
Fanxieye *Folium Sennae* ······ 130
3.2 Moistening purgatives ······ 131
Huomaren *Fructus Cannabis* ······ 131
Yuliren *Semen Pruni* ······ 132
3.3 Drastic purgatives ······ 132
Gansui *Radix Euphorbiae Kansui* ······ 133
Daji *Radix Euphorbiae Pekinensis* ······ 134
Yuanhua *Flos Genkwa* ······ 135
Qianniuzi *Semen Pharbitidis* ······ 136
4 Dampness Removing Chinese Medicinal Herbs ······ 138
4.1 Antirheumatic Chinese medicinal herbs ······ 138
Duhuo *Radix Angelicae Pubescentis* ······ 139

紫花地丁 …… 104
板蓝根 …… 105
青黛 …… 106
穿心莲 …… 108
半边莲 …… 109
贯众 …… 110
白头翁 …… 111
鱼腥草 …… 112
金荞麦 …… 113
红藤 …… 114
败酱草 …… 115
第五节 清虚热药 …… 116
青蒿 …… 117
地骨皮 …… 118
白薇 …… 119
胡黄连 …… 120
银柴胡 …… 122
第三章 泻下药 …… 123
第一节 攻下药 …… 123
大黄 …… 124
芒硝 …… 127
芦荟 …… 129
番泻叶 …… 130
第二节 润下药 …… 131
火麻仁 …… 131
郁李仁 …… 132
第三节 峻下逐水药 …… 132
甘遂 …… 133
大戟 …… 134
芫花 …… 135
牵牛子 …… 136
第四章 祛湿药 …… 138
第一节 祛风湿药 …… 138
独活 …… 139

Weilingxian *Radix Clematidis* ······ 141
Chuanwu *Radix Aconiti* ······ 142
Fangji *Radix Stephaniae Tetrandrae* ······ 143
Qinjiao *Radix Gentianae Macrophyllae* ······ 144
Qishe *Agkistrodon Acutus* ······ 145
Sangjisheng *Ramulus Taxilli* ······ 146
Wujiapi *Cortex Acanthopanacis Radicis* ······ 147
4.2 Dampness resolving Chinese medicinal herbs ······ 148
Huoxiang *Herba Agastachis* ······ 149
Peilan *Herba Eupatorii* ······ 151
Cangzhu *Rhizoma Atractylodis* ······ 151
Houpo *Cortex Magnoliae Officinalis* ······ 153
Sharen *Fructus Amomi* ······ 154
4.3 Chinese medicinal herbs for promoting diuresis and resolving dampness ······ 155
Fuling *Poria* ······ 156
Zhuling *Polyporus* ······ 157
Zexie *Rhizoma Alismatis* ······ 158
Yiyiren *Semen Coicis* ······ 158
Cheqianzi *Semen Plantaginis* ······ 160
Mutong *Caulis Akebiae* ······ 161
Haijinsha *Spora Lygodii* ······ 163
Difuzi *Fructus Kochiae* ······ 163
Bixie *Rhizoma Dioscoreae Hypoglaucae* ······ 164
Jinqiancao *Herba Lysimachiae* ······ 165
Yinchenhao *Herba Artemisiae Scopariae* ······ 166
5 The Interior Warming Chinese Medicinal Herbs ······ 168
Fuzi *Radix Aconiti Lateralis Praeparata* ······ 169
Rougui *Cortex Cinnamomi* ······ 171
Ganjiang *Rhizoma Zingiberis* ······ 173
Wuzhuyu *Fructus Evodiae* ······ 174
Xiaohuixiang *Fructus Foeniculi* ······ 175
Huajiao *Pericarpium Zanthoxyli* ······ 176
6 Qi Regulating Chinese Medicinal Herbs ······ 178
Jupi *Pericarpium Citri Tangerinae* ······ 179

威灵仙 …… 141
川乌 …… 142
防己 …… 143
秦艽 …… 144
蕲蛇 …… 145
桑寄生 …… 146
五加皮 …… 147
第二节 芳香化湿药 …… 148
藿香 …… 149
佩兰 …… 151
苍术 …… 151
厚朴 …… 153
砂仁 …… 154
第三节 利水渗湿药 …… 155
茯苓 …… 156
猪苓 …… 157
泽泻 …… 158
薏苡仁 …… 158
车前子 …… 160
木通 …… 161
海金沙 …… 163
地肤子 …… 163
萆薢 …… 164
金钱草 …… 165
茵陈蒿 …… 166
第五章 温里药 …… 168
附子 …… 169
肉桂 …… 171
干姜 …… 173
吴茱萸 …… 174
小茴香 …… 175
花椒 …… 176
第六章 理气药 …… 178
橘皮 …… 179

Qingpi *Pericarpium Citri Reticulatae Viride* ······ 180
Xiangfu *Rhizoma Cyperi* ······ 181
Muxiang *Radix Aucklandiae* ······ 182
Zhishi *Fructus Aurantii Immaturus* ······ 183
Xiebai *Bulbus Alli Macrostemi* ······ 185
Wuyao *Radix Linderae* ······ 186
Binglang *Semen Arecae* ······ 187
Chuanlianzi *Fructus Meliae Toosendan* ······ 189
Dingxiang *Flos Caryophylli* ······ 190
Chenxiang *Lignum Aquilariae Resinatum* ······ 191
Shidi *Calyx Kaki* ······ 192

7 Food Retention Relieving Chinese Medicinal Herbs ······ 194

Shanzha *Fructus Crataegi* ······ 194
Shenqu *Massa Medicata Fermentata* ······ 196
Maiya *Fructus Hordei Germinatus* ······ 196
Jineijin *Endothelium Corneum Gigeriae Galli* ······ 197

8 Hemostatic Chinese Medicinal Herbs ······ 199

Daji *Radix Cirsii Japonici* ······ 200
Xiaoji *Herba Cephalanoploris* ······ 201
Diyu *Radix Sanguisorbae* ······ 201
Huaihua *Flos Sophorae* ······ 203
Cebaiye *Cacumen Biotae* ······ 203
Baimaogen *Rhizoma Imperatae* ······ 204
Baiji *Rhizoma Bletillae* ······ 205
Xianhecao *Herba Agrimoniae* ······ 207
Sanqi *Radix Notoginseng* ······ 208
Qiancaogen *Radix Rubiae* ······ 209
Puhuang *Pollen Typhae* ······ 210
Aiye *Folium Artemisiae Argyi* ······ 211
Paojiang *Rhizoma Zingiberis Praeparata* ······ 213

9 Chinese Medicinal Herbs for Invigorating the Blood and Removing Blood Stasis ······ 214

Danshen *Radix Salviae Miltiorrhizae* ······ 215
Chuanxiong *Rhizoma Chuanxiong* ······ 217

青皮 …… 180
香附 …… 181
木香 …… 182
枳实 …… 183
薤白 …… 185
乌药 …… 186
槟榔 …… 187
川楝子 …… 189
丁香 …… 190
沉香 …… 191
柿蒂 …… 192
第七章　消食药 …… 194
山楂 …… 194
神曲 …… 196
麦芽 …… 196
鸡内金 …… 197
第八章　止血药 …… 199
大蓟 …… 200
小蓟 …… 201
地榆 …… 201
槐花 …… 203
侧柏叶 …… 203
白茅根 …… 204
白及 …… 205
仙鹤草 …… 207
三七 …… 208
茜草根 …… 209
蒲黄 …… 210
艾叶 …… 211
炮姜 …… 213
第九章　活血化瘀药 …… 214
丹参 …… 215
川芎 …… 217

Yanhusuo *Rhizoma Corydalis* ······ 219
Yujin *Radix Curcumae* ······ 220
Jianghuang *Rhizoma Curcumae Longae* ······ 222
Ruxiang *Olibanum* ······ 223
Moyao *Myrrha* ······ 224
Taoren *Semen Persicae* ······ 225
Honghua *Flos Carthami* ······ 227
Yimucao *Herba Leonuri* ······ 228
Niuxi *Radix Achyranthis Bidentatae* ······ 229
Jixueteng *Caulis Spatholobi* ······ 231
Sanleng *Rhizoma Sparganii* ······ 232
Ezhu *Rhizoma Zedoariae* ······ 233
Shuizhi *Hirudo* ······ 234
Mengchong *Tabanus* ······ 235

10 Phlegm Resolving, Antitussive and Antiasthmatic Chinese Medicinal Herbs ······ 237

Banxia *Rhizoma Pinelliae* ······ 238
Tiannanxing *Rhizoma Arisaematis* ······ 241
Baiqian *Rhizoma Cynanchi Stauntonii* ······ 243
Qianhu *Radix Peucedani* ······ 243
Gualou *Fructus Trichosanthis* ······ 244
Beimu *Bulbus Fritillariae* ······ 246
Xingren *Semen Armeniacae Amarum* ······ 248
Jiegeng *Radix Platycodi* ······ 249
Zisuzi *Fructus Perillae* ······ 250
Tinglizi *Semen Lepidii seu Descurainiae* ······ 251
Xuanfuhua *Flos Inulae* ······ 252
Pipaye *Folium Eriobotryae* ······ 254
Baibu *Radix Stemonae* ······ 254

11 Tranquilizers ······ 257

Zhusha *Cinnabaris* ······ 258
Cishi *Magnetitum* ······ 259
Longgu *Os Draconis* ······ 260
Hupo *Succinum* ······ 261

延胡索 …… 219
郁金 …… 220
姜黄 …… 222
乳香 …… 223
没药 …… 224
桃仁 …… 225
红花 …… 227
益母草 …… 228
牛膝 …… 229
鸡血藤 …… 231
三棱 …… 232
莪术 …… 233
水蛭 …… 234
虻虫 …… 235
第十章 化痰止咳平喘药 …… 237
半夏 …… 238
天南星 …… 241
白前 …… 243
前胡 …… 243
瓜蒌 …… 244
贝母 …… 246
杏仁 …… 248
桔梗 …… 249
紫苏子 …… 250
葶苈子 …… 251
旋覆花 …… 252
枇杷叶 …… 254
百部 …… 254
第十一章 安神药 …… 257
朱砂 …… 258
磁石 …… 259
龙骨 …… 260
琥珀 …… 261

Suanzaoren *Semen Ziziphi Spinosae* ······ 263
Baiziren *Semen Biotae* ······ 264
Yuanzhi *Radix Polygalae* ······ 265
Hehuanpi *Cortex Albiziae* ······ 266
12 Chinese Medicinal Herbs for Calming the Liver to Stop Endogenous Wind ······ 268
Shijueming *Concha Haliotidis* ······ 269
Muli *Concha Ostreae* ······ 270
Niuhuang *Calculus Bovis* ······ 271
Daizheshi *Haematitum* ······ 273
Lingyangjiao *Cornu Saigae Tataricae* ······ 274
Gouteng *Ramulus Uncariae cum Uncis* ······ 275
Tianma *Rhizoma Gastrodiae* ······ 276
Quanxie *Scorpio* ······ 278
Wugong *Scolopendra* ······ 279
Dilong *Lumbricus* ······ 280
Baijiangcan *Bombyx Batryticatus* ······ 282
13 Chinese Resuscitative Medicines ······ 284
Shexiang *Moschus* ······ 285
Bingpian *Borneolum Syntheticum* ······ 286
Shichangpu *Rhizoma Acori Graminei* ······ 287
14 Restoratives ······ 289
14.1 Restoratives for invigorating qi ······ 290
Renshen *Radix Ginseng* ······ 290
Dangshen *Radix Codonopsis* ······ 293
Xiyangshen *Radix Panacis Quinquefolii* ······ 295
Huangqi *Radix Astragali* ······ 296
Baizhu *Rhizoma Atractylodis Macrocephalae* ······ 298
Shanyao *Rhizoma Dioscoreae* ······ 301
Gancao *Radix Glycyrrhizae* ······ 303
Fengmi *Mel* ······ 305
14.2 Restoratives for reinforcing yang ······ 306
Lurong *Cornu Cervi Pantotrichum* ······ 307
Bajitian *Radix Morindae Officinalis* ······ 308

酸枣仁 …… 263
柏子仁 …… 264
远志 …… 265
合欢皮 …… 266
第十二章　平肝熄风药 …… 268
石决明 …… 269
牡蛎 …… 270
牛黄 …… 271
代赭石 …… 273
羚羊角 …… 274
钩藤 …… 275
天麻 …… 276
全蝎 …… 278
蜈蚣 …… 279
地龙 …… 280
白僵蚕 …… 282
第十三章　开窍药 …… 284
麝香 …… 285
冰片 …… 286
石菖蒲 …… 287
第十四章　补益药 …… 289
第一节　补气药 …… 290
人参 …… 290
党参 …… 293
西洋参 …… 295
黄芪 …… 296
白术 …… 298
山药 …… 301
甘草 …… 303
蜂蜜 …… 305
第二节　补阳药 …… 306
鹿茸 …… 307
巴戟天 …… 308

Yinyanghuo *Herba Epimedii* ······ 309
Roucongrong *Herba Cistanchis* ······ 310
Yizhiren *Fructus Alpiniae Oxyphyllae* ······ 311
Buguzhi *Fructus Psoraleae* ······ 313
Tusizi *Semen Cuscutae* ······ 314
Dongchongxiacao Cordyceps ······ 315
Duzhong *Cortex Eucommiae* ······ 316
Shayuanzi *Semen Astragali Complanati* ······ 318
14. 3 Restoratives for nourishing the blood ······ 319
Danggui *Radix Angelicae Sinensis* ······ 319
Shudihuang *Radix Rehmanniae Praeparata* ······ 322
Heshouwu *Radix Polygoni Multiflori* ······ 323
Baishaoyao *Radix Paeoniae Alba* ······ 325
Ejiao *Colla Corii Asini* ······ 327
14. 4 Restoratives for nourishing yin ······ 329
Beishashen *Radix Glehniae* ······ 329
Maimendong *Radix Ophiopogonis* ······ 331
Tianmendong *Radix Asparagi* ······ 332
Huangjing *Rhizoma Polygonati* ······ 333
Yuzhu *Rhizoma Polygonati Odorati* ······ 335
Shihu *Herba Dendrobii* ······ 336
Gouqizi *Fructus Lycii* ······ 337
Hanliancao *Herba Ecliptae* ······ 338
Nüzhenzi *Fructus Ligustri Lucidi* ······ 339
Guiban *Carapax et Plastrum Testudinis* ······ 340
Biejia *Carapax Trionycis* ······ 342
15 Astringent Chinese Medicinal Herbs ······ 344
Mahuanggen *Radix Ephedrae* ······ 345
Fuxiaomai *Fructus Tritici Levis* ······ 346
Wuweizi *Fructus Schisandrae* ······ 347
Wumei *Fructus Mume* ······ 349
Roudoukou *Semen Myristicae* ······ 350
Chishizhi *Halloysitum Rubrum* ······ 351
Shanzhuyu *Fructus Corni* ······ 353

淫羊藿 …… 309
肉苁蓉 …… 310
益智仁 …… 311
补骨脂 …… 313
菟丝子 …… 314
冬虫夏草 …… 315
杜仲 …… 316
沙苑子 …… 318
第三节 补血药 …… 319
当归 …… 319
熟地黄 …… 322
何首乌 …… 323
白芍药 …… 325
阿胶 …… 327
第四节 补阴药 …… 329
北沙参 …… 329
麦门冬 …… 331
天门冬 …… 332
黄精 …… 333
玉竹 …… 335
石斛 …… 336
枸杞子 …… 337
旱莲草 …… 338
女贞子 …… 339
龟版 …… 340
鳖甲 …… 342
第十五章 收敛固涩药 …… 344
麻黄根 …… 345
浮小麦 …… 346
五味子 …… 347
乌梅 …… 349
肉豆蔻 …… 350
赤石脂 …… 351
山茱萸 …… 353

Lianzi *Semen Nelumbinis* ······ 354
Jinyingzi *Fructus Rosae Laevigatae* ······ 355
Haipiaoxiao *Os Sepiellae seu Sepiae* ······ 356
16 Chinese Medicinal Herbs for External Application ······ 359
Liuhuang *Sulphur* ······ 359
Shengyao *Hydrargyri Oxydum* ······ 360
Luganshi *Calamina* ······ 361
Mingfan *Alumen* ······ 362
Pengsha *Borax* ······ 364
Fengfang *Nidus Vespae* ······ 365
Maqianzi *Semen Strychni* ······ 366
Shechuangzi *Fructus Cnidii* ······ 367
Index: Herbs by Latin Names ······ 369
Postscript ······ 377

莲子 …… 354
金樱子 …… 355
海螵蛸 …… 356
第十六章　外用药 …… 359
硫黄 …… 359
升药 …… 360
炉甘石 …… 361
明矾 …… 362
硼砂 …… 364
蜂房 …… 365
马钱子 …… 366
蛇床子 …… 367
附录：拉丁名索引 …… 369
后记 …… 377

General Introduction

总 论

1 Properties and Actions of Chinese Medicinal Herbs

第一章 中药的性能

The reason that Chinese medicinal herbs can prevent and treat diseases is due to their various internal natures. The properties and actions of Chinese medicinal herbs refer to their natures and effects relating to treatments.

中药能防治疾病是由其内在的各种特性所决定的。药物的性能就是指药物与治疗有关的性质和功能。

The occurrence and development of all kinds of diseases are caused by pathogenic factors acting on human body, which result in the pathologic phenomena such as imbalance between yin and yang, mutual growth and reduction between pathogenic factors and healthy qi, and the disorders of zang and fu organs. The basic principle of treating diseases with Chinese medicinal herbs is to eliminate causes of disease, dispel pathogenic factors or restore the coordination of the functions of zang and fu organs so that excess and deficiency of yin or yang can be corrected and the diseases can be cured.

任何疾病的发生和发展都是由致病因素作用于人体，由此引起机体发生阴阳失调、邪正消长或脏腑功能失常等病理现象。中药治病就是利用药物的特性来去除病因，消除病邪，或恢复脏腑功能的协调，从而纠正阴阳的偏盛偏衰，使疾病得以痊愈。

The properties and actions of Chinese medicinal herbs, which are the essential basis of the analyses and clinical usage of Chinese medicinal herbs, are summarized in medical practice and on the basis of the theories of yin-yang, zangfu, meridians, and therapeutic principles of traditional Chinese medicine, etc..

中药的性能是以中医的阴阳、脏腑、经络、治疗法则等理论为基础，从医疗实践中予以归纳总结出来的，是分析药物及临床用药的基本依据。

The theories of their properties are mainly summarized as the four natures and five flavors, floating and sinking, meridian tropism, and toxicity, etc..

中药药性理论主要有四气五味、升降浮沉、归经及毒性等。

1.1 Four natures and five flavors

Four natures and five flavors are also known as the properties and tastes of Chinese medicinal herbs.

1.1.1 Four natures

Four properties of Chinese medicinal herbs, cold, hot, warm and cool, are also called the four natures or four xing in TCM. Cold-cool and warm-hot are two completely different categories of natures, cold-cool belonging to yin, and warm-hot to yang, whereas cold and cool or hot and warm are only different, to some degrees, in their variance. Chinese medicinal herbs with cold-cool nature can clear away heat, purge fire and eliminate toxic materials, which are mainly used for heat-syndrome; Chinese medicinal herbs with warm-hot nature have the actions of expelling cold and restoring yang, which are mainly used for cold-syndrome.

In addition, there are also some Chinese medicinal herbs known as neutral ones whose cold or hot nature is not so remarkable and whose action is relatively mild. But actually they still have differences in the tendency to cool or warm so that they are still in the range of four natures.

The four natures — cold, hot, warm and cool are summarized mainly from the body's response after Chinese medicinal herbs are taken, which are so defined in relation to the properties, cold or heat of the diseases treated. After Huanglian (*Rhizoma Coptidis*) and Shigao (*Gypsum Fibrosum*) are taken, the manifestations of heat-syndromes such as high fever, dysphoria, thirst and profuse perspiration can be eliminated, which indicates that Huanglian (*Rhizoma Coptidis*) and Shigao (*Gypsum Fibrosum*) are cold in nature. According to the same reason, after Fuzi (*Radix Aconiti Lateralis Praeparata*) and

第一节 四气五味

四气五味，又称气味，也就是药物的性味。

1. 四气

指药物的寒、热、温、凉四种药性，也称为四性。寒凉与温热是两种不同的属性，寒凉属阴，温热属阳，而寒与凉、热与温仅是程度上的不同。寒凉之性的药物有清热、泻火、解毒等作用，主要适用于热性病证；温热之性的药物有散寒、助阳的作用，主要适用于寒性病证。

另外，有些药物寒热之性不明显，而称为平性。所谓“平性”，实际上仍有偏凉、偏温的区别，所以仍属四气的范围。

四气主要是从药物作用于人体所发生的反应加以概括而形成的，是与所治疾病的寒热性质相对应的。服用黄连、石膏之后，能使高热、烦躁、口渴、大汗出等热象得以解除，说明黄连、石膏是寒性的。同理，服用附子、干姜等后，能使恶寒肢冷、胃脘冷痛、泻下稀水等寒证得以缓解，说明附子、干姜等是热性的。药

Ganjiang (*Rhizoma Zingiberis*) are taken, the manifestations of cold-syndromes such as aversion to cold and cold limbs, cold and painful sensation in gastric region and diarrhea can be relieved, which indicates that Fuzi (*Radix Aconiti Praeparata*) and Ganjiang (*Rhizoma Zingiberis*) are hot in nature. Treating diseases with Chinese medicinal herbs is to make use of their cold or hot nature to correct the phenomena of overabundance of heat or cold in the body to restore them as much as possible to the normal state. Therefore, on the base of syndrome differentiation, you must distinguish heat or cold nature of disease, and have a good understanding of the cold or hot property of Chinese medicinal herbs, and then selectively apply corresponding medicinal herbs so that you can achieve the desired results. Ganjiang (*Rhizoma Zingiberis*) and Huanglian (*Rhizoma Coptidis*) can both be used to treat diarrhea but Ganjiang (*Rhizoma Zingiberis*) is hot in nature, therefore, used to treat diarrhea of cold type while Huanglian (*Rhizoma Coptidis*) cold in nature is indicated for diarrhea of heat type. If you don't consider their properties, cold or hot, when you apply medicinal herbs to treat heat or cold syndromes respectively with hot or cold medicinal herbs, you cannot achieve desired results of treatment and even bring about harmful results.

物治病就是利用药物的寒热之性来纠正疾病属热、属寒的病理改变。因此，治疗疾病必须在辨证的基础上，辨清疾病的属热、属寒和掌握药物寒热属性，有选择地应用相应的药物，才能收到预期效果。干姜和黄连都可以治泄泻，但干姜是热性药，治寒性泄泻；而黄连则属寒性，可治热性泄泻。如果用药不辨寒热，以热药治热证或寒药治寒证，就不能达到治疗目的，甚至会产生不良后果。

1.1.2 Five flavors

The five flavors of Chinese medicinal herbs refer to the five different tastes, pungent, sweet, sour, bitter and salty, which can be tasted by the tongue. With the development of the theory dealing with the medicinal properties, some flavors are summarized out of clinical actions of Chinese medicinal herbs, therefore, there is a little difference between the flavors of medicinal herbs and the tastes got by tongue. The Chinese medicinal herbs with same flavor mostly possess similar actions while the

2. 五味

五味是指药物辛、甘、酸、苦、咸五种不同的滋味。药物的滋味主要是通过口尝得出来的。随着药性理论的发展，不少药物的味是从药物的临床功效归纳出来的，药物的味与实际口尝之味也就不尽相同。味相同的药物，它们的作用大多相近；而味不同的药

medicinal herbs with different flavors show different actions in the treatment, which are shown as follows.

物,所表现出的治疗作用也不同。具体如下:

Pungent: Pungent is a flavor of medicinal herbs that has an action of dispersing and promoting circulation of qi and blood. Pungent medicinal herbs are generally indicated for exterior syndromes due to invasion of exogenous factors and syndromes of stagnation of qi and blood. For example, Zisuye (*Folium Perillae*) and Bohe (*Herba Menthae*) can produce the effects of inducing sweating to expel the exogenous pathogenic factors from the exterior, and Muxiang (*Radix Aucklandiae*) can circulate qi and Honghua (*Flos Carthami*) can promote blood circulation.

辛:具有发散、行气、行血作用。辛味药物,可用来治疗外感表证、气血郁滞证等。如紫苏叶、薄荷解表,木香行气,红花活血。

Sweet: Sweet flavor has the nourishing, harmonizing and moistening actions. Those sweet in flavor are generally indicated for deficiency syndromes, incoordination between the spleen and stomach, certain pain syndromes, constipation due to intestine-heat, cough due to lung-heat, etc.. For instance, Huangqi (*Radix Astragali*) and Shudihuang (*Rhizoma Rehmanniae Praeparatae*) have nourishing action, Gancao (*Radix Glycyrrhizae*) can relieve spasm and pain, and Fengmi (*Mel*) can moisten the intestine and promote purgation.

甘:具有滋补、缓和、润燥作用。甘味药物,可治虚证、脾胃不和、疼痛、肠燥便秘、肺燥咳嗽等。如黄芪、熟地黄滋补,甘草缓急止痛,蜂蜜润肠通便。

Sour: Sour flavor has absorbing, consolidating and astringent actions. Those sour in flavor are often used to treat incessant perspiration, chronic cough, chronic diarrhea, emission, spermatorrhea, enuresis, frequent micturition, prolonged metrorrhagia and metrostaxis, and prolonged leukorrhea, etc., caused by loss of essence due to asthenia of healthy qi. For example, Wumei (*Fructus Mume*) and Wuweizi (*Fructus Schisandrae*) are used to relieve cough and diarrhea; Shanzhuyu (*Fructus Corni*) and Jinyingzi (*Fructus Rosae Laevigatae*) are used to relieve emission and enuresis.

酸:具有收敛固涩作用。具有酸味的药物常用于治疗正虚精气耗散所致的虚汗、久咳、久泻、遗精、滑精、遗尿、尿频、崩带日久等证。如乌梅、五味子能止咳、止泻,山茱萸、金樱子能止遗精、遗尿。

Bitter: Bitter flavor has the actions of drying or

苦:具有燥湿、泄降等作

resolving dampness, purging and lowering. Those bitter in flavor are used in wide range and often used for constipation due to fire-heat, dysphoria, cough due to adverse rising of lung-qi, damp-heat or cold-damp syndrome. For example, Huanglian (*Rhizoma Coptidis*) can clear away heat and dry dampness, and Cangzhu (*Rhizoma Atractylodis*) can dry dampness due to its bitter flavor and warm nature, Dahuang (*Radix et Rhizoma Rhei*) can cause downward discharge, Xingren (*Semen Pruni Armeniacae*) can lower and disperse lung-qi and Zhizi (*Fructus Gardeniae*) can clear away heat and purge fire.

用。苦味药物适用范围较广，多用于治疗火热便秘，心烦，肺逆咳喘，湿热或寒湿证。如黄连能清热燥湿，苍术能苦温燥湿，大黄能通泄泻下，杏仁能降泄肺气，栀子能清热泻火。

Salty: Salty flavor has the effects of softening hard nodes or masses and promoting defecation, etc., so salty medicinal herbs are often used for the syndromes such as scrofula, superficial nodule, abdominal mass and internal accumulation with dry stool. For example, Haizao (*Sargassum*) and Kunbu (*Thallus Laminariae et Eckloniae*) can disperse scrofula, and Mangxiao (*Natrii Sulfas*) can relieve constipation by purgation.

咸：具有软坚、泻下作用。咸味药多用治瘰疬、瘿瘤、痰核、癥瘕、燥屎内结等病证。如海藻、昆布能消散瘰疬，芒硝能泻下通便。

In addition to the five flavors that are the basic tastes of Chinese medicinal herbs, there are also astringent and bland flavors. TCM holds that astringent flavor falls under the sour flavor category and bland flavor falls under the sweet, so they are still included in the five flavors. The actions of astringent flavor are very similar to those of sour flavor, which all have astringent action. For example, Longgu (*Os Draconis*) and Muli (*Concha Ostreae*) can stop nocturnal emission, leucorrhea and profuse perspiration; Chishizhi (*Halloysitum Rubrum*) and Yuyuliang (*Limonitum*) can arrest diarrhea. Those bland in flavor such as Zhuling (*Polyporus*) and Fuling (*Poria*) possess the actions of removing dampness and promoting diuresis, and are often used for edema and dysuria.

五味是药物的基本滋味，此外，还有涩味和淡味。中医认为，涩附于酸，淡合于甘，所以仍然称五味。涩味和酸味相似，都有收敛固涩作用，如龙骨、牡蛎可以涩精、止带、敛汗，赤石脂、禹余粮可以止泻。淡味具有渗湿利尿作用，多用于水肿、小便不利，如猪苓、茯苓等。

The nature and flavor are two kinds of medicinal properties that every Chinese herb possesses, and each of Chinese medicinal herbs must have the both properties. The natures and flavors deal with the pharmacological properties separately in different aspects. Only when you have a good understanding of the actions of both the natures and flavors, and combine them with each other, can you correctly understand their medicinal effects. Those with same natures and flavors possess essential similar actions. Therefore, different natures and flavors of medicines result in their different actions. For instance, Huanglian (*Rhizoma Coptidis*) and Huangqin (*Radix Scutellariae*) bitter in flavor and cold in nature, both can clear away heat and relieve toxic materials, purge fire and dry dampness; Huanglian (*Rhizoma Coptidis*) and Ganjiang (*Rhizoma Zingiberis*), of which Huanglian (*Rhizoma Coptidis*) is a kind of Chinese medicinal herbs bitter in flavor and cold in nature but Ganjiang (*Rhizoma Zingiberis*) is pungent in flavor and warm in nature are completely different in their actions. Ganjiang (*Rhizoma Zingiberis*) can expel cold, warm the middle energizer, restore yang, stop bleeding and warm the lung to resolve fluid retention, whose actions are completely different from those of Huanglian (*Rhizoma Coptidis*). If the Chinese medicinal herbs are similar in nature but different in flavor; or similar in flavor but different in nature, their actions are both similar and different. For instance, both Huanglian (*Rhizoma Coptidis*) and Shengdihuang (*Radix Rehmanniae*) are cold in nature and both can clear away heat, but being bitter in flavor, Huanglian (*Rhizoma Coptidis*) possesses the action of drying dampness while Shengdihuang (*Radix Rehmanniae*), sweet in flavor, can promote the production of the body fluids. Therefore, Huanglian (*Rhizoma Coptidis*) can clear away heat and dry dampness and is indicated for damp-heat syndrome.

气、味是每一药物均有的两种药性，任何一种药物不可能只有气而没有味，也不可能只有味而没有气。气和味分别从不同角度说明药物的药理作用，只有同时掌握气和味的作用，并相互结合才能正确掌握其药物的功效。药物的气与味相同，其作用基本相同，气味不同则作用不同。如黄连与黄芩皆为苦寒，都能清热解毒，清热泻火，清热燥湿；黄连与干姜，黄连苦寒，干姜辛热，气味完全不同，其作用也就完全不同，干姜能散寒、温中、回阳、止血、温肺化饮，与黄连完全不同。气同而味异或味同而气异，其作用既有相同的一面，又有不同的一面。如黄连与生地黄皆为寒性，都有清热作用，但黄连味苦有燥湿作用，生地黄味甘有生津之功。因此，黄连能清热燥湿，适用于湿热证，而生地黄则清热生津，适用于热甚津伤证。再如解表的生姜与薄荷，二者皆为辛味，都具发散作用，但生姜性温，能祛寒邪，而薄荷性凉能清热，所以生姜适用于风寒表证，而薄荷适用于风热表证。所以说，在辨别药性时，不能把气和味割裂开来。

Whereas, Shengdihuang (*Radix Rehmanniae*) can clear away heat and promote the production of the body fluids so it is indicated for consumption of the body fluids due to heat. Another example, both Shengjiang (*Rhizoma Zingiberis Recens*) and Bohe (*Herba Menthae*) are pungent in nature and possess dispersing action. But being warm in nature, Shengjiang (*Rhizoma Zingiberis Recens*) can eliminate cold while Bohe (*Herba Menthae*), cool in nature, can clear away heat. Therefore, Shengjiang (*Rhizoma Zingiberis Recens*) is indicated for exterior syndrome due to wind-cold while Bohe (*Herba Menthae*) for exterior syndrome due to wind-heat. In a word, when the properties of Chinese medicinal herbs are distinguished, their natures and flavors cannot be separately considered.

1.2 Lifting, lowering, floating and sinking

Lifting, lowering, floating and sinking refer to four different directions of actions of Chinese medicinal herbs in human body when they are taken.

Varying diseases often appear to bear a tendency to move upward, downward, towards the exterior or the interior. And for the state of a disease, they are distinguished into those due to adverse ascending of pathogenic factors and those due to invasion of pathogenic factors sinking deeply into the interior and lowering down to the lower energizer. Corresponding to the above, the directions of actions of medicinal herbs on human body also have the lifting, lowering, floating and sinking distinction. While treating a disease, according to its different causes, a doctor should select corresponding medicinal herbs and make the best use of their lifting, lowering, floating or sinking actions to help dispel pathogenic fac-

第二节　升降浮沉

升降浮沉是药物作用于人体的四种不同趋向。

各种疾病，从病位上来说，有上下表里之分，病势有上逆和下陷之别。与之相对应，药物作用的趋向也有升、降、浮、沉的不同。治疗疾病时，应针对不同的病机，选择相应的药物，利用或升、或降、或浮、或沉的作用，因势利导，祛除病邪，或调整脏腑功能，使之恢复正常。

tors, correct the disorder of the body' functions and restore them to the normal.

By "lifting" of Chinese medicinal herbs we mean that the direction of Chinese herbal action is toward the upper parts. Those that possess the lifting action are indicated for a disease in a lower and deeper parts. For example, Huangqi (*Radix Astragali*) and Shengma (*Rhizoma Cimicifugae*) can raise splenic qi and are indicated for syndrome of visceroptosis with hyposplenic qi such as chronic diarrhea and lingering dysentery, prolapse of the rectum, prolapse of uterus and gastroptosis. By "lowering" of Chinese medicinal herbs we mean that they function toward the lower parts and possess the action of descending adverse qi and are indicated for the disease due to adverse ascending of pathogenic factors. For example, Daizheshi (*Haematitum*), Chenxiang (*Lignum Aquilariae Resinatum*) and Shijueming (*Concha Haliotidis*) can descend adverse flow of qi and fire, subdue exuberant yang of the liver and descend adverse qi of the lung and stomach and are indicated for bleeding, painful swollen gum and aphthae due to ascendancy of rebellious qi and fire; dizziness due to exuberance of liver-yang, cough and dyspnea due to abnormal rising of lung-qi, nausea and vomiting and eructation due to abnormal rising of stomach-qi. By "floating" of Chinese medicinal herbs we mean that they function toward the upper and outward parts, generally exert the effects of sweating and dispersing and are indicated for the disease in the upper and superficial parts. For instance, Mahuang (*Herba Ephedrae*), Zisu (*Folium Perillae*), Fangfeng (*Radix Saposhnikoviae*) and Duhuo (*Radix Angelicae Pubescentis*) can dispel wind-cold and dampness from the exterior and are indicated for wind and cold exterior-syndrome, wind-damp type of Bi-syndrome, etc.. By "sinking" of Chinese medicinal

“升”是指药物作用趋势向上，具有升提作用，适用于病势向下的疾病。如黄芪、升麻能升提中气，治疗久泻久痢、脱肛、子宫脱垂、胃下垂等中气下陷之证。“降”是指药物作用趋于向下，具有降逆作用，适用于病势向上的疾病。如代赭石、沉香、石决明能降上逆之气火，潜降肝阳，降肺、胃气逆，适用于气火炎上之出血、牙龈肿痛、口舌生疮，肝阳上亢之头痛眩晕，肺气上逆之咳嗽气喘，胃气上逆之恶心呕吐、嗳气呃逆等证。“浮”是指药物作用趋势向外、向上，具有上浮、发散功能，适用于病位在表、在上的疾病。如麻黄、紫苏、防风、独活能发散风寒湿邪，用治外感表证、风湿痹痛等证，“沉”是指药物作用趋势向下、向内，具有下行、泄利功能，适用于病位在下、在里的疾病。如大黄、木通分别具有泻下、利尿作用，治疗大便不通、腹胀腹痛、小便不利等证。

herbs we mean that they function toward the lower and inward parts, have the effects of lowering the adverse flow of qi and relaxing bowels and are indicated for the disease in the lower and interior. For instance, Dahuang (*Radix et Rhizoma Rhei*) and Mutong (*Caulis Akebiae*) separately have the effects of relaxing the bowels and promoting diuresis and are used to treat constipation, abdominal distention and pain, and dysuria, etc..

Lifting and lowering, floating and sinking medicinal properties are the two couples whose direction of actions is opposite. Lifting and floating are similar in their actions, so are sinking and lowering. Therefore lifting and floating may be called concurrently, so may sinking and lowering. The lifting and floating medicinal herbs moving in ascending and outward directions generally exert the effects of invigorating splenic yang, relieving superficies, dispelling wind and cold, and resuscitation, etc.; the lowering and sinking medicinal herbs moving in descending and inward directions generally have the effects of clearing away heat, lowering the adverse flow of qi, purging, promoting diuresis, tranquilizing the mind, suppressing the hyperactive yang and stopping wind, and astringing, etc..

升与降,浮与沉是两对作用趋向相反的药性。而升与浮、沉与降作用相似,故常升浮与沉降并称。升浮的药物主上行而趋外,一般具有升阳、发表、祛风、散寒、开窍等作用;沉降的药物主下行而内敛,一般具有清热降逆、泻下、利尿、安神、潜阳息风、收敛固涩等作用。

The lifting, lowering, floating and sinking of medicinal herbs are generally based upon their natures, flavors and qualities. Generally speaking, Chinese medicinal herbs pungent and sweet in flavor, warm and heat in nature are mostly lifting and floating in their actions while those bitter, sour and salty in flavor, and cold or cool in nature are mostly sinking and lowering in their actions. Chinese medicinal herbs of flowers, leaves, and branches, etc., which are light in property are mostly lifting and floating in their actions while those of fruits, seeds, and minerals, etc., which are heavy in property are mostly

药物的升降浮沉作用与药物的性味、质地有一定的关系。一般来说,味辛、甘,性温热的药物大多升浮,而味苦、酸、咸,性寒凉的药物大多沉降;花、叶、枝等质轻的药物大多升浮,种子、果实及矿物等质重的药物大多沉降。但有少数例外,如厚朴性味虽为辛、苦、温,但能下气平喘。旋覆花虽为花类,但能降气。川

sinking and lowering. But there is an additional small number of Chinese medicinal herbs, for example, Houpo (*Cortex Magnoliae Officinalis*), a bark kind, pungent, bitter and warm in its flavor and nature can lower qi and relieve dyspnea. Xuanfuhua (*Flos Inulae*), a flower kind, can lower qi and Chuanxiong (*Rhizoma Chuanxiong*), a root kind, can move in upper direction even to the head and eyes and yet in descending direction to uterus.

芎则既可上行头目,又可下行血海等。

Besides, the lifting, lowering, floating and sinking actions of medicinal herbs may be affected by some medicinal processing or medicinal combination. For instance, the sinking or lowering medicinal herbs can turn into the lifting or floating ones when they are stir-baked with wine; in the same way, the lifting or floating herbs will turn into the sinking or lowering ones, which enter the kidney when they are stir-baked with a salt solution, and when they are used in combination with a variety of strong sinking or lowering herbs, their lifting or floating actions are changed into obscurity.

此外,药物的升降浮沉还受炮制影响。酒炒能使药物上行,盐水炒能使药物下降入肾等。复方应用中配伍也影响着药物的升降浮沉,如升浮药配在大队沉降药中则升浮作用不明显。

1.3 Meridian tropism of Chinese medicinal herbs

第三节 归 经

Meridian tropism refers to that medicinal herbs may often produce their therapeutic effects on some portion of a human body in preference, in other words, their therapeutic action is mainly related to some viscus or channel or some channels in predominance but it may seem to produce fewer effects on or seem not related to the other viscera and channels. Meridian tropism takes the theory of viscera and meridians, and the indication of syndromes as a basis. For instance, Mahuang (*Herba Ephedrae*) and Xingren (*Semen Armeniacae Amarum*) effective to syndromes of the disorder of the lung meridian marked by

归经是指某药对人体某脏腑经络病变有明显和特殊的治疗作用,而对其他脏腑经络起的作用较小或不起作用,体现了药物对人体各部位治疗作用的选择性。归经是以脏腑经络理论为基础,以主治病证为依据的。如麻黄、杏仁用于咳嗽气喘等肺经病证有效,便将其归入肺经;青皮、香附用于乳房、胁肋胀痛及疝气

cough and dyspnea are attributed to the lung-meridian; Qingpi (*Pericarpium Citri Reticulatae Viride*) and Xiangfu (*Rhizoma Cyperi*) indicated for syndromes of the disorder of the liver-meridian marked by distending pain of breast and hypochondrium and hernia pain are attributed to the liver-meridian. So generally speaking, what meridian or meridians a medicinal herb is attributed to is just related to the certain meridian or meridians on which the herb may work. If certain medicinal herb can work on several meridians, which means the medicinal herb can be used widely to treat the disorders of these meridians. From the above, we can see that meridian tropism of Chinese medicinal herbs is summerized from the therapeutic effects through a long time of clinical observation, and being practiced repeatedly, gradually develops into a theory.

痛等肝经病证有效，便将其归入肝经。故一般而论，某一药物能治何经之病，即可归入何经。如果某味药能归数经，就说明该药治疗范围较广，对数经病证都能发挥治疗作用。由此可见，中药的归经，是从临床疗效观察中总结出来，经过反复实践，逐步发展而上升为理论。

The theory of meridian tropism plays a certain role in clinical selection of Chinese medicinal herbs according to syndromes, giving a rise of direction and strengthening the therapeutic effects. For instance, medicinal herbs cold in nature have effects of clearing away heat, which also have the differences in tendency towards clearing away heat in the heart, liver, lung, or stomach; those hot in nature can all warm the interior to expel cold, but their effects also have the differences in warming the spleen, stomach, lung or kidney. Therefore, when you prescribe medicinal herbs, you should select those that work on the diseased viscus or meridian or some viscera or meridians in the light of their properties of meridian tropism to achieve desired therapeutic effects. In addition, you can take meridian tropism of Chinese medicinal herbs as a clue to probe their potential effects of some medicinal herbs and to extend their applying range.

归经理论，对指导临床随证选药，提高针对性和增强疗效，具有一定意义。例如寒性药物虽然均具清热作用，但有偏于清心、清肝、清肺、清胃等区分；热性药物都能温里散寒，亦有温脾（胃）、温肺、温肾等差异。因此，在处方用药时，应根据药物归经的特性，选择与病变脏腑经络相应的药物，方能获得理想疗效。此外，以药物归经为线索，还可探索某些药物的潜在功能，扩大其应用范围。

The theories such as meridian tropism, four natures

归经与四气五味、升降浮

and five flavors, lifting, lowering, floating and sinking all explain the properties of Chinese medicinal herbs from various points of view, which jointly constitute their properties and actions. Whereas pathological changes in the same viscus or meridian are different in cold, heat, asthenia or sthenia, and in adverse ascending or descending, and the medicinal herbs which are attributed to the same meridian also have the difference in cold, warm or cool, tonifying or reducing and adverse descending or ascending. For example, Mahuang (*Herba Ephedrae*), Huangqin (*Radix Scutellariae*) and Shashen (*Radix Adenophorae Strictae*) are all attributed to lung-meridian and can all treat cough, but Mahuang (*Herba Ephedrae*) pungent and slightly bitter in flavor and warm in nature tends to lifting and floating in actions, so it can disperse the lung to relieve cough and asthma and is indicated for cough and asthma due to exogenous wind and cold; Huangqin (*Radix Scutellariae*) bitter in flavor and cold in nature tends to sinking and lowering in actions, so it can clear away heat, and purge excessive fire and relieve cough and asthma due to lung-heat; Shashen (*Radix Adenophorae Strictae*) sweet in flavor and cold in nature tends to sinking and lowering in the action, therefore, it can nourish yin to promote secretion of the body fluids and is indicated for cough due to insufficiency of lung-yin. Therefore when you apply medicinal herbs in clinic, you must combine their various properties and effects to give them an all-round consideration so that you can select and apply them correctly and avoid one-sidedness.

沉等理论,是从不同角度来说明药性的,它们共同构成了中药的性能。而同一脏腑经络的病变有寒热虚实以及上逆、下陷等不同,归入同一经的药物也有寒热温凉补泻以及降逆、升提等的区别。如麻黄、黄芩、沙参都归肺经,皆可治疗咳嗽病证,但麻黄味辛、微苦,性温,其作用趋向为升浮,故能宣肺止咳平喘,治外感风寒之咳嗽气喘;黄芩味苦,性寒,其作用趋向为沉降,故能清热泻火,治肺热咳嗽气喘;沙参味甘,性寒,其作用趋向亦为沉降,故能养阴生津,治疗肺阴不足之咳嗽。因此,临床用药时需将药物的各种性能结合起来,全面考虑,才能正确用药,避免片面性。

But in clinical practice, owing to frequent occurrence of transmission of a disease between zangfu-organs or meridians in addition to the Chinese medicinal herbs only for one viscus or meridian, those for the other viscera or meridians are also usually used together. For instance, when

由于脏腑经络病变可以相互影响,所以在临床用药时要考虑到某一脏腑的病变可以影响到其他脏腑经络。不能单用治某一脏腑经络病变

treating lung disorders affects the spleen, both the medicinal herbs for treating lung disorders and invigorating the spleen should be used, which is called supplementing the spleen to nourish the lung. For the same reason, a syndrome with hyperactivity of liver-yang due to insufficiency of kidney-yin should be treated in combination with the medicinal herbs nourishing kidney-yin to have the liver nourished and deficiency of yang calmed, which is the method of nourishing renal yin to tonify liver yin.

的药物，如肺病影响到脾病时，除用治肺病药物外，还需应用补脾的药物，可使肺病渐愈，此即培土生金法。同理，肾阴不足而肝阳上亢者，治疗时则配伍滋肾阴药物，使肝有所养，而虚阳自潜，此即滋水涵木法。

1.4 Toxicity

第四节 毒 性

Toxicity refers to a harmful effect of a medicinal herb to the human body, a poisonous medicinal material being known as a toxin. The medicinal herbs drastic or poisonous in nature, if used improperly, can do harm to the body for the light and can cause death for the severe. In order to ensure safety in the use of medicinal herbs, their toxicity must be thoroughly understood.

Dosage of poisonous medicinal herbs in the treatment is close or same to poisoning dosage, so the safety margin is small and poisoning is easily resulted. Whereas the dosage of non-poisonous medicinal herbs in treatment is much farther from the poisoning dosage, and the safety margin is also larger. But it is not absolute whether they can result in poisonous reaction or not. In order to ensure the safety in administration of medicinal herbs and bring therapeutic effects into play and avoid poisonous reaction, you should pay attention to the follows as you use the poisonous ones.

毒性是指药物对人体的危害作用，有毒性的药物称有毒药。有毒药物及性质猛烈的药物使用不当，轻者可引起机体的损害，重者可导致死亡。为了保证用药安全，必须认识中药的毒性。

有毒药物的治疗剂量与中毒剂量比较接近或相当，因而安全度小，易引起中毒。无毒药物治疗量与中毒量相距较大，安全度亦较大，但也并非绝对不会引起中毒反应。

为了保证用药安全并发挥其治疗作用，避免毒性反应的产生，应用有毒药物应注意以下几点：

1.4.1 Strictly processing

The toxicity of poisonous Chinese medicinal herbs can be reduced by being processed. Therefore, you must strictly follow the process rules of preparing raw medicinal

1. 严格炮制

有毒药物可以通过炮制以降低毒性。因此，必须严格遵循炮制规程对药物进行炮

materials. For instance, Badou (*Fructus Crotonis*), a kind of drastic purgatives that is poisonous in nature, easily results in poisoning if not prepared into Badoushuang (*Semen Crotonis Pulveratum*) which is taken orally. After Fuzi (*Radix Aconiti*) is prepared through soaking, its toxicity decreases and it can be widely used and meanwhile does not easily cause poisoning.

制,如巴豆有毒,为强烈的泻下药,若不制成巴豆霜内服,则易引起中毒。附子炮制后,毒性降低,应用广泛而不易中毒。

1.4.2 Control of dosage

Poisonous occurrence is related to the excessive dosage of administration. So the dosage of toxic medicinal herbs, especially those with extreme toxin, must be strictly controlled and their dosage can not be increased at will. They should be used from small dose and increased according to patient's condition after they are taken. But they are not used for a long time in order to prevent the body from being poisoned due to accumulation of toxicity.

2. 控制剂量

中毒的产生与药物用量过大有关。因此,对毒药特别是有大毒的药物,用量应严格掌握,不能任意加大剂量。使用时应从小剂量开始,然后根据服药后的情况酌情加量。不能长期应用,以防蓄积中毒。

1.4.3 Notes of application

The poisonous medicinal herbs, their toxicity being extreme or mild, are not used in completely common way. Some can be applied exteriorly and can't be taken orally, such as Shengyao (Coarsely prepared mercuric oxide) and Maoliang (*Herba et Radix Ranunculi*); some can be added to pill or bolus and powder, not to decoction, such as Chansu (*Venenum Bufonis*) and Banmao (*Mylabris*); some cannot be prepared into pill or tablet with wine, such as Chuanwu (*Radix Aconiti*). If some are put into a complex prescription, their toxicity is weakened and if a single dose is taken orally, the toxicity is severer. For instance, Fuzi (*Radix Aconiti Lateralis Praeparata*) has an extreme toxin if taken singly and its toxicity will decrease if taken with Shengjiang (*Rhizoma Zingiberis Recens*).

3. 注意用法

有毒药物,毒有大小,用法不尽相同。有的只能外用,不能内服,如升药、毛茛等;有的宜入丸散,不入汤剂,如蟾酥、斑蝥等;有的不能制成酒剂,如川乌等。有的入复方毒性减弱,单服则毒性较大,如附子单用毒性大,与生姜同用则毒性减少。

In addition, TCM always holds that there is a theory of "treating virulent pathogen with poisonous agents",

此外,中医历来有"以毒攻毒"之说,是指某些有毒药

that is, some poisonous medicinal herbs with obvious therapeutic effects, under the safety of administration, may be used properly for such serious intractable diseases as malignant boil with swelling, scabies, scrofula, goiter, cancer tumor and abdominal mass.

物有着显著的治疗作用，在保证用药安全的前提下，可用适宜的有毒药物来治疗恶疮肿毒、疥癣、瘰疬瘿瘤、癌肿癥瘕等病情深重、顽固难愈的疾病。

2 Processing of Chinese Medicinal Herbs

第二章 中药的炮制

By processing of medicinal herbs, termed as Paozhi in TCM, we refer to various processes of preparing crude medicinal materials according to the theories of TCM and requirements of therapy, prescription, preparation of forms, and storage of Chinese medicinal herbs. It includes common or special treatment of crude or part of crude medicinal materials. Since most Chinese medicinal herbs come from the crude plants, of which some are mixed with impurity in the collecting process, some may easily change their properties and are not to be stored for a long time, some are violently toxic and are not to be taken directly and may need to be treated in special way so as to tally with the needs of treatment. Therefore, it is necessary for them to be processed so as to produce satisfactory medicinal effects and ensure safety in clinical practice before their use and preparation.

炮制是药物在使用前，根据中医药理论，按照医疗、调剂、制剂和贮藏的需要，对药材进行加工处理的工艺过程。它包括对药材进行的一般修治和部分药材的特殊处理。由于中药大多是生药，有的在采集过程中混有杂质，有的易变质而不能久贮，有的毒烈之性较强而不能直接服用，还有的需要特定的方法处理才能符合治疗需要。因此，中药在应用或制成制剂以前，都必须经过加工处理，才能充分发挥药效，保证用药安全。

2.1 Purposes of processing Chinese medicinal herbs

第一节 炮制的目的

The purposes of processing Chinese medicinal herbs are briefly summarized as follows.

中药炮制的目的主要有以下几点：

2.1.1 Removing or reducing the toxicity, drastic properties and side effects of some Chinese medicinal herbs. For instance, the toxicity of medicinal herbs, such as Chuanwu (*Radix Aconiti*), Caowu (*Radix Aconiti Kusnezoffii*), Gansui (*Radix Euphorbiae*

1. 消除或减低某些药物的毒性、烈性和副作用。如川乌、草乌、甘遂、天南星等有毒的药物，经炮制后可减低毒性；常山服后易致呕吐，若用

Kansui), and Tiannanxing (*Rhizoma Arisaematis*), will be reduced when they are processed; Changshan (*Radix Dichroae*), after taken, easily induce vomiting and if used to prevent recurrence of malaria, the side effects can be reduced after stir-baked with wine.

于截疟，经酒炒后即可减低这一副作用等。

2.1.2 Promoting therapeutic effects. For instance, Baibu (*Radix Stemonae*) and Pipaye (*Folium Eriobotryae*) roasted with honey can promote nourishing the lung to relieve cough; Chuanxiong (*Rhizoma Chuanxiong*) and Danggui (*Radix Angelicae Sinensis*) stir-baked with wine can promote warming channels to circulate the blood; Yanhusuo (*Rhizoma Corydalis*) prepared with vinegar can strengthen the effects of relieving pain; the effect of invigorating the spleen to relieve diarrhea will be strengthened after Baizhu (*Rhizoma Atractylodis Macrocephalae*) is stir-baked with earth; Xiangfu (*Rhizoma Cyperi*) prepared with vinegar can promote soothing the liver and regulating liver-qi.

2. 增强药物的疗效。如百部、枇杷叶蜜炙后能增强润肺止咳的功效；川芎、当归用酒炒后，能增强温经活血作用；延胡索经醋制后能加强止痛之功；白术土炒后能加强健脾止泻作用；香附醋制后能加强疏肝理气的作用等。

2.1.3 Modifying the natures and actions of Chinese medicinal herbs so as to make them suitable for therapeutic requirements. For instance, Shengdihuang (*Radix Rehmanniae*) cool in nature has the effect of eliminating blood-heat, but after processed, it can be warm and good at nourishing the blood; Heshouwu (*Radix Polygoni*) in raw form has moistening-purging effect, but after processed, it can be good at invigorating the liver and kidney; Dahuang (*Radix et Rhizoma Rhei*) in raw form has strong effect of purging, whereas after processed, its purging effect can decrease and after stir-baked into charcoal, it hardly has purging effect but is good at stopping bleeding.

3. 改变药物的性能，使其适合治疗需要。如地黄生用性凉，能清热凉血；制熟后性温，则以补血见长。何首乌生用有润下作用，制熟后则善于补肝肾。大黄生用泻下力强，制熟后则泻下力缓，炒炭后几无泻下作用而长于止血等。

2.1.4 Facilitating decocting and taking medicine, making preparation and storing medicine. Most botanical medicinal herbs after cut into segments or pieces

4. 便于煎服、制剂和贮藏。一般植物药经切制后便于煎煮，使有效成分易于溶

will be easily decocted in water and their effective components will be easily dissolved out or the forms of medicines will be easily prepared. And most minerals and shells of Chinese medicinal herbs, after calcined or quenched with vinegar, will be easy to be ground into powder. Some medicinal herbs are to be stir-baked and fully dried so as to be kept for a long time from being moldy and rot.

出;或便于粉碎、制剂。矿物、贝壳类药物经火煅醋淬后易于粉碎。某些药物需经充分干燥而便于贮存,不致霉变、腐烂等。

2.1.5 Taking away the impurity, non-pharmaceutical parts and unpleasant tastes, thus making the medicinal herbs clean and pure, and convenient for patients to take. The pharmaceutical herbs which are generally mixed with mud and sand must be washed and the impurity in the plants must be cleared away, thus they are convenient for patients to take. Some pharmaceutical plants need to be softened so as to be easily cut or prepared. The hair of some plants must be brushed away; heads, feet or wings of some pharmaceutical animals must be taken out; and the salty or offensive taste or smell of some sea products must be eliminated by rinsing with water.

5. 除去杂质、非药用部分及不良的味道,使药物清洁纯净,便于服用。一般植物药混有杂质、泥沙,需经处理,才能使用;有些药材需使其软化,以便于切制。有的植物药需刮皮去毛;某些动物药需去头、足、翅;某些海产品需漂去咸腥味等。

2.2 Methods of processing medicinal materials

第二节 炮制的方法

There are several commonly-used methods of processing medicinal materials which are listed briefly as follows:

炮制的方法很多,大致可分为以下几类:

2.2.1 Purifying and cutting

1. 修制

2.2.1.1 Discarding impurity: Taking away the mud and impurity and non-pharmaceutical parts, thus making the herbs clean and pure.

(1) 纯净处理:将药物中的泥土、杂质及非药用部分除去,使其清洁纯净。

2.2.1.2 Breaking into fine pieces: Some medicinal materials should be pounded or ground into powder for convenience in decocting, making preparations or administrating.

(2) 粉碎处理:将药物压碎或碾成粉末,便于进一步炮制、制剂和服用。

2.2.1.3 Cutting: According to different requirements, cut medicinal materials into pieces, parts or tiny bit, etc., for convenience in decocting or further preparing, drying, and storing, etc..

(3) 切制处理：按照不同的要求，将药物切成片、段、块、丝等，便于煎煮和进一步炮制，并利于干燥、贮藏和调剂。

2.2.2 Processing with water

2. 水制

Processing herbs with water is a kind of method of treating pharmaceutical materials for the purposes of cleaning, softening, or making them easy to cut or regulate medicinal properties, reducing their toxicity, or making mineral drugs pure, fine and smooth, etc.. The commonly-used methods are listed as follows.

是用水处理药物的一种方法。水制的目的主要是清洁、软化药材，以便于切制或调整药性，以及减低毒性，使矿物类药物纯净、细腻等。常用的方法有：

2.2.2.1 Washing: Mud and impurity on the surface of the pharmaceutical materials should be washed with water.

(1) 洗：用水洗去药材表面的泥土、杂质或淘去杂质等。

2.2.2.2 Softening: Softening is a method for making the medicinal materials soft gradually through permeable actions such as sprinkling, washing, soaking-with-sealing with clean water so as to make them easy to cut.

(2) 润：用少量清水反复淋洒药物，并覆盖湿物，使药材软化以便于切制。

2.2.2.3 Rinsing: Rinsing is a method for removing the salty elements, offensive smell, poisonous substances from the medicinal materials by putting them a certain time in a large container with water which must be running or changed frequently.

(3) 漂：将药材放入清水或长流水中，以漂去其咸味、腥味或毒性成分，便于制剂和应用。

2.2.2.4 Powder-refining method with water: This is a method for refining and getting the fine powder by grinding the insoluble and mineral medicinal minerals in water. This method is first applied to crush the medicinal materials into particles, and then to grind them in a mortar which contains a certain amount of clean water (its level above the drugs). During grinding, the supernatant suspension is decanted and then water is added again. The procedures above may be repeated until all the coarse particles are ground into fine particles. The sediment of coarse particles will be left when the supernatant fluid of

(4) 水飞：是将不溶于水的矿物类药物与水同研制细粉的一种方法。取药物粉碎成粗粒，入容器内加水同研，倾出混悬液，再加水反复研磨至无沉渣，将混悬液澄清，去上清液晒干。水飞的药物，纯洁细腻，易于吸收，外用刺激性小；加工中又能减少药物的损失。

suspension is decanted, from which fine powder is precipitated, separated and then dried in the sun for use. The medicinal herbs through powder-refining method with water are pure, fine and smooth, easily absorbed and light stimulative when used exteriorly; during the process, the loss of medicinal materials can also be reduced.

2.2.3 Processing with fire

3. 火制

Processing with fire is a method which is used in treating crude medicinal materials by heating with fire. This method includes the following commonly used ones, such as parching, stir-baking with adjuvants, calcining, and roasting in ashes, etc..

是用火加热处理药物的方法。常用的有炒、炙、煅、煨等。

2.2.3.1 Parching: By parching, some of the pharmaceutical components can be destroyed or eliminated, their properties and effects can be properly changed, their irritant properties and side-effects can be reduced and their side-nature of coldness or dryness may be moderated. Parched medicinal materials have the actions of checking offensive odor and tastes and invigorating the spleen, and they are easy to be pounded into pieces or powder and stored, and their effective components may be dissolved easily in decoction. Parching may be divided into two procedures with adjuvants or without adjuvants.

(1) 炒：药物经炒后，可以破坏或清除其中的某种成分，适当改变其性能，减低药物的刺激性或副作用，缓和过寒、过燥的偏性，有矫臭、矫味、健脾等作用，且便于粉碎、贮藏和有效成分的煎出。根据是否加辅料分为清炒和辅料炒两种。

2.2.3.1.1 Simple parching: It is the procedure of stir-baking without adjuvants. According to the degrees required, parching may be divided into three kinds, parching medicinal materials until they become yellowish, burnt-color or carbonized. By parching them into yellowish we mean that they are stir-baked into yellow surface or till they bulge while there is no change in their interior. The medicinal materials parched into yellowish can reduce the coldness and check the tastes. By parching them into burnt-color we mean that they are toasted into burnt-yellow or burnt-brown surface and yellow interior with

①清炒：不加任何辅料，将药物炒至所需程度。有炒黄、炒焦和炒炭三种方法。炒黄，是将药物炒至表面黄色或鼓起，内部无变化。药物炒黄，能减轻寒性并能矫味。炒焦，是将药物表面炒至焦黄或焦褐色，内部黄色，并有焦香气味。药物炒焦后，可增强健脾、消食作用。炒炭，将药物表面炒至焦黑，内部焦黄，部

burnt odor. After they are parched into those with burnt-color, they can promote the action of invigorating the spleen and digestion. By parching them into carbonized one we mean that their surface becomes burnt black and the interior is burnt yellow while their medicinal properties still exist. After parching, their effect of arresting hemorrhage can be reinforced.

分炭化而存性为度。药物制炭后,止血作用增强。

2.2.3.1.2 Complex parching: It is the procedure of stir-baking with certain amount of solid adjuvants until the degrees needed. The commonly-used adjuvants are mud, bran, rice, talc or powder of surf clam shell, etc..

② 辅料炒:将药物加一定量的固体辅料同炒至所需程度。常用的辅料有灶心土、麦麸、大米、滑石、蛤粉等。

2.2.3.2 Stir-baking with liquid adjuvants: This procedure is a method for the purpose of correcting their pharmaceutical properties, increasing their therapeutic actions or reducing their side effects through gradual increase of permeation of the liquid adjuvants into the medicinal materials during processing. The commonly used liquid adjuvants include honey, wine, vinegar, salt solution, ginger and juice, etc.. The procedures are respectively known as stir-baking with honey, wine, vinegar, salt solution and ginger juice. Since the used adjuvants are different, their effects are also different. For example, honey-stir-baked Chinese medicinal herbs have better effects on moistening the lung and relieving cough, invigorating the stomach and spleen, or can moderate the pharmaceutical properties and reduce the toxic effects; wine-stir-baked ones can promote the blood circulation and reduce the side-effects of some pharmaceutical herbs; vinegar-stir-baked ones can exert more remarkable effects on soothing the liver and relieving pain and reducing the toxic effects; salt-solution-baked ones will strengthen the effects on tonifying the kidney, nourishing yin and lowering the fire, etc.; ginger juice-stir-baked ones can get more obvious effects on relieving cold, vomiting and re-

(2) 炙:加入一定量的液体辅料与药物同炒,使其渗入药物内部,能起到改变药性,增强疗效,或减低毒副作用等。常用的辅料有蜂蜜、酒、醋、盐水、姜汁等,其方法分别称为蜜炙、酒炙、醋炙、盐水炙、姜汁炙等。由于所用的辅料不同,其作用亦有区别。如蜜炙可增强润肺止咳、补中益气的作用,或缓和药性,减低毒副作用;酒炙可加强活血作用,减低某些药物的副作用;醋炙可加强疏肝止痛作用,减低毒性;盐水炙加强补肾、滋阴降火等功能;姜汁炙能制药之寒性,加强止呕功效和减低毒副作用。

ducing the toxic effects.

2.2.3.3 Calcining: It is a method of treating crude medicinal materials by direct or indirect burning with strong fire. The purposes are to make them pure, clean, crispy, easy to be powdered and their effective components decocted out or their natures change to produce better therapeutic effects. Some crude medicinal herbs of hard minerals or shells may be burned directly till they are thoroughly reddish, then they are quickly put into vinegar or clean water, which is called tempering. Some medicinal herbs as Xueyutan (*Crini Carbonisatus*), Zonglütan (*Trachycarpi Carbonisatus*) should be burned and carbonized in a sealed refractory container till its bottom gets fully flushed.

(3) 煅：将药物直接或间接用火煅烧，使药物纯净、松脆，易于粉碎，便于有效成分煎出，或改变药物性能，加强疗效。一般矿物类、贝壳类药物直接火上煅烧至红透，或马上放入醋或清水内，后者称为煅淬。某些需制炭的药物，如血余炭、棕榈炭等，应在耐火容器中密闭煅烧。

2.2.3.4 Roasting in hot ashes: The process requires to wrap the raw medicinal materials with wet paper or dough and roast them in smouldering ashes till the coat becomes burnt black so as to eliminate some oil, irritant materials or reduce toxic side effects.

(4) 煨：用湿纸或湿面粉将药物包裹，置于热的火灰中加热，至表面焦黑，以除去部分油脂或刺激性物质，减低毒副作用等。

2.2.4 Processing with both fire and water

4. 水火共制

It is a method for treating medicinal materials with fire and water or sometimes with other adjuvants added. These frequently used methods are as follows.

是既用火又用水，或加入其他液体辅料加工处理的方法。常用的有：

2.2.4.1 Steaming: Steaming is a method of processing crude medicinal materials by putting them in a steaming pot or the like so as to heat them with steam.

(1) 蒸：即用蒸气或隔水加热的方法。

2.2.4.2 Boiling: Boiling is a method of treating the crude by heating them in clean water or other liquid adjuvants at boiling temperature.

(2) 煮：用水或液体辅料对药物进行加热处理的方法。

2.2.4.3 Scalding: Scalding is a method of treating the crude by putting them into boiling water, and stirring them for a short while before taking them out.

(3) 燀：是将药物快速入沸水中潦过，然后快速取出的方法。

The medicinal materials through the above treatments can promote therapeutic effects, reduce their

药物通过以上处理，可以增强疗效，减低毒性，改变性

toxicity, change their nature and effects and are easily stored.

2.2.5 Other processing methods

There are some other special processing methods according to different requirement of pharmaceutical herbs, such as germination, fermentation, and frost-like powder, etc.. Germination means that pharmaceutical crude seeds are germinated to certain highness, which are then dried. Fermentation means that pharmaceutical crude materials are fermented at certain temperature with a series of procedures. Frost-like powder means pharmaceutical crude seed is frosted on the surface of defatted herbal seed with a series of procedures.

能，便于贮藏。

5. 其他制法

根据药物的不同要求进行的一些特殊加工方法，如发芽、发酵、制霜等。发芽，是将种子类药物发芽至一定长度，然后干燥。发酵，即将药物置于一定温度下发酵。制霜，即将种子类药物去掉部分油脂，或将芒硝放入西瓜中置于通风处，使表面析出白霜。

3 Compatibility of Chinese Medicinal Herbs

Compatibility of Chinese medicinal herbs refers to the combination of more than two herbs with purpose in the light of the clinical requirement and medicinal properties and actions. It is the main method of medicinal application in clinic and also the basis of making up formulae of Chinese medicinal herbs.

During clinical practice, we only use a single to treat a disorder and fulfill its therapeutic purpose if the case condition is simple and light. But on occasions when a disease is accompanied by other diseases, or it is due to invasion of both superficies and interior by pathogenic factors, or asthenic syndrome is complicated with sthenic syndrome, or cold syndrome accompanied by heat syndrome alternatively, a single formula can fail to achieve desired effects. Furthermore, some medicinal herbs used in single form may produce toxic side-effects or may be harmful to a patient. Therefore several Chinese medicinal herbs must be used in combination according to their specific properties so as to extend the circulation of their treatment, decrease their toxic side-effects and gain better therapeutic effects.

Chinese medicinal herbs may have complicated changes by combination. Some may reinforce or decrease their effects, moderate or eliminate their original toxic side-effects, whereas others may produce toxicity and poor reactions. The relationship between a single and the compatible ingredients was generalized previously by ancient

第三章 中药的配伍

中药的配伍就是根据病情需要和药物性能，有目的地将两种以上的药物配合在一起使用。配伍是临床用药的主要方式，也是组成方剂的基础。

病情单纯，病势较轻者，只用一味药就能达到良好的治疗效果。但病情往往是复杂多变的，或数病相兼，或表里同病，或虚实并见，或寒热错杂，在这种情况下，应用单味药物就无法取得理想的效果。再者，某些药物单用时能产生毒副作用，于病人不利。因此，必须选用多种药物配合应用，以扩大治疗范围，降低药物的毒副作用，提高疗效。

药物通过配伍之后，可发生复杂的变化。有的增强药效，有的减低药效，有的能抑制和消除原有的毒副作用，而有的却能产生毒性和不良反应。前人把中药配伍后产生

physicians as seven aspects, namely, singular application, mutual reinforcement, mutual assistance, mutual restraint, mutual detoxication, mutual inhibition and incompatibility. Except that singular application means using a single medicinal herb, the other six aspects mainly denote the relationship of compatibility between Chinese medicinal herbs.

的不同效应总结为“七情”,即单行、相须、相使、相畏、相杀、相恶、相反七个方面。除单行为单味药物应用外,其余都是药物之间的配伍关系。

Mutual reinforcement: That is, two or more ingredients with similar properties and effects are used in combination to reinforce each other's action. For example, Dahuang (*Rhizoma et Radix Rhei*) and Mangxiao (*Natrii Sulfas*) which are both purgative, after they are used in combination, can reinforce each other's original purgating action; Honghua (*Flos Carthami*) and Taoren (*Semen Persicae*) of blood invigorating herbs used in combination can reinforce their action of invigorating the blood and removing blood obstruction.

相须:即将药性、功效相近的药物配合同用,可起协同作用,以增强药效。如同为泻下药中的大黄与芒硝,配伍后可加强原有的泻下作用;活血药中的红花配伍桃仁,活血化瘀作用得以加强。

Mutual assistance: That is, Chinese medicinal herbs that are not certainly similar but have some relationship in the aspect of medicinal properties and actions are used in combination, in which one herb is taken as the dominate factor and the others as its assistants to raise its therapeutic effects. For example, Huangqi (*Radix Astragali*) with the effect of tonifying qi and promoting the flow of water is used in combination with Fangji (*Radix Stephaniae Tetrandrae*) with the effects of promoting the flow of water and permeating the dampness, the latter reinforcing the former's action of promoting the flow of water, so their combination can be used for edema due to spleen-deficiency; Shigao (*Gypsum Fibrosum*) with the effect of clearing away heat and purging fire in combination with Xixin (*Herba Asari*) can purge fire to relieve pain and treat toothache due to stomach-fire.

相使:即以一种药物为主,配合其他药物,来提高主药的疗效。相配的药物性能与主药不一定相同,但存在着某些联系。如补气利水的黄芪配伍利水渗湿的防己,后者可加强前者的利水作用,而治脾虚水肿;清热泻火的石膏配伍散寒止痛的细辛,可泻火止痛,治胃火牙痛等。

Mutual restraint: That is, mutual restraining effect

相畏:即一种药物的毒

of different medicines to weaken or neutralize each other's harmfulness, such as toxicity or side-effects. For example, the poisonous action of Banxia (*Rhizoma Pineliae*) or Nanxing (*Rhizoma Arisaematis*) may be decreased or eliminated by Shengjiang (*Rhizoma Zingiberis Recens*), therefore we say there is mutual restraint between Banxia (*Rhizoma Pineliae*) or Nanxing (*Rhizoma Arisaematis*) and Shengjiang (*Rhizoma Zingiberis Recens*).

性或副作用,能被另一种药物减轻或消除。如半夏或南星的毒性能被生姜所减弱,就称为半夏或南星畏生姜。

Mutual detoxication: That is, one medicinal herb can relieve or remove toxic properties and side-effects of the other. For instance, Shengjiang (*Rhizoma Zingiberis Recens*) can be used to relieve or eliminate the toxicity or side effects of Banxia (*Rhizoma Pineliae*), Nanxing (*Rhizoma Arisaematis*), etc., therefore it is said that Shengjiang (*Rhizoma Zingiberis Recens*) can detoxicate the toxicity or eliminate the side effects of these medicinal herbs. From the mentioned above, we can see that mutual restraint and mutual detoxication actually refer to same thing, yet each one is putting its constraint into the others.

相杀:即一种药物能减轻或消除另一种药物的毒性和副作用。如生姜能减轻半夏、南星的毒性等,就称为生姜杀半夏、南星毒。相畏、相杀实际上是同一配伍关系的两种提法。

Mutual inhibition: That is, when two herbs are used together, one herb and the other act on each other, resulting in their original actions being weakened, even lose of their medicinal effects. For instance, the qi-tonifying effect of Renshen (*Radix Ginseng*) can be weakened by Laifuzi (*Semen Raphani*). So we say there is mutual inhibition between Renshen (*Radix Ginseng*) and Laifuzi (*Semen Raphani*).

相恶:即两种药物同用,一种药物的功效能被另一种药物降低,甚则丧失。如人参的补气作用,能被莱菔子削弱等。就称人参恶莱菔子。

Incompatibility: That is, toxic reaction or side-effects may result when two incompatible ingredients are used in combination. For instance, there are eighteen incompatible medicaments which are believed to give rise to serious side effects if given in combination.

相反:即两种药物合用,能产生或增强毒性反应和副作用。如"十八反"中的药物。

In clinical application of medicinal herbs, we should

临床应用药物,应尽量用

make the widest possible use of the two kinds of ingredients with the relation of mutual reinforcement or mutual assistance so as to make full use of their coordination and reinforcing each other's action and to raise their therapeutic effects and extend the range of their treatment. When we use medicinal herbs with toxicity or severe side-effects, we should choose the herbs with the relation of mutual restraint or mutual detoxication with the purpose of weakening or eliminating each other's toxic action or side-effects. The medicinal herbs with the relation of mutual inhibition and incompatibility should be avoided as much as possible to use in combination so as to prevent the therapeutic effects from decreasing or losing, or to stop producing toxin and side effects.

相须和相使的配伍，这样可充分利用其协同作用和增效作用，以提高疗效，扩大治疗范围；在应用有毒药物或药性剧烈具有副作用的药物时，可有意选择有“相畏”、“相杀”关系的配伍，以制约其毒副作用；而对“相恶”和“相反”的药物，则尽量避免同用，以防止药物疗效的降低或丧失，甚或产生的毒副作用。

4 Contraindication of Chinese Medicinal Herbs

第四章 用药禁忌

Herbal medicine can not only produce actions of treating and preventing disorders but also have the harmful effect to human beings. When learning medicinal properties, we should not only know their therapeutic effects but also grasp their harmful actions produced after taking. For instance, cool or cold Chinese medicinal herbs having the effect on clearing away heat may be likely to damage yang; warm or hot ones having the effect on dispersing pathogenic cold may damage yin; drastic ones having the effect on removing pathogenic factors may damage healthy qi; tonics having the effect on invigorating healthy qi may linger the pathogenic factors; ones with lifting yang used in the patient with exuberance of yang may produce the side-effect of lifting yang seriously; ones with the action of lowering the adverse-rising qi can make it worse for the patient with qi-collapse, etc.. For example, Huanglian (*Rhizoma Coptidis*) cold in nature and bitter in flavor is indicated for diarrhea due to damp-heat, but it is not suitable for diarrhea due to spleen-yang deficiency. Ganjiang (*Rhizoma Zingiberis*) hot in nature and pungent in flavor is indicated for cough due to lung-cold, but contraindicated for dry cough due to lung-heat. In a word, the preponderant properties of these medicinal herbs which have an unfavorable aspect on human body should be corrected or avoided, which is essential to understand the contraindications of medicinal herbs.

药物有防治疾病，对人体有利的一面，但也有毒副作用，对人体不利的一面。学习药性，既要了解其防治疾病的作用，也要了解其可能产生的不良反应。如寒凉药虽能清热，但能伤阳；温热药虽可散寒，但易耗阴；攻伐药固然可以祛邪，但每致伤正；滋补药虽能扶正，但可恋邪；升阳药阳亢者用之阳升更甚；降逆药气陷者投之反致增剧；等等。例如苦寒的黄连，能治湿热泻痢，但不宜用于脾阳虚的泄泻。辛热的干姜，能治肺寒的咳嗽，但肺热燥咳者忌用。总之，从药性之偏，认识其对人体的不利的一面，避其所短，是掌握用药禁忌的关键。

The contraindications are divided into caution and

用药禁忌，按其程度不

abstention from some disorders according to their degree. Some herbs are not suitable for some cases as for their medicinal natures, but when they are processed, combined with other or given improvement of their administration, they can also be used.

同,有禁用(或忌用)和慎用之分。有些药物,就其本身具有的药性来说,对某些病证是不宜使用的,但是通过炮制、配伍、改进给药方法等还是可以应用的。

Besides, the contraindication in pregnant women and in compatibility should be known well.

用药禁忌,除了上述内容外,还应掌握妊娠用药禁忌及配伍禁忌。

4.1 Prescription incompatibility

1. 配伍禁忌

Prescription incompatibility refers to that some medicinal herbs can not be used together in a prescription, otherwise the toxic effect will be produced harming the patient's health, and even his life. Incompatibility also denotes incompatible medicinal herbs, especially denotes "the 18 incompatible medicaments". and "19 medicaments of mutual antagonisms".

配伍禁忌是指某些药物不能配伍应用,否则会产生毒副作用,危害患者的健康,甚则危及生命,也就是指相反的药物,具体是指"十八反"和"十九畏"。

In the 18 incompatible medicaments the following herbs are believed to be incompatible in their actions if given in combination: Wutou (*Radix Aconiti*) being incompatible with Banxia (*Rhizoma Pinelliae*), Gualou (*Fructus Trichosanthis*), Beimu (*Bulbus Fritillariae*), Bailian (*Radix Ampelopsis*) and Baiji (*Rhizoma Bletinae*); Gancao (*Radix Glycyrrhizae*) incompatible with Haizao (*Sargassum*), Daji (*Radix Euphorbiae Pekinensis*), Yuanhua (*Flos Genkwa*) and Gansui (*Radix Euphorbiae Kansui*); Lilu (*Rhizoma et Radix Veratri*) incompatible with Renshen (*Radix Ginseng*), Shashen (*Radix Adenophorae Strictae*), Danshen (*Radix Salviae Miltiorrhizae*), Xuanshen (*Radix Scrophulariae*), Kushen (*Radix Sophorae Flavescentis*), Xixin (*Herba Asari*) and Shaoyao (*Radix Paeoniae*). Nineteen medicaments of mutual antagonisms include Liuhuang (*Sulfur*) being antagonistic Qianniuzi (*Semen Pharbitidis*),

"十八反"的内容是:乌头反半夏、瓜蒌、贝母、白蔹、白及;甘草反海藻、大戟、芫花、甘遂;藜芦反人参、沙参、丹参、玄参、苦参、细辛、芍药。"十九畏"的内容是:硫黄畏牵牛子,丁香畏郁金,川乌、草乌畏犀角,牙硝畏三棱,官桂畏五灵脂。必须说明,这里所说的"畏"是相恶之意,与中药配伍关系中的"相畏"涵义不同。

Dingxiang (*Flos Caryorphylli*) antagonistic to Yujin (*Radix Curcumae*), Chuanwu (*Radix Aconiti*) and Caowu (*Radix Aconiti Kusnezoffii*) to Xijiao (*Cornu Rhinocerotis Asiatici*), Yaxiao (*Crystallized Mirabilite*) to Sanleng (*Rhizoma Sparganii*) and Guangui (*Cortex Cinnamomi*) to Wulingzhi (*Faeces Trogopterorum*). It must be denoted that "being antagonistic" here means "being loath" or "being dislike", which is different from "Mutual Restraint" in the compatibility of Chinese medicinal herbs.

As to the 18 incompatible medicaments and 19 medicaments of mutual antagonisms, they are regarded as ingredients which are incompatible, but some of them were still used in combination by some physician in various dynasties. The conclusion of the 18 incompatible medicaments and 19 medicaments of antagonisms got in modern experiments and research is not completely similar. Therefore, the conclusion has not been confirmed and further research will be made. So we should use them cautiously and generally we should avoid using them in combination.

"十八反"和"十九畏"中的药物不宜同用,但有部分内容与实际应用并不完全相同,历代医家也有所论及,"畏"、"反"药物同用的方剂也不乏其例。现代实验研究,结论亦不完全一致。因此,尚难给予肯定和否定,还有待于进一步研究。但在未得出结论之前,应慎重应用,一般情况下,仍遵循传统习惯,避免配伍同用。

4.2 Contraindication of Chinese medicinal herbs in pregnancy

2. 妊娠用药禁忌

Some medicinal herbs should be regarded as those that are contraindicated or used with cautions in pregnant women, otherwise, side effects of damaging fetus, inducing abortion or miscarriage may be brought about. They may be divided into two kinds, one being contraindicated in pregnancy, which involve poisonous medicinal herbs and drastic purgatives; the other being used with caution, which mainly includes those for eliminating blood stasis and promoting circulation of qi, the purgatives and part of herbs warming the interior. If this kind of medicinal herbs are used improperly, the fetus may be damaged or abortion (miscarriage) may be induced.

妇女妊娠期间,有些药物不能使用,而又有些药物应谨慎使用,否则会损伤胎元或引起坠胎。妊娠用药禁忌一般分为两类:一类为禁用药,多是毒性强烈或药性峻猛药;一类为慎用药,主要是活血祛瘀药、行气药、攻下药、温里药中的部分药,这些药物应用不当亦可损伤胎气,引起坠胎。

Chinese medicinal herbs contraindicated are Shuiyin (*Hydrargyrum*), Pishuang (*Arsenicum*), Xionghuang (*Realgar*), Qingfen (*Calomelas*), Banmao (*Radix Sacchari Arundinacei*), Wugong (*Scolopendra*), Maqianzi (*Semen Strychni*), Chansu (*Venenum Bufonis*), Chuanwu (*Radix Aconiti*), Caowu (*Radix Aconiti Kusnezoffii*), Lilu (*Radix et Rhizoma Veratri*), Danfan (*Chalcanthium*), Guadi (*Pedicellus Melo Fructus*), Badou (*Fructus Crotonis*), Gansui (*Radix Euphorbiae Kansui*), Daji (*Radix Euphorbiae Pekinensis*), Yuanhua (*Flos Genkwa*), Qianniuzi (*Semen Pharbitidis*), Shanglu (*Radix Phytolaccae*), Shexiang (*Moschus*), Ganqi (*Resina Rhois Praeparata*), Shuizhi (*Hirudo*), Mengchong (*Tabanus*), Sanleng (*Rhizoma Sparganii*), and Ezhu (*Rhizoma Curcumae*), etc..

禁用药：水银、砒霜、雄黄、轻粉、斑蝥、蜈蚣、马钱子、蟾酥、川乌、草乌、藜芦、胆矾、瓜蒂、巴豆、甘遂、大戟、芫花、牵牛子、商陆、麝香、干漆、水蛭、虻虫、三棱、莪术等。

Chinese medicinal herbs used with caution are Niuxi (*Radix Achyranthis Bidentatae*), Chuanxiong (*Rhizoma Chuanxiong*), Honghua (*Flos Carthami*), Taoren (*Semen Persicae*), Jianghuang (*Rhizoma Curcumae Longae*), Mudanpi (*Cortex Montan Radicis*), Zhishi (*Fructus Aurantii Immaturus*), Zhike (*Fructus Aurantii*), Dahuang (*Radix et Rhizoma Rhei*), Fanxieye (*Folium Cassiae*), Luhui (*Aloe*), Tiannanxing (*Tuber Arisaematis*), Mangxiao (*Natrii Sulfas*), Fuzi (*Radix Aconiti Lateralis Praeparata*), and Rougui (*Cortex Cinnamomi*), etc..

慎用药：牛膝、川芎、红花、桃仁、姜黄、牡丹皮、枳实、枳壳、大黄、番泻叶、芦荟、天南星、芒硝、附子、肉桂等。

No matter whether the medicinal herbs are regarded as forbidden herbs or cautiously used ones, they should be avoided in pregnancy if there is no special need so as to avoid unexpected results. But if the pregnant woman is dangerously ill, and no other choices are available, those mentioned above may be used with great care. If the patient in pregnancy has been unconscious due to severe illness, the medicinal herbs for regaining consciousness like Shexiang (*Moschus artifactus*) may be still used to make her conscious.

凡是妊娠禁忌或慎用的药物，若无特殊需要。孕妇应尽量避免使用，以防发生意外，造成不良后果。但如遇到孕妇患者有严重疾病，不用禁忌或慎用类药物不能治愈时，亦可慎重地酌情使用。如孕妇患病已神志昏迷时，仍可使用麝香等开窍药物，以苏醒神志。

4.3 Dietetic restraint

Dietetic restraint is that some sorts of foods are prohibited or limited to be eaten for therapeutic purpose during taking certain medicinal herbs.

Generally speaking, a patient should abstain from raw, cold, greasy and irritant foods and foods with smelling of fish or mutton during taking medicinal herbs. In addition, dietetic restraint differs in different diseases. For example, pungent, greasy or fried food is prohibited while a patient is affected with heat-syndrome; raw and cold foods should be avoided while a patient is affected with cold-syndrome; fatty or greasy foods, smoking and drinking spirits should be prohibited while a patient with such syndromes as retention of phlegm in the chest, chest distress and cardiac pain; pungent foods should be avoided in a patient with syndromes of headache and dizziness due to hyperactivity of liver-yang; fried and greasy foods should be prohibited in a patient with deficiency of the stomach and spleen; fish, shrimp, crab and pungent foods should be prohibited in a patient with pathogenic infection and ulcerous disease of skin and other skin troubles.

In ancient medical classic books, onion is prohibited while Changshan (*Radix Dichroae*) is taken; green Chinese onion, garlic or turnip is prohibited while Dihuang (*Radix Rehmanniae*) or Heshouwu (*Radix Polygoni Multiflori*) is taken; soft-shelled turtle is prohibited while Bohe (*Herba Menthae*) is taken; vinegar is prohibited while Fuling (*Poria*) is taken; three-colored amaranth is prohibited while Biejia (*Carapax Trionycis*) is taken and taking honey should abstain from onion. From the above, we can see that some medicinal herbs cannot be taken together with some foods, otherwise, there can be no benefits to the cure of a disease and even toxic effects can be brought about. We should take all the above for reference when we take Chinese medicinal herbs.

3. 服药时的饮食禁忌

饮食禁忌，又叫忌口、食忌，就是指服药期间对某些食物的禁忌。

一般而言，凡病人在服药期间都应忌食生冷、油腻、腥膻和有刺激性的食物。另外，根据不同的疾病，饮食禁忌也不相同。如热性疾病忌食辛辣、油腻、煎炸类食物；寒性疾病忌食生冷；痰阻胸阳，胸闷心痛者，忌食肥腻及烟、酒；肝阳上亢、头痛眩晕者，忌食辛辣之品；脾胃虚弱者忌食油炸黏腻等物；疮疡、皮肤病患者，忌食鱼、虾、蟹及辛辣食品。

在古代文献中还有服常山忌食葱；服地黄、何首乌忌食葱、蒜、萝卜；服薄荷忌食鳖肉；服茯苓忌服醋；服鳖甲忌苋菜，以及蜜反生葱等记载。说明服用某些药物时不能和某些食物同食，食之则不利于疾病的治愈，甚则产生毒副作用。这些都应作为用药时的参考。

5 Dosage and Administration

第五章 剂量与煎服法

5.1 Dosage

第一节 剂 量

The amount of medicinal herbs to be taken is called dosage, which signifies the daily amount of one particular herb by adults, and secondly shows the comparative measurements of medicinal herbs in the same prescription and is also known as relative dosage. Generally speaking, the amount following each herb refers to the daily amount of one dried raw herb by adults in making decoction or the daily amount of powder by adults, which is ground from dry raw herbs. As to the amount of Chinese medicinal herbs to be taken, we mostly take weight as the unit of measurement, and take quantity and capacity as the unit for the special ones. Now we take the metric system (g) as the unit of measurement, which is now stipulated in the mainland of China.

剂量,即用药量。主要是指每一味药的成人一日量;其次是指方剂中药与药之间的比较用量,即相对剂量。一般而言,各药下所标明的用量是指干燥后的生药在汤剂中的成人一日内服量及干燥后生药研作末后成人一次服用量。中药的用量,大多以重量计算,个别以数量、容量表示。现在中国内地规定的重量计算单位是以公制克为单位。

As the dosage of a medicinal herb has direct relationship with its therapeutic effect, a medicinal herb when used below its level of effective dosage, will not achieve desired results; the dose of a certain herb when used beyond its limit, may often damage the healthy qi and is also wasted. Since most Chinese medicinal herbs are generally crude plants with fairly moderate nature and a wide-safety range of dosage, their doses may not be used so strictly as those of chemicals. But some of them are also drastic or extremely poisonous, so their doses must be used properly to get the best therapeutic effects and meanwhile prevent

药物剂量的大小与疗效有着直接的关系,如病重药轻,则不能达到预期的治疗效果;病轻药重,又常常伤及正气,并浪费药材。中药大都是原生药,安全幅度较大,用量没有化学药品那样严格,但其中也有一些性质猛烈和剧毒的药物,使用时应恰当地掌握剂量,以取得最好的治疗效果,并防止发生中毒。

patients from poisoning.

The dosage of Chinese medicinal herbs is yet affected by the following factors, and it is used flexibly.

中药的用量还受下列因素的影响，有一定的灵活性。

5.1.1 Properties of medicinal herbs

1. 药物的性质

The medicinal herbs moderate in nature can be used in a large amount; those drastic or poisonous in nature must be used in a small amount; those light in property should be used in a small amount; those heavy in property, such as mineral and shell but without toxin can be used in a large amount; fresh plant medicinal herbs, since they contain water, should be used in amount about twice as much as dry ones.

性质平和者，用量可大些；有毒、药性峻猛者，用量宜小；质轻者，用量宜小；质重者（如矿物药、贝壳类药）、无毒者，用量宜大；新鲜植物药，因含水分，用量应比干燥药大 1 倍左右。

5.1.2 Compatibility and dosage

2. 配伍、剂型

The amount of a singly used herb is usually large than that applied in a prescription; the amount of a main ingredient in a prescription larger than that of an accessory one; the amount of a medicinal herb in making decoction larger than that in pills or powder. For instance, Rougui (*Cortex Cinnamomi*) used in decoction usually weights 3 g, but if used in pill or powder, it is only needed 0.5 - 1 g.

单味药物的用量宜大，复方的用量相对较小，药物在方中作为主药的用量较辅药用量大些。在剂型方面，汤剂的用量比丸、散剂用量大，如肉桂入汤剂一般用 3 克，而入丸、散剂则只需 0.5～1 克即可。

5.1.3 The condition of illness, the patients' physique and age

3. 病情、体质、年龄

The amount of a medicinal herb used in the treatment of serious and acute disease must be fairly larger while the amount used in the treatment of the mild or chronic comparatively smaller. The amount used for those with strong physique must be larger while for those with weak physique, the old and children, the dose generally smaller. For children over 6 years, half the dose of an adult's is used; for the children below 5 years, 1/3 - 1/2 dose of an adult's is used; for an infant, the dose should be much smaller.

重病、急性病用量宜大，病轻、慢性病用量宜小；体质虚弱者用量宜小，体质壮实者宜大；儿童及老人用量一般较小。一般小儿的用量，6 岁以上者，可用成人的 1/2，5 岁以下，可用成人的 1/3～1/2；婴幼儿用量应更小。

Besides, the dose of expensive medicines under

除此以外，价格昂贵的药

ensurance of medicinal effects should be small, such as, Shexiang (*Moschus Artifactus*), Niuhuang (*Calculus Bovis*), etc., that we should avoid waste of medicinal materials and economic burden on the patient; the dose must be used flexibly according to the differences of patient's physique and areas, climates, and seasons, etc..

物,在保证药效的前提下,用量宜小。如麝香、牛黄等,以免浪费药材和增加病人的经济负担;还要根据病人的个体差异,地域的不同,及气候、季节的具体情况,灵活掌握药物的用量。

5.2 Administration

第二节 煎服法

The common administration of Chinese medicinal herbs may be oral, external or local. Forms of decoction, pill, powder, soft extract, and wine, etc., are prepared for oral use, while application, moxibustion, pigmentum, lotion, laryngeal insufflation of medicinal powder, eye drops, thermotherapy, and suppository, etc. are used exteriorly. Whereas the form of decoction is still most widely used at present, which are generally prepared by patients. Therefore doctors should tell their patients or patient's relatives how to decoct medicinal herbs in order to ensure achieving desired effects in clinical application of medicinal herbs.

药物的用法有内服和外用之分,内服多制成汤、丸、散、膏、酒等剂型,外用有敷、灸、涂搽、洗浴、吹喉、点眼、温熨、坐药等。但汤剂,仍然是目前中医应用最广的剂型,并且大多由患者自制。为了保证临床用药能获得预期的效果,医生应将汤剂的正确煎煮和服用方法向患者或亲属交待清楚。

5.2.1 Methods of decocting Chinese medicinal herbs

1. 煎药法

Stewing utensils available are a clay pot or earthen jar or a piece of enamelware. The water available must be clean and without peculiar smell. First put Chinese medicinal herbs into the enamelware and add water to it, the water being usually over the surface of the herbs. Before being decocted, the Chinese medicinal herbs need immersing in water for half an hour so as to make their medicinal components easily dissolve in the solution. Fire used in decocting the herbs should be controlled in the light of medicinal properties and qualities. The medicinal herbs with

煎药的器皿宜用砂锅或砂罐。煎药用水必须无异味,洁净澄清。将药物倒入器皿中加入洁净的水,以淹没药物为度,浸泡半小时左右即可煎煮。火候的控制可根据药物的性质和质地而定,气味芳香者,宜武火急煎,煮沸数分钟后,改用文火略煮即可,否则药效减弱;滋补药物质地滋

aromatic smell should be decocted with strong fire until the solution is boiled for several minutes, then a small fire is followed until the decoction is done, otherwise the medicinal effects will reduce; nourishing medicinal herbs, since their qualities are greasy, should be decocted with a small fire for a long time or the effective factors are not easily decocted out. A dose of Chinese medicinal herbs is taken daily, which is usually decocted twice while nourishing ones may be decocted three times, the decocted juice being about 250 - 300 ml.

腻,宜文火久煎,否则有效成分难以煎出。一般每日 1 剂,煎煮 2 次,滋补药可煎 3 次。煎成药汁 250 ~ 300 毫升即可。

Since their qualities and properties are usually obviously different, different medicinal herbs should be given different treatment in decocting method and time. When a prescription is made out, the methods should be noted, so as to be followed by drug store or patients when the solution is decocted. The chief methods are shown as follows.

各种药物的质地、性质往往有显著差异,因此,煎煮方法或煎煮时间常不相同。处方时应予写明,以便药房配药及患者煎煮时遵循,主要有以下几种方法。

Being decocted first: some kinds of minerals and shell medicines, such as Shigao (*Gypsum Fibrosum*), Cishi (*Magnetium*), Shijueming (*Concha Haliotidis*) and Biejia (*Carapax Trionycis*) must be decocted first for 10 - 30 minutes, then the other kinds are put in, since they are hard in qualities and their effective components are not easily decocted out. The method is also indicated for decocting or boiling poisonious medicinal herbs, such as Wutou (*Radix Aconiti*) and Fuzi (*Radix Aconiti Lateralis Praeparata*) thus their poisonous effects may be lessened or eliminated.

先煎:将药物放入器皿中,加水煎煮 10～30 分钟后,再放入其他药物煎煮。主要适用于矿物、介壳类等质地较硬,有效成分不易煎出的药物,如石膏、磁石、石决明、鳖甲等。也适用于煎煮能降低毒性的有毒药物,如乌头、附子等。

Being decocted later: Some aromatic medicinal herbs such as Bohe (*Herba Menthae*), Sharen (*Fructus Amomi*), Gouteng (*Ramulus Uncariae cum Uncis*) and Shengdahuang (*Radix et Rhizoma Rhei*) with volatile components must be added after the solution of the other medicinal herbs has been boiled 10 - 30 minutes, and then boiled another 5 minutes or so.

后下:先煎煮其他药物 10～30 分钟,再加入后下的药物,煎煮 5 分钟左右即可。主要适用于气味芳香或久煎有效成分易于破坏的药物。如薄荷、砂仁、钩藤、生大黄等。

Boiling of wrapped herbs: Some medicinal herbs must be wrapped in a piece of cloth or of gauze, and then put together with others in an enamelware to which water is added . The method is mainly indicated for the following medicinal herbs : the herbs, if decocted directly in water will make their decoction turbid which is difficult to be taken orally; some small seed medicinal herbs, after boiled, will float on the decoction and not be removed easily; some downy herbs, if decocted directly in water, will make their decoction mixed with soft hairs, which can not be removed easily and can irritate the throat when the decoction is taken. For instance, Chishizhi (*Halloysitum Rubrum*), Feihuashi (*Talcum*), Cheqianzi (*Semen Plantaginis*) and Xuanfuhua (*Flos Inulae*).

包煎：将药物用纱布包后，和其他药物一同放入器皿中加水煎煮。主要适用于下列药物：入煎后会使药液混浊，难以入口；细小种子类药物，煎后会浮于液面；附有绒毛的药物，对咽喉有刺激。如赤石脂、飞滑石、车前子、旋覆花等。

Decocting or boiling singlely: The Chinese medicinal herbs, such as Renshen (*Radix Ginseng*) and Lingyangjiao (*Cornu Saigae Tataricae*) must be decocted or boiled separately, which is mainly indicated for some precious medicines in order to prevent them being absorbed by other ingredients when they are decocted or boiled with other medicinal herbs.

另炖或另煎：将另炖或另煎的药物单独炖或煎，而不和其他药物一同煎煮。主要适用于贵重药物，避免与其他药物同煎时其有效成分被其他药物吸附。如人参、羚羊角等。

Melting: Put the medicinal herbs to be melted into the decoction that has been boiled well and hasn't contained dregs of decoction and the medicinhal herbs being stirred together until they are melted well for oral use. Besides, the medicines can also be melted by steaming in the container with water, and then the melted ones are mixed with the decocted juice without dregs for oral use. The method is mainly indicated for the medicine containing a lot of mucilage and easily soluble ones, such as Ejiao (*Colla Corii Asini*), Guibanjiao (*Colla Plastri Testudinis*) and Yitang (*Saccharum Granorum*). If decocted directly together with other herb medicines in water, they will be deposited at the bottom of the pot or

烊化：将要烊化的药物放入煎好去渣的药液中微煮，同时搅拌使其溶解后服用。亦可将要烊化的药物放入器皿中加水蒸化，然后倒入已煎好去渣的药液中搅匀服用。主要适用于胶类及性黏而易于溶解的药物，以防与其他药物同煎时粘附其他药物，或粘锅煮焦。如阿胶、龟版胶、饴糖等。

stick to the other ingredients and not be easily filtered.

Infusions for oral taking: Some medicines that are dissolved as soon as they are put in water, such as Mangxiao (*Natrii Sulfas*). Some kinds of juice medicine such as Zhuli (*Succus Phyllostachydis Henonis*), Fengmi (*Mel*) and Yitang (*Saccharum Granorum*), and those that are got by grinding such kinds of medicines as Lingyangjiao (*Cornu Saigae Tataricae*), Chenxiang (*Lignum Aquilariae Resinatum*) with water do not need decocting and are suitable to be mixed directly with water or the decocted juice for oral use.

冲服：入水即化的药，如芒硝；汁液类药物，如竹沥、蜂蜜、饴糖等，以及羚羊角、沉香等加水磨取的药汁，不需入煎，宜直接用开水或药汁冲服。

5.2.2 Methods of taking Chinese medicinal herbs

2. 服药法

Generally speaking, decoction must be taken warm. Chinese medicinal herbs in a prescription or a dose may be decocted twice, and the decocted juice is mixed together, being divided into two parts for daily use. An acute case must take two doses a day or even three doses, that is, once for every four hours. A chronic patient may take a dose a day or two days. Those used for stopping vomiting should be taken frequently in small amount; a patient with unconsciousness or trismus may be fed through his nose; diaphoretics should be taken warmly so as to promote the medicinal actions until sweating; purging Chinese medicinal herbs are taken until reducing diarrhea or vomiting. Pill or powder may be taken with warm water. As far as treatments are concerned, Chinese medicinal herbs warm in nature should be taken in cold or those cold in nature should be taken in warm.

中药汤剂一般宜温服，每日 1 剂，煎 2 次，每服 1 煎。病情急重者可 1 日 2 剂，甚或 3 剂，即每 4 小时煎服一次；慢性病可隔日 1 次，或 1 剂分 2 日服，即每日服 1 煎。止吐药宜少量多次服；昏迷病人或牙关紧闭者可予鼻饲；发汗药宜热服，以助药力，以出汗为宜；泻下药以下为度，否则泻下太过损伤正气。丸、散等药可用温开水送服。若用从治法，则热药冷服，或冷药热服。

As for the time of taking medicine, tonics should be taken before meals, paraciticides and purging medicinal herbs should be taken when stomach is empty, those for calming the mind should be taken before sleeping and those for stopping malaria should be taken two hours

从服药时间来说，滋补药宜食前服，驱虫药和泻下药宜空腹服，安神药宜在睡前服，截疟药宜在疟发前 2 小时服。对胃肠有刺激性的药物宜在

ahead when the disease has an attack. Those irritant to the stomach and intestine should be taken after meals. A patient with an acute disease may take medicine as soon as the disease attacks without limits of time.

饭后服。急性病则可以不拘时间,随时服用。

Specific Discussions 各论

1 Diaphoretics or Exterior Syndrome Relieving Chinese Medicinal Herbs

第一章 解表药

Any Chinese medicinal herb that has the actions of dispersing or expelling pathogens from the superficies and relieving the exterior syndrome by means of perspiration is considered to be a diaphoretic medicinal herbs.

凡以发散表邪，解除表证为主要作用的药物，称解表药，又叫发表药。

This kind of medicinal herbs are mainly attributed to the lung and bladder meridians. They can promote sweating in varying degree and disperse pathogenic factors from the superficies. They are mainly indicated for the superficies-syndrome caused by exogenous pathogenic factors attacking the body, such as aversion to cold, fever, headache, general soreness, anhidrosis or unsmooth perspiration and floating pulse, etc. Some of them are also accompanied with the actions of inducing diuresis to reduce edema, relieving cough and dyspnea, letting out skin eruption, dispelling wind and dampness to relieve arthralgia-pain and eliminating sore. They are suitable for edema, cough and dyspnea, measles with inadequate eruption at the early stage, rheumatic arthralgia and initial syndrome of sore or ulcer with the exterior-syndrome.

本类药物以入肺经与膀胱二经为主。具有透发毛窍，发汗解表之作用。主治外感表证恶寒，发热，头痛，身痛，无汗或有汗不畅，脉浮。部分药物兼有利尿消肿，止咳平喘，透疹，祛风湿止痹痛，消疮作用，可用于水肿，喘咳，麻疹初起，透发不畅，风湿痹证，疮疡初起兼有表证者。

Diaphoretics are divided into two kinds: pungent-warm herbs relieving superficies, also termed as the herbs for dispersing wind-cold, and pungent-cool herbs relieving superficies, also termed as herbs for dispersing wind-

解表药分辛温解表药（又称发散风寒药）和辛凉解表药（又称发散风热药）两类，临床应辨证选用并注意配伍。兼

heat, which should be selected according to the differentiation of syndrome and their compatibility should be paid attention to in clinic. If the exterior syndrome is accompanied with interior heat, it should be treated with diaphoretics combined with the herbs for clearing away heat; if accompanied with dampness, it should be treated in combination with those for expelling dampness; if accompanied with pathogenic dryness, it should be combined with those for moisturizing. If a weak patient is attacked by exogenous pathogenic factors, he should be treated with diaphoretics combined with tonics so as to strengthen healthy qi and eliminate pathogenic factors.

内热者，配清热药；挟湿者，配祛湿药；兼燥邪者，与润燥药同用。若虚弱者外感，应配伍补益药，以扶正祛邪。

When diaphoretics are used, their dosage should be controlled and the application should be stopped as soon as the syndrome disappears, otherwise, profuse-sweating will consume yang and the body fluids. Therefore, they should be contraindicated or used with great care for spontaneous perspiration due to superficial asthenia, night sweat due to yin-deficiency, and prolonged pyocutaneous disease, stranguria or blood loss with exterior syndrome.

使用解表药时，应控制用量，中病即止，否则发汗太多，易耗伤阳气，损及津液。表虚自汗，阴虚盗汗，以及疮疡日久、淋证、失血者，虽有表证，均当忌用或慎用。

Diaphoretics mostly with active volatile oil, if added to decoction, should not be decocted or boiled for a long time to prevent effective constituents from volatilizing so as to decrease the therapeutic results.

解表药多含挥发油，入汤剂不宜久煎，以免有效成分挥发而降低疗效。

1.1 Diaphoretics with pungent-warm property

第一节 辛温解表药

This kind of herbs are most pungent in taste and warm in nature and have remarkable action of dispersing wind-cold from superficies. They are indicated in patients with the exterior syndrome caused by wind-cold, which are characterized by chills, fever, anhidrosis or unsmooth perspiration, headache, general soreness, thin and white

本类药物性味多辛温，以发散风寒为主要作用。用于外感风寒表证之恶寒发热，无汗或汗出不畅，头痛，身痛，舌苔薄白，脉浮。部分药物还可用治痹证及咳喘，水肿，麻疹，

tongue coating, floating pulse. Besides, some of them may be used to treat Bi-syndrome, cough and dyspnea, edema, measles and sores at the early stage accompanied with the exterior syndrome of wind-cold.

以及疮疡初起兼表证者。

Mahuang *Herba Ephedrae*

麻黄

The source is from the herbaceous stem of *Ephedra sinica* stapf, *Eintermedia schrenk* et C. A. Mey, and *E. equisetina* Bunge, family Ephedraceae. The producing areas are mainly in Hebei, Shanxi, Gansu provinces and Inner Mongolia Autonomous Region, etc.. The medicinal material is collected in autumn, dried in shade and cut into pieces. Its commonly used form is crude one or the one prepared with honey.

为麻黄科植物草麻黄、木贼麻黄和中麻黄的草质茎。主产于河北、山西、内蒙古、甘肃等地。秋季采收,阴干,切段。生用、蜜炙或捣绒用。

Medicinal Properties Pungent and slightly bitter in flavor, warm in nature, and attributive to the lung and bladder meridians.

【药性】 味辛、微苦,性温。归肺、膀胱经。

Actions Induce sweating to relieve superficies disperse the lung to relieve asthma and promote diuresis to subside edema.

【功效】 发汗解表,宣肺平喘,利水消肿。

Application

【临床应用】

1. It is used for superficial syndrome due to wind and cold. Since the medicinal herb can strongly promote sweating, it is often used for superficial sthenia-syndrome due to wind and cold, which is manifested as aversion to cold, fever, anhidrosis, headache, stuffy nose, floating and tight pulse. It is often used in combination with Guizhi (*Ramulus Cinnamomi*), such as Mahuang Tang (Decoction).

1. 用于外感风寒证。本品发汗作用最强,多用于外感风寒表实证,症见恶寒发热,无汗,头痛,鼻塞,脉浮紧,常与桂枝相须配伍,如麻黄汤。

2. For sthenia-syndromes with cough and dyspnea. It is indicated for all syndromes such as cough and dyspnea due to stagnation of lung-qi, or cold, heat, phlegm or retention of fluids whether they have superficial syndrome or not. It is combined with Xingren (*Semen Pruni Armeniacae*) and Gancao (*Radix Glycyrrhizae*), such as

2. 用于咳喘实证。邪壅于肺,肺气不宣之咳嗽气喘,无论寒、热、痰、饮,有无表证均可应用。风寒郁肺之咳喘,与杏仁、甘草配伍,如三拗汤。肺有寒饮,痰多清稀者,可配

San'ao Tang (Decoction) for cough and dyspnea due to accumulation of wind and cold in the lung. It is combined with Ganjiang (*Rhizoma Zingiberis*), Xixin (*Herba Asari*), Banxia (*Rhizoma Pinelliae*), etc., like Xiaoqinglong Tang (Decoction) for retention of cold-fluid in the lung manifested as profuse watery sputum. It may also be combined with Shigao (*Gypsum Fibrosum*), Xingren (*Semen Pruni Armeniacae*) and Gancao (*Radix Glycyrrhizae*) to treat syndrome with asthma and yellowish-thick sputum due to stagnancy of lung-heat, such as Mahuang Xingren Gancao Shigao Tang (Decoction) to clear away lung heat and relieve dyspnea and cough.

伍干姜、细辛、半夏等，如小青龙汤。肺有郁热，喘息痰黄稠者，也可以与石膏、杏仁、甘草配伍以清肺平喘止咳，如麻黄杏仁甘草石膏汤。

3. For wind edema with exterior syndromes, it is often combined with Shengjiang (*Rhizoma Zingiberis Recens*), Baizhu (*Rhizoma Atractylodis Macrocephalae*), Gancao (*Radix Glycyrrhizae*), etc., such as Yuebi Jia Zhu Tang (Decoction).

3. 用于风水而兼有表证者。常与生姜、白术、甘草等配伍，如越婢加术汤。

Besides, it is also indicated for wind-cold Bi-syndrome, deep-rooted carbuncle of yin type, subcutaneous nodule, etc.. It is often combined with Shudihuang (*Radix Rehmanniae Praeparatae*), Rougui (*Cortex Cinnamomi*), Lujiaojiao (*Colla Cornu Cervi*), etc., such as Yanghe Tang (Decoction) to treat the deep-rooted carbuncle of yin type.

此外，还可治风寒痹证、阴疽、痰核等，治阴疽，常与熟地黄、肉桂、鹿角胶等同用，如阳和汤。

Usage and Dosage 3 -9 g is used in decoction for oral use; the crude form is suitable for inducing sweating to relieve superficies and the prepared form with honey for relieving cough and dyspnea.

【用法用量】 水煎服，3～9 克。发汗解表宜生用，止咳平喘多蜜炙用。

Notes It is not used excessively and contraindicated in conditions of spontaneous perspiration due to exterior deficiency, night sweating due to yin deficiency, asthenia-dyspnea and high blood pressure.

【使用注意】 不可过量使用，表虚自汗、阴虚盗汗、虚喘及高血压患者禁用。

Guizhi *Ramulus Cinnamomi*

桂 枝

The source is from the tender branch of *Cinnamo-*

为樟科植物肉桂的嫩枝。

mum cassia Presl, family Lauraceae. Its producing areas are mainly in the provinces of Guangdong, Guangxi and Yunnan. The medicinal material is collected in spring and summer, and dried either in shade or in the sun, then is cut into pieces or segments for use.

主产于广东、广西及云南。春、夏季割取嫩枝，晒干或阴干，切片或切段。生用。

Medicinal Properties Pungent and sweet in flavor, warm in nature, and attributive to the heart, lung and bladder meridians.

【药性】 味辛、甘，性温。归心、肺、膀胱经。

Actions Induce sweating to relieve superficies and activate yang and circulate qi by warming meridian.

【功效】 发汗解表，温通经脉，通阳化气。

Application

【临床应用】

1. It is used for the superficial syndrome due to wind and cold whether the syndrome is asthenic or sthenic. For the wind-cold syndrome with spontaneous perspiration due to superficial deficiency, it is often combined with Baishaoyao (*Radix Paeoniae Alba*), etc., such as Guizhi Tang (Decoction) to keep the actions of yingqi and weiqi in balance. It is combined with Mahuang (*Herba Ephedrae*) to treat sthenia-syndrome of the superficies with anhidrosis.

1. 用于风寒表证，无论表实或表虚证均可用。感受风寒，表虚自汗，常与白芍药等同用，以调和营卫，如桂枝汤。表实无汗者，常与麻黄同用。

2. It is used for pains due to blood stagnancy due to stagnation of cold. It is often combined with Zhishi (*Fructus Aurantii Immaturus*), Xiebai (*Allii Macrostemi*), etc., such as Gualou Xiebai Guizhi Tang (Decoction) for the treatment of the weakness of thoracic yang, the obstruction in heart channel and thoracic pain due to thoracic obstruction; combined with Fuzi (*Radix Aconiti Lateralis Praeparata*), such as Guizhi Fuzi Tang (Decoction) for the treatment of arthralgia due to stagnation of wind-cold-damp; combined with Taoren (*Semen Persicae*), Mudanpi (*Cortex Moutan Radicis*), etc., such as Guizhi Fuling Wan (Pill) for the treatment of irregular menstruation, dysmenorrhea, amenorrhea or abdominal mass due to blood stagnation caused by invasion of

2. 用于寒凝血滞诸痛证。胸阳不振，心脉瘀阻，胸痹心痛，常与枳实、薤白等同用，如瓜蒌薤白桂枝汤；还可用于风寒湿邪痹阻，关节疼痛，常配附子同用，如桂枝附子汤；妇女寒凝血滞，月经不调，痛经，经闭或腹部有积块，常与桃仁、牡丹皮等同用，如桂枝茯苓丸。

cold.

3. It is combined with Fuling (*Poria*), Baizhu (*Rhizoma Atractylodis Macrocephalae*), etc., such as Ling Gui Zhu Gan Tang (Decoction) for the treatment of palpitation, dizziness and fullness in the chest due to retention of fluids; combined with Zhuling (*Polyporus*), Zexie (*Rhizoma Alismatis*), etc., such as Wuling San (Powder) for dysuria and edema.

Usage and Dosage 3 -9 g is used in decoction for oral use.

Notes Since it is pungent and warm in nature and easily damages yin and blood, it is contraindicated for the syndromes such as exuberant heat impairing yin in seasonal febrile disease, hyperactivity of yang due to yin-deficiency in miscellaneous diseases and bleeding due to blood-heat, and must be used with caution in pregnant women.

Explanation Both Guizhi (*Ramulus Cinnamomi*) and Mahuang (*Herba Ephedrae*) are diaphoretics for dispersing wind-cold, whereas Guizhi (*Ramulus Cinnamomi*) is moderate in action and weaker than Mahuang (*Herba Ephedrae*) in inducing sweating. It can be used for spontaneous perspiration due to superficial deficiency and can be combined with Baishaoyao (*Radix Paeoniae Alba*) to warm the meridians, activate yang, resolve fluid retention and induce diuresis, etc.. Since Mahuang (*Herba Ephedrae*) is a medicinal herb mainly attributive to the lung meridian and has the strong action of perspiration, it is often used for exterior sthenia syndrome with anhidrosis due to wind and cold and can disperse the lung and relieve asthma, promote diuresis to relieve edema.

3. 用于痰饮心悸，头眩，胸胁胀满。可与茯苓、白术同用，如苓桂术甘汤；若小便不利、水肿者，与猪苓、泽泻等同用，如五苓散。

【用法用量】 水煎服，3～9 克。

【使用注意】 本品辛温，易伤阴动血，凡温热病热盛伤阴及杂病阴虚阳亢，血热妄行诸证忌用。孕妇慎用。

【说明】 桂枝与麻黄均为发散风寒药，桂枝发汗力不及麻黄，作用缓和，可用于表虚自汗者，多与白芍药配伍，并有温通经脉，通阳化饮利水等功效。麻黄为肺经主药，发汗之力较强，多用于风寒表实无汗者，还能宣肺平喘，利水消肿。

Zisuye *Folium Perillae*

The source is from the leaf of *Perilla frutescens* (L.) Britt. var. *acuta* (Thunb.) Kudo., family Labiatae. The producing areas are in all parts of China. The

紫苏叶

为唇形科植物紫苏的叶。产于中国各地。夏、秋季采收，阴干。生用。

medicinal material is collected in summer and autumn, dried in shade and the crude form is used for medication.

Medicinal Properties Pungent in flavor, warm in nature, and attributive to the lung and spleen meridians.

【药性】 味辛,性温。归肺、脾经。

Actions Relieve superficial pathogenic factors to dissipate cold, and promote the circulation of qi and regulate the function of the stomach.

【功效】 解表散寒,行气和胃。

Application

【临床应用】

1. It is used for superficial syndrome of wind and cold type with anhidrosis and cough. It is often combined with Xingren (*Semen Pruni Armeniacae*), such as Xingren San (Powder); it can circulate qi as well, so it can be used for wind-cold syndrome due to exogenous attack, with sensation of fullness and oppression in the chest and epigastric region due to qi stagnation. It is often combined with Xiangfu (*Rhizoma Cyperi*), such as Xiang Su San (Powder) to expel exterior wind and cold and interior qi-stagnation.

1. 用于风寒表证,无汗兼咳嗽。常配伍杏仁同用,如杏苏散;又兼能行气,所以外感风寒,兼见胸脘痞闷等气滞之象者,常配香附等以外散风寒,内疏气滞,如香苏散。

2. It is used for the stagnation of spleen-qi and stomach-qi with fullness in the chest and vomiting. It is often combined with Jupi (*Pericarpium Citri Tangerinae*), Banxia (*Rhizoma Pinelliae*), Huoxiang (*Herba Agastachis*), etc., such as Huoxiang Zhengqi San (Powder); for excessive heat syndrome, combined with Huanglian (*Rhizoma Coptidis*); for morning sickness, vomiting and no appetite or feeling of oppression in the thorax during pregnancy, combined with Jupi (*Pericarpium Citri Tangerinae*), Sharen (*Fructus Amomi*), etc.

2. 用于脾胃气滞,胸闷呕吐。常配伍橘皮、半夏、藿香等,如藿香正气散;偏热者,可与黄连同用。治妊娠恶阻,呕吐不食,或妊娠胎气上逆,常与橘皮、砂仁等同用。

In addition, it can also relieve fish and crab poisoning. It can be used in single or combined with Shengjiang (*Rhizoma Zingiberis Recens*), Jupi (*Pericarpium Citri Tangerinae*), and Huoxiang (*Herba Agastachis*), etc. to treat poisoning with vomiting and diarrhea after intake of fish and crab.

此外,还能解鱼蟹毒。凡食鱼蟹中毒,呕吐,腹泻,可单用水煎服,或配伍生姜、橘皮、藿香等同用。

Usage and Dosage 3 -10 g is used in decoction for oral use. But it is not suitable to be decocted for a long time.

【用法用量】 水煎服，3～10克。不宜久煎。

Explanation During treatment, either its leaves or its stems are often used in separation. Its stems are pungent in flavor and warm in nature, can promote the circulation of qi and regulate the function of the stomach and spleen, therefore, it is often used for stagnation of spleen-qi and stomach-qi, and depression of liver-qi, and not used for superficial syndrome.

【说明】 紫苏的老茎为紫苏梗。性味辛温。功能行气和中。多用于脾胃气滞及肝郁不舒诸证，而无解表之功。

Xiangru *Herba Elsholtziae*

香 薷

Its source is from the aerial parts of the perennial herbaceous plants, herb of *Elsholtzia splendens* Nakai ex F. Maekawa, family Labiatae. The medicinal material is mainly produced in Jiangxi, Anhui and Henan provinces. It is collected when the leaves and stems are vigorous and the fruits are ripe in summer or autumn, dried in the sun and cut into pieces for use.

为唇形科植物石香薷的地上部分。主产于江西、安徽及河南。夏、秋季茎叶茂盛，果实成熟时割取，晒干，切段。生用。

Medicinal Properties Pungent in flavor, slightly warm in nature, and attributive to the lung, spleen and stomach meridians.

【药性】 味辛，性微温。归肺、脾、胃经。

Actions Induce sweating to relieve exterior syndrome, eliminate dampness and regulate the function of the spleen and stomach, promote diuresis and relieve edema.

【功效】 发汗解表，化湿和中，利水消肿。

Application

1. It is often combined with Houpo (*Cortex Magnoliae Officinalis*) and Biandou (*Semen Dolichoris Album*), such as Xiangru Yin (Decoction). It is indicated for the illness due to invasion of exogenous wind and cold as well as invasion of the interior by dampness in summer, which is manifested as aversion to cold and fever, headache, anhidrosis, vomiting, and diarrhea, etc..

2. It is used for wind edema with dysuria, and can be

【临床应用】

1. 用于夏季外感风寒，内伤暑湿，症见恶寒发热，头痛无汗，呕吐腹泻。常配伍厚朴、扁豆同用，如香薷饮。

2. 用于风水，小便不利。

used in single or combined with Baizhu (*Rhizoma Atractylodis Macrocephalae*), such as Ru Zhu Wan (Pill).

可单用煎服；或配伍白术同用，如薷术丸。

Usage and Dosage 3 -9 g is used in decoction for oral use.

【用法用量】 水煎服，3～9克。

Notes It is contraindicated in those with perspiration due to superficial deficiency and yang summer-heat syndrome since it is pungent and warm and can induce much sweating.

【使用注意】 本品辛温发汗之力较强，表虚有汗及阳暑证当忌用。

Jingjie *Herba Schizonepetae*

荆 芥

Its source is from aerial parts of the herbaceous plant, *Schizonepeta tenuifolia* Brig., family Labiatae. The medicinal material is mainly produced in Jiangsu, Zhejiang, and Jiangxi provinces, etc. and collected in summer or autumn, dried in shade and cut into segments, generally, either crude or stir-baked or carbonized one is used for medication.

为唇形科植物荆芥的地上部分。主产于江苏、浙江及江西等地。夏、秋季采收，阴干，切段。生用或炒黄、炒炭用。

Medicinal Properties Pungent in flavor, slightly warm in nature, and attributive to the lung and liver meridians.

【药性】 味辛，性微温。归肺、肝经。

Actions Expel wind and relieve exterior syndrome, promote eruption and alleviate itching, the carbonized one arresting bleeding.

【功效】 祛风解表，透疹，止痒，炒炭止血。

Application

【临床应用】

1. It is used for exterior syndrome due to exogenous attack, either wind-cold or wind-heat syndrome. It is often combined with Fangfeng (*Radix Saposhnikoviae*), Qianghuo (*Rhizoma et Radix Notopterygii*), etc., such as Jing Fang Baidu San (Powder) for exterior syndrome due to pathogenic wind-cold, which is manifested as fever and aversion to cold, headache, and anhidrosis, etc.; combined with Jinyinhua (*Flos Lonicerae*), Lianqiao (*Fructus Forsythiae*), and Bohe (*Herba Menthae*), etc., such as Yin Qiao San (Powder) for exterior syndrome due to pathogenic wind-heat, which is manifested

1. 用于外感表证，无论风寒、风热均可应用。风寒表证，发热恶寒，头痛无汗，常配防风、羌活等同用，如荆防败毒散；风热表证，头痛目赤，口渴咽干，多与金银花、连翘、薄荷等配伍，如银翘散。

as headache, redness of eyes, thirst, and dry throat.

2. Used for the unsmooth eruption during measles, and urticaria. It is often combined with Chantui (*Periostracum Cicadae*), Bohe (*Herba Menthae*), and others pungent in flavor and cool in nature with the action of promoting eruptions to treat the unsmooth eruption during measles at the early stage; combined with Kushen (*Radix Sophorae Flavescentis*), Fangfeng (*Radix Saposhnikoviae*), Chishaoyao (*Radix Paeoniae Rubra*), such as Xiaofeng San (Powder) to treat urticaria with itching and eczema with itching and pain.

2. 用于麻疹不透,风疹瘙痒。麻疹初起,透发不畅,常与蝉蜕、薄荷等辛凉透疹之品同用。治风疹瘙痒,湿疹痒痛,常与苦参、防风、赤芍药同用,如消风散。

3. It is used for bleeding-syndrome and the carbonized one can arrest bleeding. It is often combined with Shengdihuang (*Radix Rehmanniae*), Baimaogen (*Rhizoma Imperatae*), and Cebaiye (*Cacumen Biotae*), etc. to treat symptoms of hematemesis and epistaxis; combined with Diyu (*Radix Sanguisorbae*), Huaihua (*Flos Sophorae*), etc. to treat symptoms of bloody stool and bleeding due to hemorrhoids; combined with Zonglütan (*Trachycarpi Carbonisatus*), Lianfang (*Receptaculum Nelumbinis*), etc. for metrorrhagia and metrostaxis.

3. 用于出血证。炒炭后能止血。治吐血,衄血,常配伍生地黄、白茅根、侧柏叶等。治便血、痔血,与地榆、槐花等同用。治妇女崩漏下血,可配伍棕榈炭、莲房等。

4. Used for sores at the early stage accompanied with exterior syndrome. For that being a bit on the wind-cold side, it is combined with Qianghuo (*Rhizoma et Radix Notopterygii*), Chuanxiong (*Rhizoma Chuanxiong*), and Duhuo (*Radix Angelicae Pubescentis*), etc., such as Baidu San (Powder); for that being a bit on the wind-heat side, combined with Jinyinhua (*Flos Lonicerae*), Chaihu (*Radix Bupleuri*) and others, such as Yin Qiao Baidu San (Powder).

4. 用于疮疡初起见有表证。偏于风寒者,与羌活、川芎、独活等同用,如败毒散;偏于风热者,与金银花、柴胡等配伍,如银翘败毒散。

Usage and Dosage 3 -9 g is used in decoction for oral use. It is not suitable to be decocted for a long time. The crude form is used for expelling exogenous pathogenic

【用法用量】 水煎服,3~9克。不宜久煎。发表透疹消疮宜生用,止血宜炒炭用。

factors to promote eruption during measles and treat sores, and the carbonized form for arresting bleeding.

Notes Contraindicated in patients with headache due to yin-deficiency.

【使用注意】表虚自汗，阴虚头痛者禁服。

Fangfeng　*Radix Saposhnikoviae*

防　风

The source is from the root of *Saposhnikoviae divaricata* (Turcz.) Schischk, family Umbelliferae. Its producing areas are mainly in those of Northeast China, Hebei, Sichuan, and Yunnan, etc.. The medicinal material is collected in spring or autumn, dried in the sun and cut into pieces, generally, either crude one or carbonized one is used for medication.

为伞形科植物防风的根。主产于东北及河北、四川、云南等地。春、秋季采挖，晒干，切片。生用或炒炭用。

Medicinal Properties Pungent and sweet in flavor, slightly warm in nature, and attributive to the bladder, liver and spleen meridians.

【药性】 味辛、甘，性微温。归膀胱、肝、脾经。

Actions Expel wind and relieve exterior syndrome, eliminate dampness, relieve convulsion and diarrhea.

【功效】 祛风解表，胜湿，止痉，止泻。

Application

【临床应用】

1. It can be used for exterior syndrome due to exogenous attack, whether the syndrome is caused by wind-cold or wind-heat or it belongs to exterior asthenia or exterior sthenia. It is most suitable to be used for exterior syndrome due to wind-cold, which is manifested as severe headache and general pain, it is often used together with Jingjie (*Herba Schizonepetae*), Qianghuo (*Rhizoma et Radix Notopterygii*), etc., such as Jing Fang Baidu San (Powder). For a disease caused by exogenous wind, cold and dampness manifested as severe headache, general heaviness and painful limbs, it can be used together with Qianghuo (*Rhizoma seu Radix Notopterygii*), Duhuo (*Radix Angelicae Pubescentis*), and Chuanxiong (*Rhizoma Chuanxiong*), etc., such as Qianghuo Shengshi Tang (Decoction).

1. 用于外感表证，不论风寒、风热、表虚、表实证均可使用。风寒表证见头身痛甚者，用之尤宜。常配荆芥、羌活等同用，如荆防败毒散。如外感风寒湿邪，头痛如裹、身重肢痛者，可与羌活、独活、川芎等同用，如羌活胜湿汤。

2. It is suitable for arthralgia of wind-cold-dampness, arthrodynia of the extremities and stiffness of tendon and can be used together with Qianghuo (*Rhizoma et Radix Notopterygii*), Guizhi (*Ramulus Cinnamomi*), and Jianghuang (*Rhizoma Curcumae Longae*), etc., such as Juanbi Tang (Decoction).

2. 用于风寒湿痹,肢节疼痛,筋脉挛急。可配伍羌活、桂枝、姜黄等同用,如蠲痹汤。

3. It is used for tetanus and infantile convulsion. For the treatment of tetanus, it can be used together with Tiannanxing (*Rhizoma Arisaematis*), Baifuzi (*Rhizoma Typhoni*), and Tianma (*Rhizoma Gastrodiae*), etc., such as Yuzhen San (Powder); for high fever and convulsion in children, it is often used together with Gouteng (*Ramulus Uncariae cum Uncis*), Niuhuang (*Calculus Bovis*), and Qingdai (*Indigo Naturalis*), etc..

3. 用于破伤风及小儿惊风。治破伤风,可配伍天南星、白附子、天麻等同用,如玉真散。治小儿高热惊风,常与清热熄风止痉之钩藤、牛黄、青黛等同用。

In addition, for spleen disorder due to liver stagnation marked by abdominal pain with diarrhea, it is often used together with Jupi (*Pericarpium Citri Tangerinae*), Baishaoyao (*Radix Paeoniae Alba*), and Baizhu (*Rhizoma Atractylodis Macrocephalae*), etc., such as Tongxie Yaofang (Decoction).

此外,还可用于肝郁侮脾,腹痛泄泻,常配伍橘皮、白芍药、白术同用,如痛泻要方。

Usage and Dosage 3 -9 g is used in decoction for oral use.

【用法用量】 水煎服,3～9 克。

Notes Contraindicated in the patient with convulsion due to blood-deficiency and hyperactivity of fire due to yin deficiency.

【使用注意】 血虚发痉及阴虚火旺者忌用。

Explanation The herb is slightly warm in nature but not dry, and moderate in medicinal property with mild actions, and considered as one of the medicines for dispersing wind but with moisturizing effect. It is often combined with Jingjie (*Herba Schizonepetae*). Compared with Jingjie (*Herba Schizonepetae*), Fangfeng (*Radix Saposhnikoviae*) has better effect to expel wind and relieve pain, and is suitable for exterior syndrome with gen-

【说明】 本品温而不燥,药性缓和,有"风药中润剂"之称。常与荆芥相须同用。与荆芥相比,防风祛风止痛作用较好,表证身痛者宜用之;荆芥发汗之力较强,且能透疹,止血。

eral pain; Jingjie can promote eruption during measles and arrest bleeding as well as has larger action of promoting sweating.

Qianghuo *Rhizoma et Radix Notopterygii*

Its source is from the dried rhizomes and roots of the perennial herbaceous plant, Rhizome of *Notopterygium incisum* Ting ex H. T. Chang or the Rhizome and root of *N. forbesii* Boiss, family Umbelliferae. The producing areas are mainly in the provinces of Sichuan, Gansu, and Yunnan, etc.. The medicinal material is collected in the early stage of spring and autumn, dried and cut into pieces for being used in crude form.

Medicinal Properties Pungent and bitter in flavor, warm in nature, and attributive to the bladder and kidney meridians.

Actions Expel wind and dampness, dispel cold to relieve pain.

Application

1. It is used for the syndrome of exogenous wind-cold with dampness marked by aversion to cold with fever, painful head and nape, sore and heavy feelings of extremities with pain. It is often used together with Fangfeng (*Radix Saposhnikoviae*), Duhuo (*Radix Angelicae Pubescentis*) and so on, such as Duhuo Shengshi Tang (Decoction).

2. It is used for headache of wind-damp type, and Bi-syndrome of wind-cold-dampness type. For the former involving the nape and back, it is often used together with Fangfeng (*Radix Saposhnikoviae*), Chuanxiong (*Rhizoma Chuanxiong*), etc.; for the latter or arthralgia, especially in the upper part of the body, usually used together with Fangfeng (*Radix Saposhnikoviae*), Jianghuang (*Rhizoma Curcumae Longae*) and Danggui (*Radix Angelicae Sinensis*).

羌 活

为伞形科植物羌活及宽叶羌活的根茎及根。主产于四川、甘肃、云南等地。初春及秋季采挖，干燥，切片。生用。

【药性】 味辛、苦，性温。归膀胱、肾经。

【功效】 祛风胜湿，散寒止痛。

【临床应用】

1. 用于外感风寒挟湿证，症见恶寒发热，头项疼痛，肢体酸重而疼者。常与防风、独活等同用，如羌活胜湿汤。

2. 用于风湿头痛，风寒湿痹。风湿头痛，痛连项背，常配伍防风、川芎等同用；治风寒湿痹，关节疼痛，尤能解上半身痹痛，多配防风、姜黄、当归同用。

Usage and Dosage 3 -10 g is used in decoction for oral use.

【用法用量】 水煎服，3～10 克。

Notes Contraindicated in the patient with yin-deficiency or in-sufficiency of blood due to its warm and dryness in nature.

【使用注意】 性温燥，阴虚或气血不足者忌用。

Explanation Either Fangfeng (*Radix Saposhnikoviae*) or Qianghuo (*Rhizoma et Radix Notopterygii*) is the medicinal herb for expelling wind and eliminating dampness. Since it is pungent and bitter in flavor, warm and dry in nature, and has stronger actions of expelling wind, cold and dampness, Qianghuo (*Rhizoma et Radix Notopterygii*) is especially used for headache involving the nape and back or limbs due to wind-cold or wind-dampness, while Fangfeng (*Radix Saposhnikoviae*) is pungent with sweet flavor and has nourishing property and is good at expelling wind, therefore, it is often used for the syndrome caused by pathogenic wind whether the wind is exterior or interior, and it can also relieve convulsion and diarrhea.

【说明】 防风与羌活均为祛风胜湿之品。羌活辛苦温燥之性和祛风散寒胜湿止痛之功较著，尤适用于风寒或风湿所致的头痛连及项背或肢体疼痛者；防风之味兼甘，性偏润，善于祛风，多用于风邪为患之证，无论外风、内风均可，并能止痉、止泻。

Xixin *Herba Asari*

细 辛

Its source is from the dried entire herb of the perennial herbaceous plant, *Asarum heterotropoides* Fr. Schmidt var. *mandshuricum* (Maxim) Kitag., and *A. sieboldii* Miq., family Aristolochiaceae. The producing areas are mainly in the provinces of Liaoning, Jilin, Heilongjiang, Shandong, Anhui, and Shanxi, etc. The Medicinal material is collected in summer and autumn, dried in shade and the crude form is used for medication.

为马兜铃科植物北细辛、汉城细辛、华细辛的全草。前两种习称“辽细辛”，主产于辽宁、吉林、黑龙江；后一种产于山东、安徽、陕西等地。夏、秋季采收，阴干。生用。

Medicinal Properties Pungent in flavor, warm in nature, mildly toxic and attributive to the lung, kidney and heart meridians.

【药性】 味辛，性温。有小毒。归肺、肾、心经。

Actions Expel wind and dispel cold, remove the obstruction of the nose, relieve pain and warm the lung to remove the retention of fluids.

【功效】 祛风散寒，宣通鼻窍，止痛，温肺化饮。

Application

1. For exterior syndrome of wind-cold type manifested as headache and general pain, it can be used together with Qianghuo (*Rhizoma et Radix Notopterygii*), Fangfeng (*Radix Saposhnikoviae*), etc., such as Jiuwei Qianghuo Tang (Decoction); for yang-deficiency exterior syndrome marked by aversion to cold with anhidrosis, fever and sinking pulse, used together with Mahuang (*Herba Ephedrae*) and Fuzi (*Radix Aconiti Lateralis Praeparata*), such as Mahuang Fuzi Xixin Tang (Decoction).

2. It is indicated for headache, toothache, Bi-syndrome of wind-cold-dampness type, etc.. For wind-syndrome of headache, it is often used together with Chuanxiong (*Rhizoma Chuanxiong*) and Fangfeng (*Radix Saposhnikoviae*); for toothache of wind-cold type, Xixin (*Herba Asari*) is singly decocted as gargle, or combined with Baizhi (*Radix Angelicae Dahuricae*), Ruxiang (*Olibanum*), etc.; for Bi-syndrome of wind-cold-damp type, or arthralgia, used together with Duhuo (*Radix Angelicae Pubescentis*), Fangfeng (*Radix Saposhnikoviae*), and Qinjiao (*Radix Gentianae Macrophyllae*), such as Duhuo Jisheng Tang (Decoction).

3. For retention of cold in the lung, cough with plenty of thin and clean sputum, it is often combined with Mahuang (*Herba Ephedrae*), Ganjiang (*Rhizoma Zingiberis*), and Wuweizi (*Fructus Schisandrae*), etc., such as Xiao Qinglong Tang (Decoction).

4. For the obstruction of nose, headache, and episodes of running nose, it is used together with Xinyi (*Flos Magnoliae*), Baizhi (*Radix Angelicae Dahuricae*), and Cang'erzi (*Fructus Xanthii*), etc..

Usage and Dosage 1-3 g is used in decoction for oral use; 0.5-1 g can be used in pill or powder.

【临床应用】

1. 用于风寒表证,头身疼痛。可与羌活、防风等同用,如九味羌活汤;与麻黄、附子同用,还可治恶寒无汗,发热脉沉的阳虚外感,如麻黄附子细辛汤。

2. 用于头痛、牙痛、风寒湿痹等痛证。治头风痛,常与川芎、防风等同用;治风寒牙痛,单味煎汤含漱有效,或配白芷、乳香等同用;治风寒湿痹,关节疼痛,可与独活、防风、秦艽等同用,如独活寄生汤。

3. 用于寒饮伏肺,咳喘痰多清稀。常配麻黄、干姜、五味子等同用,如小青龙汤。

4. 用于鼻渊不通,头痛流涕者,可配辛夷、白芷、苍耳子等。

【用法用量】 水煎服,1～3 克;入丸、散剂,0.5～

1克。

Notes The dosage should not be excessively large, contraindicated in the patient with headache caused by hyperactivity of yang due to yin deficiency and dry cough due to yin-damage resulting from lung-dryness. It is incompatible with Lilu (*Rhizoma et Radix Veratri*).

【使用注意】 用量不可过大。阴虚阳亢头痛,肺燥伤阴干咳者忌用。反藜芦。

Cang'erzi *Fructus Xanthii*

苍耳子

Its source is from the fruit and involucre of *Xanthium sibiricum* Patr., family Compositae. The producing areas are in all parts of China. The medicinal material is collected in autumn, dried in the sun, and are stir-baked for being used as medicine after its thorns are removed.

为菊科植物苍耳的果实。产于中国各地。秋季采收,晒干。炒去硬刺用。

Medicinal Properties Pungent and bitter in flavor, warm in nature, mildly toxic and attributive to lung meridian.

【药性】 味辛、苦,性温。有小毒。归肺经。

Actions Expel wind and dampness, clear the nasal passage and alleviate pain.

【功效】 散风除湿,通窍止痛。

Application

【临床应用】

1. It is indicated for headache due to affection of wind-cold and arthralgia of wind-damp type. For the disease due to exterior wind and cold marked by aversion to cold with anhidrosis, headache and stuffy nose, it is often combined with Fangfeng (*Radix Saposhnikoviae*), Qianghuo (*Rhizoma et Radix Notopterygii*), Baizhi (*Radix Angelicae Dahuricae*), etc.; for arthralgia of wind-damp type and spasm of limbs, it can be used in single or together with Qianghuo (*Rhizoma et Radix Notopterygii*), Duhuo (*Radix Angelicae Pubescentis*), and Weilingxian (*Radix Clematidis*), etc..

1. 用于风寒头痛,风湿痹痛。治外感风寒,恶寒无汗,头痛鼻塞,多与防风、羌活、白芷等同用;治风湿痹证,四肢拘挛,可单用,或与羌活、独活、威灵仙等同用。

2. For headache due to sinusitis, loss of smelling due to stuffy nose and episodes of running nose, it is often combined with Xixin (*Herba Asari*), Bohe (*Herba Menthae*), etc., such as Cang'erzi San (Powder).

2. 用于鼻渊头痛,鼻塞不闻香臭,浊涕时流。常配细辛、薄荷等同用,如苍耳子散。

In addition, it can be also used for itching due to ru-

此外,还可用于风疹瘙

bella, scabies, etc., and combined with Difuzi (*Fructus Kochiae*), Baixianpi (*Cortex Dictamni Radicis*), etc. which are decocted together for exterior use, washing.

痒、疥癣等。可配地肤子、白鲜皮等用于外洗。

Usage and Dosage 3-10 g is used in decoction for oral use; or in pill or powder. It can be also used exteriorly with suitable amount.

【用法用量】 水煎服，3～10 克；或入丸、散。外用，适量。

Notes Contraindicated in the patient with headache due to blood-deficiency and not be taken excessively.

【使用注意】 血虚头痛患者忌用。内服不可过量。

Xinyi *Flos Magnoliae*

辛 夷

The source is from the flower bud of *Magnolia biondii* Pamp, *M. denudata* Desr. and *M. liliflore* Desr., family Magnoliaceae. The medicinal material is collected when its flower bud does not open in the early stage of spring, dried in shade after the stem is picked out and the crude can be used.

为木兰科植物望春花或武当玉兰的花蕾。春初花未开放时采收，除去枝梗，阴干。生用。

Medicinal Properties Pungent in flavor, warm in nature and attributive to the lung and stomach meridians.

【药性】 味辛，性温。归肺、胃经。

Actions Expel wind and cold and clear the nasal passage.

【功效】 发散风寒，宣通鼻窍。

Application

【临床应用】

1. For the headache due to sinusitis, it is often used together with Xixin (*Herba Asari*), Baizhi (*Radix Angelicae Dahuricae*), etc., such as Xinyi San (Powder); for that being a bit on the wind-heat side and manifested as episodes of running nose with yellow color and foul smell, it can be used together with Juhua (*Flos Chrysanthemi*), Lianqiao (*Fructus Forsythiae*), Huangqin (*Radix Scutellariae*), and Bohe (*Herba Menthae*), etc..

1. 用于鼻渊头痛。常与细辛、白芷等同用，如辛夷散；若偏于风热，鼻流浊涕，色黄而臭者，可与菊花、连翘、黄芩、薄荷等配伍。

2. For exogenous diseases due to wind and cold manifested as headache and stuffy nose, it is often combined with Fangfeng (*Radix Saposhnikoviae*), Chuanxiong (*Rhizoma Chuanxiong*), etc. to expel wind and clear the nasal passage.

2. 用于外感风寒头痛，鼻塞。常配防风、川芎等，以散寒通窍。

Usage and Dosage 3 -9 g is used in decoction for oral use; it is wrapped with gauze and then decocted with other herbs in water since it is covered by hair that can irritate the throat.

【用法用量】 水煎服，3～9克;表面有毛，容易刺激咽喉，内服宜用纱布包煎。

Notes Contraindicated in the patient with hyperactivity of fire due to yin deficiency.

【使用注意】 阴虚火旺者忌服。

1.2 Diaphoretics with pungent-cool property

第二节 辛凉解表药

These herbs are mostly pungent and cool in nature, and take the actions of dispersing wind-heat as dominant one, but diaphoretic action is milder. They are indicated for exogenous diseases due to wind and heat, which are manifested as severe fever and slight aversion to cold, dry throat and thirst, headache, redness of eye, thin and yellow tongue coating, floating and rapid pulse, etc.. Of the herbs, some can be used for swollen and painful throat, unsmooth eruption of measles, cough , etc..

本类药物性味多辛凉，以发散风热为主，发汗作用较和缓。适用于外感风热，症见发热重、恶寒轻、咽干口渴、头痛、目赤、舌苔薄黄、脉浮数等。其中有些药物还可用于目赤、咽喉肿痛、麻疹不透及咳嗽等证。

Bohe *Herba Menthae*

薄　荷

Its source is from branch and leaf of *Mentha haplocalyx* Briqi, family Labiata. The producing areas are in all parts of China but the best in quality in Jiangsu province. The medicinal material is collected in summer and autumn, dried in shade, cut into pieces and the crude or fresh form is used for medication.

为唇形科植物薄荷的茎叶。产于中国各地，以江苏产质量最好。夏、秋季采收，阴干，切段。生用或鲜用。

Medicinal Properties Pungent in flavor, cool in nature and attributive to the lung and liver meridians.

【药性】 味辛，性凉。归肺、肝经。

Actions Expel wind and heat, clear away heat from the head and eye, ease the throat, promote eruption, soothe the liver and disperse stagnation of liver-qi.

【功效】 疏散风热，清利头目，利咽透疹，疏肝解郁。

Application

【临床应用】

1. For exterior syndrome due to wind and heat or seasonal febrile diseases at the early stage manifested as

1. 用于风热表证或温热病初起，症见发热无汗，微恶

fever and anhidrosis, slight aversion to wind and cold and headache, it is often combined with Jingjie (*Herba Schizonepetae*), Jinyinhua (*Flos Lonicerae*), and Lianqiao (*Fructus Forsythiae*), etc., such as Yin Qiao San (Powder).

风寒,头痛者,常配荆芥、金银花、连翘等同用,如银翘散。

2. For the syndrome of wind and heat attacking upwards manifested as headache and redness of eyes, swollen and painful throat, it is used together with Sangye (*Folium Mori*), Juhua (*Flos Chrysanthemi*) and others that can clear away heat from head and eye.

2. 用于风热上攻,头痛目赤,咽喉肿痛。可配桑叶、菊花等清利头目之品同用。

3. For unsmooth eruption of measles and rubella with itching, it is usually used together with Chantui (*Periostracum Cicadae*), Jingjie (*Herba Schizonepetae*), and Niubangzi (*Fructus Arctii*), etc. so as to promote eruption of measles; it can be combined with Kushen (*Radix Sophorae Flavescentis*), Baixianpi (*Cortex Dictamni Radicis*), and Fangfeng (*Radix Saposhnikoviae*), etc. to expel wind and relieve itching and treat rubella with itching, too.

3. 用于麻疹不透,风疹瘙痒。常配蝉蜕、荆芥、牛蒡子等以增强透疹之力;与苦参、白鲜皮、防风等配伍,能祛风止痒,可治风疹瘙痒。

4. For stagnation of liver-qi, oppressed feeling in the chest and hypochondriac pain, or swollen pain of breast and irregular menstruation, it can be used together with Chaihu (*Radix Bupleuri*), Baishaoyao (*Radix Paeoniae Alba*) and Danggui (*Radix Angelicae Sinensis*), such as Xiaoyao San (Powder).

4. 用于肝气郁结,胸闷胁痛,或乳房胀痛,月经不调。可配伍柴胡、白芍药、当归同用,如逍遥散。

Usage and Dosage 3-6 g is used in decoction for oral use and put in decoction later.

【用法用量】 水煎服,3~6克,宜后下。

Notes It is not suitable for spontaneous perspiration due to exterior deficiency.

【使用注意】 表虚自汗者不宜用。

Juhua *Flos Chrysanthemi*

菊　花

The source is from the capitulum of the perennial herbaceous plant, *Chrysanthemum morifolium* Ramat, family Compositae. The producing areas are mainly in the provinces of Zhejiang, Anhui, and Henan, etc.. The me-

为菊科植物菊的头状花序。主产于浙江、安徽、河南等地。秋末冬初采摘,阴干。生用。

dicinal material is collected in the end of autumn and early stage of winter, dried in shade for medication.

Medicinal Properties Pungent, bitter and sweet in flavor, slightly cold in nature and attributive to the lung and liver meridians.

【药性】 味辛、甘、苦,性微寒。归肺、肝经。

Actions Expel wind and clear away heat, clear liver-fire to treat eye disease, and eliminate toxic substances.

【功效】 疏散风热,清肝明目,清热解毒。

Application

【临床应用】

1. For exogenous disease due to wind and heat or early stage of seasonal febrile disease manifested as fever, headache and cough, it is usually used together with Sangye (*Folium Mori*), Bohe (*Herba Menthae*), and Lianqiao (*Fructus Forsythiae*), etc., such as Sang Ju Yin (Decoction).

1. 用于外感风热或风温初起,症见发热,头痛,咳嗽,多与桑叶、连翘、薄荷等同用,如桑菊饮。

2. It is used for red, swollen and painful eyes and blurred vision whether the syndrome is asthenic or sthenic. For redish, swollen and painful eyes due to wind and heat attacking liver meridian or flaming-up of the exuberant liver-fire, it is usually combined with Sangye (*Folium Mori*), Juemingzi (*Semen Cassiae*), and Longdan (*Radix Gentianae*), etc.. For deficiency of the liver and kidney with blurred vision, it can be used together with Gouqizi (*Fructus Lycii*), Shudihuang (*Radix Rehmanniae Praeparata*), and Shanzhuyu (*Fructus Corni*), etc., such as Qi Ju Dihuang Wan (Pill).

2. 用于目赤肿痛,目暗昏花,无论虚实均可应用。肝经风热或肝火上炎之目赤肿痛,常配伍桑叶、决明子、龙胆等。肝肾不足,目暗昏花,可配枸杞子、熟地黄、山茱萸等,如杞菊地黄丸。

3. For dizziness and headache due to hyperactivity of liver-yang, it can be used together with Shijueming (*Concha Haliotidis*), Baishaoyao (*Radix Paeoniae Alba*), and Gouteng (*Ramulus Uncarriae cum Uncis*), etc..

3. 用于肝阳上亢之眩晕,头痛。可与石决明、白芍药、钩藤等同用。

4. It is used for furuncle and especially for furunculosis. The fresh form can be pounded into juice for oral use and the left dregs can be covered on the affected site; or it can be combined wtih Zihuadiding (*Herba Violae*),

4. 用于疔疮肿毒,尤善治疔毒。可单用鲜品捣汁服,其渣外敷;或配紫花地丁、蒲公英等同用。

Pugongying (*Herba Taraxaci*), etc..

Usage and Dosage 5 -9 g is used in decoction for oral use; or soaked in boiling water as tea for oral use; used externally with suitable amount.

【用法用量】 水煎服，5~9克；或泡茶饮。外用，适量。

Chantui *Periostracum Cicadae*

蝉蜕

Its source is from the slough shed by the cicada, *Cryptotympana pustulata* Fabricius, family Cicadidae. The producing areas are mainly in the provinces of Shandong, Hebei, Hubei, and Jiangsu, etc.. The medicinal material is collected in summer, the clean crude form is dried in the sun for medication.

为蝉科昆虫黑蚱羽化后的皮壳。主产于山东、河北、湖北、江苏等地。夏季采收，去净泥土，晒干。生用。

Medicinal Properties Sweet in flavor, cold in nature and attributive to the lung and liver meridians.

【药性】 味甘，性寒。归肺、肝经。

Actions Expel wind and heat, let out the skin eruption and alleviate itching, improve eyesight and remove nebula, and stop wind and relieve convulsion.

【功效】 疏散风热，透疹止痒，明目退翳，熄风止痉。

Application

【临床应用】

1. It is indicated for the wind-heat syndrome due to exogenous attack and seasonal febrile disease at the early stage marked by fever and hoarseness. For the cases with headache and fever as dominate symptom, it is usually used together with Juhua (*Flos Chrysanthemi*), Bohe (*Herba Menthae*), and Lianqiao (*Fructus Forsythiae*), etc., such as Yin Qiao San (Powder); for those with sore throat and obvious hoarseness, used together with Jiegeng (*Radix Platycodi*), Pangdahai (*Semen Sterculiae Scaphigerae*), and Niubangzi (*Fructus Arctii*), etc..

1. 用于外感风热及温病初起，发热音哑。以头痛发热为主症者，多与菊花、薄荷、连翘配伍同用，如银翘散。若咽痛音哑明显，可与桔梗、胖大海、牛蒡子等配伍。

2. It is indicated for unsmooth eruption of measles and rubella with itching. For unsmooth eruption of measles, it is usually used together with Bohe (*Herba Menthae*), Niubangzi (*Fructus Arctii*) and Zicao (*Radix Arnebiae seu Lithospermi*); for rubella, eczema and skin itching, used together with Jingjie (*Herba Schizonepetae*), Fangfeng (*Radix Saposhnikoviae*), and Kushen

2. 用于麻疹不透，风疹瘙痒。治麻疹不透，常与薄荷、牛蒡子、紫草同用。治风疹，湿疹，皮肤瘙痒，可与荆芥、防风、苦参等同用。

(*Radix Sophorae Flavescentis*), etc..

3. For conjunctivitis and pterygium, it is often combined with Juhua (*Flos Chrysanthemi*), Sangye (*Folium Mori*), and Juemingzi (*Semen Cassiae*), etc..

3. 用于目赤翳障。常与菊花、桑叶、决明子等同用。

4. For infantile convulsion and tetanus, it can be singly grounded into powder that is taken with millet wine or used together with Gouteng (*Ramulus Uncariae cum Uncis*), Quanxie (*Scorpio*), and Baijiangcan (*Bombyx Batryticatus*), etc..

4. 用于小儿惊痫，破伤风。可单用研末，黄酒冲服；或与钩藤、全蝎、白僵蚕等同用。

Usage and Dosage 3-6 g is used in decoction for oral use; or it is pounded into powder to be taken with water. Large dosage is used for stopping wind and relieving convulsion.

【用法用量】 水煎服，3～6 克；或研末冲服。熄风止痉用量宜大。

Notes It is used in a pregnant woman with caution.

【使用注意】 孕妇慎用。

Niubangzi *Fructus Arctii*

牛蒡子

The source is from the fruit of *Arctum lappa* L., family Compositae. The producing areas are mainly in the provinces of Hebei, Zhejiang, etc.. The medicinal material is collected in autumn, dried in the sun. The crude or stir-baked form can all be used.

为菊科植物牛蒡的成熟果实。主产于河北、浙江等地。秋季采收，晒干。生用或炒用。

Medicinal Properties Pungent and bitter in flavor, cold in nature and attributive to the lung and stomach meridians.

【药性】 味辛、苦，性寒。归肺、胃经。

Actions Expel wind and heat, let out the skin eruption, ease the throat, remove toxic materials and dissipate nodules.

【功效】 疏散风热，透疹利咽，解毒散结。

Application

【临床应用】

1. For exterior syndrome of wind and heat type with sore and swollen throat, it can be used together with Bohe (*Herba Menthae*), Jinyinhua (*Flos Lonicerae*), and Lianqiao (*Fructus Forsythiae*), etc., such as Yin Qiao San (Powder); for those with sore and swollen throat of heat type, used together with Dahuang (*Radix et Rhizoma*

1. 用于风热表证，咽喉肿痛。可与薄荷、金银花、连翘等同用，如银翘散。若咽喉肿痛热毒较甚者，可与大黄、黄芩等清热解毒之品同用。

Rhei), Huangqin (*Radix Scutellariae*) and other herbs that can clear away heat and remove toxic materials.

2. For unsmooth eruption of measles, usually combined with Bohe (*Herba Menthae*), Jingjie (*Herba Schizonepetae*), and Chantui (*Periostracum Cicadae*), etc..

3. It is used for carbuncle or pyogenic infection of the skin and mumps, and especially suitable for the carbuncle due to either wind-heat syndrome due to exogenous attack or stasis of toxic heat in the interior accompanied with constipation. It is often used together with Dahuang (*Radix et Rhizoma Rhei*), Mangxiao (*Natrii Sulfas*), and Zhizi (*Fructus Gardeniae*), etc.. It is combined with Xuanshen (*Radix Scrophulariae*), Huangqin (*Radix Scutellariae*), Banlangen (*Radix Isatidis*), etc. to treat mumps and pharyngalgia.

Usage and Dosage 6 -12 g is used in decoction for oral use. It is pounded into pieces that is used in decoction, and the stir-baked one can reduce its cold nature.

Notes Contraindicated in the patient with diarrhea due to qi deficiency.

Sangye *Folium Mori*

The source is from the leaf of *Morus alba* L., family Moraceae. The producing areas are in all parts of China. The medicinal material is collected after frost, dried in the sun and the raw or the one stir-baked with honey can be used for medication.

Medicinal Properties Sweet and bitter in flavor, cold in nature and attributive to the lung and liver meridians.

Actions Expel wind and heat, clear away lung-heat and moisturize dryness, and clear away liver-fire to treat eye disease.

Application

1. For the wind-heat syndrome due to exogenous at-

2．用于麻疹透发不畅。常配薄荷、荆芥、蝉蜕等同用。

3．用于痈肿疮毒，痄腮。对于风热外袭或热毒内结之痈肿疮毒，兼有便秘者用之尤宜。常与大黄、芒硝、栀子等同用。治痄腮、喉痹，可与玄参、黄芩、板蓝根等同用。

【用法用量】 水煎服，6～12克。入汤剂宜捣碎。炒用可减轻寒性。

【使用注意】 性寒滑利，气虚便溏者忌用。

桑叶

为桑科植物桑树的叶。产于中国各地。霜后采收，晒干。生用或炙用。

【药性】 味甘、苦，性寒。归肺、肝经。

【功效】 疏散风热，清肺润燥，清肝明目。

【临床应用】

1．用于外感风热之发

tack manifested as headache, cough, and sore throat, it is usually combined with Juhua (*Flos Chrysanthemi*), Bohe (*Herba Menthae*), etc., such as Sang Ju Yin (Decoction).

热，头痛，咳嗽，咽痛。常与菊花、薄荷等同用，如桑菊饮。

2. For the damage to the lung due to dryness and heat marked by dry cough with little sputum and dry throat, it can be combined with Xingren (*Semen Armeniacae Amarum*), Beimu (*Bulbus Fritillariae Cirrhosae*), Shashen (*Radix Adenophorae*), and Maimendong (*Radix Ophiopogonis*), etc., such as Qingzao Jiufei Tang (Decoction).

2. 用于燥热伤肺，干咳少痰，咽干。可与杏仁、贝母、沙参、麦门冬等同用，如清燥救肺汤。

3. It is indicated for conjunctivitis and dizziness due to liver-heat, etc.. It can be combined with Juhua (*Flos Chrysanthemi*), Juemingzi (*Semen Cassiae*), and Cheqianzi (*Semen Plantaginis*), etc., to treat conjunctivitis due to liver-heat. For hyperactivity of liver-yang manifested as headache and dizziness, often combined with Juhua (*Flos Chrysanthemi*), Shijueming (*Concha Haliotidis*), and Baishaoyao (*Radix Paeoniae Alba*), etc..

3. 用于肝热目赤、眩晕等。治肝热目赤，可与菊花、决明子、车前子等配伍。治肝阳上亢，头痛眩晕，常配伍菊花、石决明、白芍药等同用。

In addition, it can be used for bleeding due to blood-heat manifested as hematemesis and epistaxis.

此外，还可用治血热妄行之吐血、衄血。

Usage and Dosage 5 -10 g is used in decoction for oral use; or it is added to pill or powder, and can be stir-baked with honey, which is often used for cough due to lung-dryness.

【用法用量】 水煎服，5～10 克；或入丸、散。肺燥咳嗽多蜜炙用。

Chaihu *Radix Bupleuri*

柴 胡

Its source is from the dried root or the herb of the Perennial herbaceous plant, *Bulpleurum chinense* Dc. or *B. scorzonerifolium* Willd., family Umbelliferae. The former is mainly produced in the provinces of Liaoning, Gansu, Hebei, and Henan, etc.; the latter in Hubei, Jiangsu, and Sichuan, etc.. The medicinal material is collected in spring and autumn, dried in the sun and cut into

为伞形科植物柴胡(北柴胡)和狭叶柴胡(南柴胡)的根。前者主产于辽宁、甘肃、河北、河南等地；后者主产于湖北、江苏、四川等地。春秋两季采挖，晒干，切段。生用或醋炙用。

pieces. The raw or the one fried with vinegar is used for medication.

Medicinal Properties Bitter and pungent in flavor, slightly cold in nature and attributive to the liver and gallbladder meridians.

【药性】 味苦、辛，性微寒。归肝、胆经。

Actions Regulate the functional relation of internal organs to relieve fever, disperse the stagnated liver-qi and uplift yang-qi to raise sinking.

【功效】 和解退热，疏肝解郁，升阳举陷。

Application

【临床应用】

1. It is used for fever due to exogenous pathogenic factors with alternating episodes of chills and fever. It is effective in eliminating the pathogenic factors located in the half-superficial and half-interior, hence it is an indispensable medicine for treating shaoyang disease, which is manifested as feeling of fullness and oppression in the chest and hypochondrium, bitter taste in the mouth and dry throat. It is usually combined with Huangqin (*Radix Scutellariae*), Banxia (*Rhizoma Pinelliae*), etc., such as Xiao Chaihu Tang (Decoction). For fever due to exogenous pathogenic factors, it can be combined with Gegen (*Radix Puerariae*), Huangqin (*Radix Scutellariae*), and Shigao (*Gypsum Fibrosum*), etc., such as Chai Ge Jieji Tang (Decoction).

1. 用于外感发热，寒热往来。善于疏散少阳半表半里之邪，为治疗邪在少阳、寒热往来、胸胁苦满、口苦咽干等少阳证之要药。常与黄芩、半夏等同用，如小柴胡汤。治外感发热，可与葛根、黄芩、石膏等同用，如柴葛解肌汤。

2. For depression and stasis of liver-qi manifested as irregular menstruation, pain in the chest, hypochondria and breast, it can be combined with Baishaoyao (*Radix Paeoniae Alba*), Chuanxiong (*Rhizoma Chuanxiong*), and Zhike (*Fructus Aurantii*), etc., such as Chaihu Shugan San (Powder).

2. 用于肝郁气滞，月经不调，胸胁乳房疼痛。可与白芍药、川芎、枳壳等配伍，如柴胡疏肝散。

3. It is used for the treatment of prolapses due to deficiency of qi, such as prolapse of rectum, or uterus, or gastroptosis, and shortness of breath and weakness, etc. since it is effective in uplifting qi of the stomach and spleen. It can be combined with Shengma (*Rhizoma*

3. 用于气虚下陷诸证。本品善于升举脾胃清阳之气，可治气虚下陷之脱肛、子宫下垂、胃下垂、短气乏力等，可与升麻、黄芪等升提中气之品同

Cimicifugae), Huangqi (*Radix Astragali*) and other herbs that can uplift the qi of middle energizer, such as Buzhong Yiqi Tang (Decoction).

用,如补中益气汤。

Usage and Dosage 3 -10 g is used in decoction for oral use. The raw is suitable for reconciliation and relieving fever and uplifting yang-qi, and the stir-fried with vinegar for dispersing the stagnated liver-qi. Small dosage is suitable for uplifting yang and soothing the liver, 3 - 5 g being generally used; large dosage for reconciliation to relieve fever, 10 g being generally used.

【用法用量】 水煎服,3~10克。和解退热,升举阳气宜生用,疏肝解郁宜醋炙。升阳、疏肝,用量宜小,一般3~5克;和解退热,用量宜大,一般10克。

Notes Contraindicated for the syndromes of sthenia of liver-yang, liver-wind stirring inside, hyperactivity of fire due to yin-deficiency or adverse flow of qi.

【使用注意】 肝阳上亢,肝风内动,阴虚火旺及气机上逆者忌用。

Gegen *Radix Puerariae*

葛 根

The source is from the roots of *Pueraria lobata* (Willd.) ohwi, family Leguminosae. The producing areas are in all parts of China. The medicinal material is collected in spring and autumn, cut into pieces, dried in the sun and the raw or the stewed form is used for medication.

为豆科植物野葛或甘葛藤的根。产于中国各地。春秋两季采挖,切片,晒干。生用,或煨用。

Medicinal Properties Sweet and pungent in flavor, cool in nature and attributive to the spleen and stomach meridians.

【药性】 味甘、辛,性凉。归脾、胃经。

Actions Expel pathogenic factors in the muscles to abate heat, let out the skin eruptions, promote the production of body fluid to relieve thirst and uplift yang to relieve diarrhea.

【功效】 解肌退热,透发麻疹,生津止渴,升阳止泻。

Application

【临床应用】

1. It is used for exterior syndrome due to exogenous attack. For wind-heat syndrome due to exogenous attack manifested as aversion to cold and fever, headache and dryness of nose, it is often used together with Chaihu (*Radix Bupleuri*), Huangqin (*Radix Scutellariae*) and Baizhi (*Radix Angelicae Dahuricae*), such as Chai Ge Jieji Tang (Decoction). It is also a common medicine for

1. 用于外感表证。外感风热,恶寒发热,头痛鼻干,常与柴胡、黄芩、白芷同用,如柴葛解肌汤。又为治项背强痛常用之药,多用于风寒表证见有项背强痛者,可与麻黄、桂枝等散寒解表药同用,如葛

treating stiffness and pain of the nape and back and mostly used for superficial syndrome of wind-cold type manifested as stiffness and pain of the nape and back, and used together with Mahuang (*Herba Ephedrae*), Guizhi (*Ramulus Cinnamomi*), and others that expel cold from the exterior, such as Gegen Tang (Decoction).

根汤。

2. It is used for measles at the early stage with unsmooth eruption. It is usually used together with Shengma (*Rhizoma Cimicifugae*), Jingjie (*Herba Schizonepetae*), and Niubangzi (*Fructus Arctii*), etc..

2. 用于麻疹初起，透发不畅。常与升麻、荆芥、牛蒡子等同用。

3. Used for febrile disease with excessive thirst and internal heat with diabetes, it is often combined with Lugen (*Rhizoma Phragmitis*), Tianhuafen (*Radix Trichosanthis*), and Maimendong (*Radix Ophiopogonis*), etc..

3. 用于热病烦渴，内热消渴。常与芦根、天花粉、麦门冬等同用。

4. It is used for dysentery. For dysentery of damp-heat type, it is often combined with Huangqin (*Radix Scutellariae*), Huanglian (*Rhizoma Coptidis*), etc., such as Gegen Huangqin Huanglian Tang (Decoction). For diarrhea due to spleen-deficiency, often used together with Renshen (*Radix Ginseng*), Baizhu (*Rhizoma Atractylodis Macrocephalae*), and Fuling (*Poria*), etc., such as Qiwei Baizhu San (Powder).

4. 用于泻痢。治湿热泻痢，多配伍黄芩、黄连等同用，如葛根黄芩黄连汤。若为脾虚泄泻，常与人参、白术、茯苓等同用，如七味白术散。

Usage and Dosage 10 -15 g is used in decoction for oral use. The raw is suitable for reducing fever and promoting the production of the body fluids and the stewed form for uplifting yang and relieving diarrhea.

【用法用量】 水煎服，10~15克。退热生津宜生用，升阳止泻宜煨用。

Explanation The research has shown that the pharmacological action of Gegen (*Radix Puerariae*) is to reduce blood pressure and dilate blood vessels, therefore it is indicated for high blood pressure with headache and stiffness of the nape, coronary heart disease, etc..

【说明】 药理研究葛根有降压、扩血管等作用。可用于治疗高血压病头痛项强、冠心病等。

Gehua (*Flos Puerariae*): The flower of the perennial deciduous liana consists of flower bud and is sweet in

葛花：为葛的花蕾。味甘性平。功能解酒醒脾，为治饮

flavor and neutral in nature. It can relieve alcoholism and activate the spleen-qi and it is effective in treating over-drinking of alcohol.

酒过度的良药。

Shengma *Rhizoma Cimicifugae*

Its source is from the rhizome of *Cimicifuga heracleifolia* kom., *C. dahurica* (Turcz.) Maxim. and *C. foetida* L., family Ranunculaceae. The producing areas are mainly in the provinces of Liaoning, Heilongjiang, Hunan, etc., and the medicinal material is collected in summer and autumn, dried in the sun and then cut into pieces. The crude or the one stir-baked with honey can be used for medication.

Medicinal Properties Pungent and sweet in flavor, slightly cold in nature and attributive to the spleen, stomach and large intestine meridians.

Actions Expel pathogenic factors from the superficies and promote eruption of measles, clear away heat and remove the toxic materials, and uplift yang-qi of the spleen.

Application

1. For exterior syndrome of wind-heat type manifested as fever, headache, or unsmooth eruption of measles, it can be used together with Gegen (*Radix Puerariae*), such as Gegen Shengma Tang (Decoction).

2. It is indicated for yangming-heat manifested as aphthae, toothache, sore and swollen throat. For toothache and aphthae due to stomach-fire, it can be combined with Huanglian (*Rhizoma Coptidis*), Shengdihuang (*Radix Rehmannia*), and Mudanpi (*Cortex Moutan Radicis*), etc., such as Qingwei San (Powder). For sore and swelling of throat due to wind and heat ascending, combined with Jiegeng (*Radix Platycodi*) and Xuanshen (*Radix Scrophulariae*). For pyocutaneous disease of heat type, used with Jinyinhua (*Flos Lonicerae*), Lian-

升 麻

为毛茛科植物大三叶升麻、兴安升麻和升麻的根茎。主产于辽宁、黑龙江、湖南等地。夏、秋两季采挖，晒干切片。生用或蜜炙用。

【药性】 味辛、甘，性微寒。归肺、脾、胃、大肠经。

【功效】 发表透疹，清热解毒，升举阳气。

【临床应用】

1. 用于风热表证发热头痛，或麻疹出而不畅，可与葛根同用，如葛根升麻汤。

2. 用于阳明热毒，口疮齿痛，咽喉肿痛。治胃火牙痛，口舌生疮，可配伍黄连、生地黄、牡丹皮等同用，如清胃散。治风热上壅之咽喉肿痛，可与桔梗、玄参同用。如用于热毒疮疡，可与金银花、连翘、蒲公英等同用。

qiao (*Fructus Forsythiae*), and Pugongying (*Herba Taraxaxi*), etc..

3. For prolapse due to qi deficiency manifested as shortness of breath, fatigue, prolapse of rectum due to chronic diarrhea, prolapse of uterus, uterine bleeding without stopping, it is usually combined with Chaihu (*Radix Bupleuri*), Huangqi (*Radix Astragali*) and others that replenish qi for lifting and ascending, such as Buzhong Yiqi Tang (Decoction).

3. 用于气虚下陷之短气、倦怠、久泄脱肛、子宫下垂、崩漏不止等。常与柴胡、黄芪等益气升提药同用,如补中益气汤。

Usage and Dosage 3 -9 g is used in decoction for oral use. The crude is suitable for expelling pathogenic factors from the superficies and promoting eruption of measles, and the prepared form for uplifting yang-qi and treating prolapse.

【用法用量】 水煎服,3～9克。发表透疹解毒宜生用,升阳举陷固脱宜制用。

Notes Contraindicated for syndrome of yin deficiency and yang floating, dyspnea, adverse rising of qi and smooth eruption of measles since it is uplifting and floating in property.

【使用注意】 本品具升浮之性,凡阴虚阳浮,喘满气逆及麻疹已透者,忌用。

Explanation Chaihu (*Radix Bupleuri*), Gegen (*Radix Puerariae*) and Shengma (*Rhizoma Cimicifugae*) can all expel pathogenic factors from the superficies and invigorate the spleen-yang, and are indicated for the disease due to exogenous pathogenic wind and heat with fever and headache. But Shengma (*Rhizoma Cimicifugae*) and Chaihu (*Radix Bupleuri*) can invigorate the spleen-yang in sending qi and nutrients upward and are used for prolapse due to qi deficiency marked by prolapse of the rectum due to chronic diarrhea and prolapse of internal organs. Shengma (*Rhizoma Cimicifugae*) and Gegen (*Radix Puerariae*) can let out eruption of measles as well, so they are indicated for early stage of measles with unsmooth eruption. In addition, Chaihu (*Radix Bupleuri*) can also mediate shaoyang meridian, soothe the liver and remove the stagnancy of liver-qi, so it is often used

【作用说明】 柴胡、葛根、升麻均能发表、升阳,用于外感风热,发热头痛等。但柴胡、升麻能升阳举陷,用于气虚下陷,久泻脱肛,内脏下垂。升麻、葛根又能透发麻疹,用于麻疹初起,透发不畅。此外,柴胡又能和解少阳,疏肝解郁,常用于少阳病寒热往来,胸胁苦满,口苦咽干;肝郁气滞,月经不调,胸胁疼痛。并且退热作用好。升麻善于清热解毒,常用于齿痛、口疮、咽喉肿痛、丹毒等热毒证。葛根能升发清阳,生津止渴,止泻止痢,用于热病烦渴,阴虚

for syndrome of the shaoyang meridians manifested as alternate spells of fever and chills, fullness in the chest and hypochondrium, bitter taste in the mouth and dryness of throat, and also for stagnancy of liver-qi with irregular menstruation, pain in the chest and hypochondrium, and is effective in abating fever. Shengma (*Rhizoma Cimicifugae*) is good at clearing away heat and relieving toxic materials and often used for heat syndromes marked by toothache, aphthae, sore and swollen throat and erysipelas. Gegen (*Radix Puerariae*) can raise lucid yang, produce the body fluids and relieve thirst, diarrhea and dysentery and is indicated for febrile disease with excessive thirst, diabetes due to yin deficiency, diarrhea and dysentery due to heat, diarrhea due to spleen-deficiency. It can expel pathogenic factors in the muscles and relieve fever as well, so it can be used for exterior syndrome manifested as stiffness and pain of the nape and back.

消渴，热泄热痢，脾虚泄泻。并能解肌退热，用于外感表证，项背强痛。

2 Heat Clearing Chinese Medicinal Herbs

第二章 清热药

Any Chinese medicinal herb that has the main action of clearing away interior heat is considered to be an antipyretic herb.

凡以清解里热为主要作用的药物，称为清热药。

Antipyretic herbs are mostly cold or cool in nature and have the actions to clear away heat, purge fire, dry dampness, cool the blood, relieve toxic materials, clear away deficiency-heat, etc.. They are chiefly used for various internal heat syndromes without exterior pathogenic factors and stagnation marked by febrile disease due to exogenous pathogenic factors with high fever, excessive thirst and dysentery due to damp and heat; maculae due to warm-toxin, carbuncle, ulcer, skin disease, and fever due to yin-deficiency.

清热药药性寒凉，有清热泻火、燥湿、凉血、解毒、清虚热等功效。主要用于外感热病，高热烦渴，湿热泻痢，温毒发斑，痈肿疮毒及阴虚发热等病证表邪已解，里热炽盛，而无积滞的各种里热证候。

Depending on different types of qifen, xuefen, asthenia and sthenia of the interior heat syndrome, and on different actions of medicinal herbs, antipyretic herbs are classified as five types, that is, heat clearing and fire purging, heat clearing and dampness drying, heat clearing and toxic materials eliminating, heat clearing and blood cooling, and deficient heat clearing ones.

针对里热证属气分还是血分，属实热还是虚热的不同类型，并根据药物功效的不同，清热药分为清热泻火药、清热燥湿药、清热解毒药、清热凉血药和清虚热药五类。

When antipyretic herbs are applied, we must first distinguish the exterior from the interior, or asthenia from sthenia and be sure of the position of heat. If the heat is in qi-fen or qi phase, heat clearing and fire purging medicinal herbs should be applied; if the heat in xue-fen or blood phase, heat clearing and blood cooling medicinal herbs should be applied. There are differences in applica-

应用清热药首先要辨清表里虚实，明确邪热所在部位。热在气分，应用清热泻火药；热在血分，当选清热凉血药。实热证有清热泻火、清营凉血、气血两清等的用药不同；虚热证用药则有清热凉

tion of medicinal herbs, that is, the medicinal herbs used for the sthenic heat-syndrome are different in clearing away heat and purging fire, or clearing away heat from yingfen and cooling blood, or clearing away heat from both qifen and xuefen; those used for deficient heat-syndrome are different in clearing away heat and cooling blood, or nourishing yin to clear away heat or cooling blood to remove steaming fever. Meanwhile, antipyretic herbs must be used in combination with others according to syndromes accompanying with or following the above syndromes. For instance, for heat-syndrome with exogenous pathogenic factors, the exogenous pathogenic factors should be first removed and then interior heat is cleared away, or they are used together with ones for relieving exterior syndrome so as to remove pathogenic factors from both the interior and exterior; for syndrome of heat stagnation in the interior, they should be used together with downward purging herbs.

血、养阴透热及滋阴清热、凉血除蒸之别。同时，须根据兼证，随证配伍用药。如热证兼有表邪者，当先解表后清里，或与解表药同用，以期表里双解；若里热积滞者，则应配伍泻下药。

Heat clearing medicinal herbs are both cold and cool in nature, easily injuring the spleen and stomach, so they are used with caution for deficiency of spleen-qi and stomach-qi, which is manifested as poor appetite and loose stool; furthermore, heat clearing and dampness drying medicinal herbs should be also used with caution for yin deficiency and consumption of the body fluids when they are used to treat febrile diseaes since they are bitter in flavor and cold in nature and easily injure yin and consume body fluids as well as remove dryness, and febrile disease easily consumes body fluids, too; for excessive yin rejecting yang and true cold and false heat syndrome, they can not be used.

清热药性均寒凉，易伤脾胃，脾胃气虚，食少便溏者慎用；热病易伤津液，清热燥湿药性味苦寒，易化燥伤阴伤津，故阴虚津伤者也应当慎用；如遇阴盛格阳，真寒假热之证，更不可妄用。

2.1 Heat clearing and fire purging Chinese medicinal herbs

This kind of medicinal herbs take the main action of clearing away and purging pathogenic heat from qifen or the qi phase. They are mostly bitter in flavor and cold in nature while some are sweet and cold, so they are mainly indicated for sthenic heat-syndrome at qifen marked by febrile disease with high fever, restlessness, thirst, perspiration, full and big pulse and even coma and delirium. They are separately indicated for fire-heat syndrome of zang and fu organs due to lung-heat, stomach-heat, heart-fire, and liver-fire, etc..

Shigao *Gypsum Fibrosum*

It is the monoclinic system of gypsum ore, containing hydrous calcium sulfate, its producing areas are in the provinces of Hubei, Gansu and Sichuan and can be mined all year round. The crude one may be pounded or calcined for being used as a medication.

Medicinal Properties Bitter and sweet in flavor, extreme cold in nature and attributive to the lung and stomach meridians.

Actions Clear away heat and purge fire, relieve restlessness and thirst, and induce astringent and promote tissue regeneration.

Application

1. It is used for high fever and excessive thirst. With strong actions of clearing away heat and purging fire, and relieving restlessness and thirst, it is the essential medicine to clear away sthenic heat in qifen of lung and stomach meridians. For sthenic-heat syndrome manifested as seasonal febrile disease in qifen, high fever, excessive thirst, and perspiration, it is often used together

第一节　清热泻火药

清热泻火药,以清泄气分邪热为主。性味大多苦寒,部分甘寒。主要适用于温热病高热烦躁,口渴,汗出,脉象洪大,甚则神昏谵语等气分实热证。又分别适用于肺热、胃热、心火、肝火等引起的脏腑火热证。

石　膏

为硫酸盐类矿物硬膏族石膏,含结晶水硫酸钙。主产于湖北、甘肃及四川。全年可采,研细。生用或煅用。

【药性】 味辛、甘,性大寒。归肺、胃经。

【功效】 清热泻火,除烦止渴,收敛生肌。

【临床应用】

1. 用于壮热烦渴。清热泻火之力强,并能除烦止渴,为清泻肺胃二经气分实热的要药。用于温病邪在气分,壮热、烦渴、汗出等实热证,常与知母相须为用,如白虎汤。若气血两燔,高热,神昏谵语,发

with Zhimu (*Rhizoma Anemarrhenae*), such as Baihu Tang (Decoction). For pyrosyndrome involving both qifen and xuefen with high fever, coma, delirium and maculae, it is usually combined with Shengdihuang (*Radix Rehmanniae*), Mudanpi (*Cortex Moutan Radicis*), Xuanshen (*Radix Scrophulariae*) and others that can cool blood.

斑疹者,配生地黄、牡丹皮、玄参等凉血药同用。

2. For stagnation of heat in the lung manifested as cough, thick sputum, fever and thirst, it is often combined with Mahuang (*Herba Ephedra*), Xingren (*Semen Armeniacae Amarum*) to strengthen its action of relieving cough and asthma, such as Ma Xing Shi Gan Tang (Decoction).

2. 用于热郁于肺,咳嗽痰稠,发热口渴。常与麻黄、杏仁等配伍以增强止咳平喘之力,如麻杏石甘汤。

3. For up-rising of stomach-fire with headache, swelling and pain of gum, it is often combined with Huanglian (*Rhizoma Coptidis*), Shengma (*Rhizoma Cimicifugae*) and others that can clear away stomach-heat, such as Qingwei San (Powder).

3. 用于胃火上炎,头痛,牙龈肿痛,常配伍黄连、升麻等清泻胃热,如清胃散。

4. Externally used for inducing astringent and promoting tissue regeneration, pyocutaneous disease, eczema, burned or boiled wounds and bleeding due to trauma. It can be used in single or together with Qingdai (*Indigo Naturalis*), Huangbai (*Cortex Phellodendri*), etc. to clear away heat and remove toxic materials, eliminate dampness and treat ulcer.

4. 外用收敛生肌,用于疮疡,湿疹,烧烫伤及外伤出血。可单用,也可配伍青黛、黄柏等同用,以清热解毒,收湿敛疮。

Usage and Dosage 15 -60 g is used in decoction for oral use and the crude is suitable to be broken and decocted early; externally used with suitable amount, calcined and then pounded into powder which is mixed with water, being covered on the wounded area.

【用法用量】 水煎服,15～60克,宜打碎先煎。外用,适量,调敷。内服宜生用,外用宜火煅研末。

Notes It is contraindicated in the patient with deficiency and cold of the spleen and stomach, or interior heat due to yin deficiency.

【使用注意】 脾胃虚寒及阴虚内热者忌用。

Zhimu *Rhizoma Anemarrhenae*

The source is from rhizome of a perennial herbaceous plant, *Anemarrhena asphodeloides* Bunge, family Liliaceae. The producing areas are mainly in the provinces of Hebei, Shanxi, and Northeast China, etc.. The medicinal material is collected in spring and autumn, the crude without hair or external skin is dried in the sun and cut into pieces or stir-baked with a salt solution for use.

Medicinal Properties Bitter and sweet in flavor, cold in nature and attributive to the lung, stomach and kidney meridians.

Actions Clear away heat and purge fire, nourish yin and moisturize dryness.

Application

1. For overabundance of pathogenic heat due to seasonal febrile disease with symptoms of high fever and excessive thirst, it is usually combined with Shigao (*Gypsum Fibrosum*), such as Baihu Tang (Decoction).

2. The medicinal herb is used for symptoms of cough due to lung-heat, dry cough due to yin deficiency, since it can nourish yin and moisten the lung as well as clear away heat and purge fire from the lung. For cough with yellow sputum due to lung-heat, it is used together with Huangqin (*Radix Scutellariae*), Beimu (*Bulbus Fritillariae*), Sangbaipi (*Cortex Mori Radicis*) and others that can clear away heat from the lung and resolve phlegm. For dry cough and dryness of throat due to dryness of the lung and yin-deficiency, it is combined with Shashen (*Radix Glehniae*), Maimendong (*Radix Ophiogonis*) and others that can nourish yin and moisten the lung.

3. For the hyperactivity of fire due to yin deficiency marked by hectic fever, night sweat and restlessness, it is often combined with Huangbai (*Cortex Phellodendri*) that is added to yin nourishing medicinal herbs so as to

知　母

为百合科植物知母的根茎。主产于河北、山西及东北等地。春、秋季采挖，除去茎苗和须根，或剥去外皮晒干，切片。生用或盐水炙用。

【药性】 味苦、甘，性寒。归肺、胃、肾经。

【功效】 清热泻火，滋阴润燥。

【临床应用】

1. 用于温热病邪热亢盛，壮热，烦渴。常与石膏相须为用，如白虎汤。

2. 用于肺热咳嗽，阴虚燥咳。既能清泻肺火，又能滋阴润肺。治肺热咳嗽痰黄，可与黄芩、贝母、桑白皮等清肺化痰药同用。如治肺燥阴虚之燥咳咽干，则配伍沙参、麦门冬等养阴润肺之品。

3. 用于阴虚火旺，骨蒸潮热，盗汗，心烦。常与黄柏配伍，加入养阴药中，以加强滋阴降火作用，如知柏地黄丸。

strengthen the action of nourishing yin to reduce fire, such as Zhi Bai Dihuang Wan (Pill).

4. For Diabetes due to yin deficiency manifested as thirst due to consumption of body fluids, constipation due to dryness of intestine, it can be combined with Tianhuafen (*Radix Trichosanthis*), Gegen (*Radix Puerariae*) and others that can clear away heat and promote the regeneration of body fluids.

4. 用于阴虚消渴,津伤口渴,肠燥便秘。可配伍天花粉、葛根等清热生津之品。

Usage and Dosage 6 - 12 g is used in decoction for oral use. The crude is suitable for clearing away heat and purging fire; the stir-baked form with salt solution for nourishing yin and reducing fire.

【用法用量】 水煎服,6～12 克。清热泻火宜生用;滋阴降火宜盐水炙用。

Notes Contraindicated in the patient with diarrhea due to spleen-deficiency since the drug is cold in nature and moistening in property, and can lubricate the intestine.

【使用注意】 本品性寒质润,能滑肠,脾虚便溏者不宜用。

Zhizi *Fructus Gardeniae*

栀　子

The source is from a fruit of *Gardenia jasminoides* Ellis var. radicans (Thunb.) Makino, family Rubiaceae. The producing areas are maily in all provinces to the south of the Yangtze River. The medicinal material is collected in autumn and the crude or the one stir-baked to brown or the carbonized can be used.

为茜草科植物栀子的成熟果实。主产于长江以南各省。秋季采收。生用,炒焦或炒炭用。

Medicinal Properties Bitter in flavor, cold in nature and attributive to the heart, liver and triple energizer meridians.

【药性】 味苦,性寒。归心、肝、三焦经。

Actions Purge sthenic fire to relieve vexation, clear away heat and remove dampness, cool blood and remove toxic materials, subside swelling to alleviate pain.

【功效】 泻火除烦,清热利湿,凉血解毒,消肿止痛。

Application

【临床应用】

1. It is used for febrile disease with irritability and can clear away fire from the triple energizer and heart, and relieve vexation. For febrile diseases with irritability, it is often combined with Dandouchi (*Semen Sojae*

1. 用于热病心烦。能清三焦火邪,清心除烦。治温热病,心烦郁闷,躁扰不宁,常与淡豆豉同用,如栀子豉汤。心

Praeparata), such as Zhizi Chi Tang (Decoction); for overabundance of heart-heat with high fever, irritability, coma and delirium, usually used together with Huanglian (*Rhizoma Coptidis*), Huangqin (*Radix Scutellariae*), Huangbai (*Cortex Phellodendri*) and others that can clear away heat and purge fire, such as Huanglian Jiedu Tang (Decoction).

火炽盛,高热烦躁,神昏谵语,多与黄连、黄芩、黄柏等清热泻火之品同用,如黄连解毒汤。

2. For stagnation of dampness and heat in the liver and gallbladder manifested as jaundice, fever and oliguria with brownish urine, it is often combined with Yinchen (*Herba Artemisiae Scopariae*), Dahuang (*Radix et Rhizoma Rhei*), etc., such as Yinchenhao Tang (Decoction).

2. 用于湿热郁结肝胆之黄疸,发热,小便短赤。常与茵陈、大黄等同用,如茵陈蒿汤。

3. For bleeding due to blood-heat manifested as hematemesis, epistaxis, and hematuria, etc.. It is often combined with Baimaogen (*Rhizoma Imperatae*), Shengdihuang (*Radix Rehmanniae*), and Huangqin (*Radix Scutellariae*), etc..

3. 用于血热妄行之吐血、衄血、尿血。常与白茅根、生地黄、黄芩等同用。

4. It is used for pyocutaneous disease with swelling and trauma. For the former due to heat-toxin with reddish swelling and heat pain, it is often combined with Jinyinhua (*Flos Lonicerae*), Lianqiao (*Fructus Forsythiae*), and Pugongying (*Herba Taraxaci*); for the latter, or trauma with local swelling and pain, the crude one can be ground into powder, which is mixed with egg white for local application.

4. 用于疮疡肿毒,跌打损伤。治热毒疮疡,红肿热痛,多配伍金银花、连翘、蒲公英等同用。治跌打损伤,瘀肿疼痛,可用生品研末,鸡蛋清调敷。

Usage and Dosage 6–9 g is used in decoction for oral use, the crude one is used for purging fire, the carbonized one for stopping bleeding.

【用法用量】 水煎服,6~9克。泻火生用,止血炒炭用。

Notes It is not suitable for loose stool due to spleen-deficiency.

【使用注意】 脾虚便溏者不宜用。

Xiakucao *Spica Prunellae*

夏枯草

The source is from spike of *Prunella vulgaris* L., family Labiatae. The producing areas are in all parts of

为唇形科植物夏枯草的果穗。产于中国各地,主产于

China, but mainly in the provinces of Jiangsu, Zhejiang, and Anhui, etc.. The medicinal material is collected in summer, dried in the sun and the raw is used for medication.

Medicinal Properties Bitter and pungent in flavor, cold in nature and attributive to the liver and gallbladder meridians.

Actions Clear away liver-fire and disperse stagnation.

Application

1. For hyperactivity of liver-fire with conjunctivitis, headache and dizziness, it is often combined with Juhua (*Flos Chrysanthemi*), Juemingzi (*Semen Cassiae*), etc.; for insufficiency of liver-yin with eye pains, it is used together with Danggui (*Radix Angelicae Sinensis*), Gouqizi (*Fructus Lycii*) so as to nourish the liver and improve eyesight. Now it is often used for the treatment of high blood pressure due to liver heat and yang hyperactivity.

2. For scrofula and goiter caused by stagnation of phlegm and fire due to stagnation of liver-qi transforming into fire, it is often combined with Beimu (*Bulbus Fritillariae Thunbergii*), Xuanshen (*Radix Scrophulariae*), and Muli (*Concha Ostreae*); for goiter, also used with Haigeke (*Concha Cyclinae*), Kunbu (*Thallus Laminariae seu Eckloniae*), and Haizao (*Sargassum*), etc..

Usage and Dosage 9 -15 g is used in decoction for oral use, or decocted into medicinal extract for oral use.

Notes Used with caution in those with deficiency of the spleen and stomach.

Lugen *Rhizoma Phragmitis*

The source is from underground rhizomes of perennial herbaceous plant, *Phragmites communis* Trin, fam-

江苏、浙江、安徽等省。夏季采收，晒干。生用。

【药性】 味苦、辛，性寒。归肝、胆经。

【功效】 清肝火，散郁结。

【临床应用】

1. 用于目赤肿痛，头痛眩晕。治肝火上炎，目赤肿痛，头痛眩晕，常与菊花、决明子等同用。肝阴不足，目珠疼痛，可与当归、枸杞子等同用，以养肝明目。现多用于治疗高血压病属肝热阳亢者。

2. 用于肝郁化火，痰火凝结之瘰疬、瘿瘤。常与贝母、玄参、牡蛎同用；治瘿瘤，还常与海蛤壳、昆布、海藻等配伍。

【用法用量】 水煎服，9～15 克，或熬膏服。

【使用注意】 脾胃虚弱者慎用。

芦　根

为禾本科植物芦苇的根茎。产于中国各地。春末夏

ily Gramineae, and the producing areas are in all parts of China. The medicinal material is collected in the end of spring and early stage of summer or in autumn, cut into segments, the fresh or the dried can be used.

初或秋季采挖,切段。鲜用或晒干用。

Medicinal Properties Sweet in flavor, cold in nature and attributive to the lung and stomach meridians.

【药性】 味甘,性寒。归肺、胃经。

Actions Clear away heat and promote the production of the body fluids, stop vomiting and relieve restlessness.

【功效】 清热生津,止呕除烦。

Application

【临床应用】

1. For the treatment of febrile disease consuming the body fluids marked by fever with restlessness, thirst, redness of the tongue and shortness of the tongue fluid, it is often combined with Tianhuafen (*Radix Trichosanthis*), Maimendong (*Radix Ophiopogonis*), etc. to clear away heat and promote the production of the body fluids together.

1. 用于热病伤津,烦热口渴,或舌红少津。常与天花粉、麦门冬等配伍,共奏清热生津之效。

2. For vomiting due to stomach-heat, it can be decocted alone into thick juice for oral use; or used together with Zhuru (*Caulis Bambusae in Taeniam*) and ginger juice so as to strengthen the action of stopping vomiting.

2. 用于胃热呕吐。可单用煎浓汁饮服;或与竹茹、姜汁等同用,以加强止呕吐作用。

3. It is used for cough due to lung-heat and pulmonary abscess and can resolve phlegm and drain pus as well as clear away lung-heat. For cough due to exogenous wind and heat, it is usually combined with Jiegeng (*Radix Platycodi*), Sangye (*Folium Mori*), and Niubangzi (*Fructus Arctii*), etc. to expel wind and heat, such as Sang Ju Yin (Decoction); For cough due to lung-heat with yellow and thick sputum, often combined with Gualou (*Fructus Trichosanthis*), Beimu (*Bulbus Fritillariae*), and Huangqin (*Radix Scutellariae*), etc.. For pulmonary absess with pus sputum, combined with Yiyiren (*Semen Coicis*), Dongguaren (*Semen Benincasae*) and

3. 用于肺热咳嗽,肺痈。既能清肺热,又能祛痰排脓。治风热外感咳嗽,常与桔梗、桑叶、牛蒡子等同用,以疏散风热,如桑菊饮;治肺热咳嗽,咯痰黄稠,多与瓜蒌、贝母、黄芩等同用。若为肺痈吐脓痰者,可与薏苡仁、冬瓜仁等清热排脓之品同用,如苇茎汤。

others that can clear away heat and disperse pus, such as Weijing Tang (Decoction).

In addition, it has certain action of clearing away heat and promoting diuresis, so it is also used for oliguria with brownish urine and pyretic stranguria with pain.

此外,有一定清热利尿作用,可治疗小便短赤,热淋涩痛。

Usage and Dosage 15 - 30 g is used in decoction for oral use. 30 - 60 g of the fresh is effective in clearing away heat and promoting the production of body fluids and diuresis.

【用法用量】 水煎服,15～30克,鲜品30～60克。清热生津,利尿鲜品效佳。

Notes Used with caution in the patient with deficiency and cold of the spleen and stomach.

【使用注意】 脾胃虚寒者慎用。

Tianhuafen *Radix Trichosanthis*

天花粉

Its source is from the root of *Trichosanthes kirilowii* Maxim., family Cucurbitaceae, the medicinal material is produced in all parts of China and collected in autumn and winter, the fresh one is used or cut into pieces, dried in the sun for medication.

为葫芦科植物栝楼或日本栝楼的块根。产于中国各地。秋冬季采挖。鲜用或切片晒干用。

Medicinal Properties Sweet and slightly bitter in flavor, slightly cold in nature and attributive to the lung and stomach meridians.

【药性】 味甘、微苦,性微寒。归肺、胃经。

Actions Clear away heat and promote the production of body fluids, resolve swelling and drain pus.

【功效】 清热生津,清肺润燥,消肿排脓。

Application

【临床应用】

1. It is used for febrile disease with thirst, diabetes and frequent drinking, since it is sweet, cold but moistening in properties, and can clear away heat and promote production of the body fluids. For febrile disease with thirst or diabetes due to consumption of the body fluids, it is often combined with Lugen (*Rhizoma Phragmitis*), Maimendong (*Radix Ophiopogonis*), etc.. For diabetes with frequent drinking due to deficiency and interior heat, combined with Gegen (*Radix Puerariae*) and Shanyao (*Rhizoma Dioscoreae*), such as Yuye Tang (Decoction).

1. 用于热病口渴,消渴多饮。本品甘寒而润,能清热生津。治热病津伤口渴、消渴,常与芦根、麦门冬等同用。治消渴多饮,证属阴虚内热者,可与葛根、山药同用,如玉液汤。

2. It can clear away lung-heat and moisturize the

2. 用于肺热燥咳。能清

lung, so it is used for dry cough due to lung-heat. For damage to the lung due to dry-heat with dry cough and scanty sputum, it is often combined with Tianmendong (*Radix Asparagi*), Maimendong (*Radix Ophiopogonis*), and Shengdihuang (*Radix Rehmanniae*), etc. to clear away heat, moisten the lung to stop cough.

肺热而润肺燥。用于燥热伤肺,干咳少痰,常与天门冬、麦门冬、生地黄等同用,以清热润肺止咳。

3. It can be used for pyocutaneous disease of heat type whether the infection is ulcerous or not. It can relieve carbuncle for the nonulcerous and can drain pus and promote the production of muscles for the ulcerous, often combined with Jinyinhua (*Flos Lonicerae*), Baizhi (*Radix Angelicae Dahuricae*), etc., such as Xianfang Huoming Yin (Decoction).

3. 用于热毒疮疡,无论未溃已溃均可应用。未溃者可消散,已溃者能排脓生肌。常与金银花、白芷等同用,如仙方活命饮。

Usage and Dosage 10 -15 g is used in decoction for oral use.

【用法用量】 水煎服,10～15 克。

Notes Contraindicated in pregnant women and it is incompatible with Wutou (*Radix Aconiti*).

【使用注意】 孕妇忌服。反乌头。

Danzhuye *Herba Lophatheri*

淡竹叶

The source is from the entire plant of a perennial herb, *Lophatherum gracile* Brongn, family Gramineae, and its producing areas are mainly in the provinces of Zhejiang, Jiangsu, Hunan, and Hubei, etc.. The medicinal material is collected in summer, dried in the sun and the crude herb is cut into segments for medication.

为禾本科植物淡竹叶的叶。主产于浙江、江苏、湖南、湖北等地。夏季采收。晒干,切段。生用。

Medicinal Properties Sweet and bland in flavor, cold in nature and attributive to the heart, stomach and small intestine meridians.

【药性】 味甘、淡,性寒。归心、胃、小肠经。

Actions Clear away heat to relieve restlessness, clear away heart-fire and promote diuresis.

【功效】 清热除烦,清心利尿。

Application

【临床应用】

1. It is used for febrile diseases with dysphoria and thirst, since it can clear away fire and heat from the heart meridian, and relieve restlessness and thirst. It is often combined with Shigao (*Gypsum Fibrosum*), Lugen

1. 用于热病心烦口渴。能清心经火热,而除烦止渴。常与石膏、芦根等同用。

(*Rhizoma Phragmitis*), etc..

2. It is used for excessive heart-fire and heat involved in the small intestine manifested as tongue sore, dysuria, edema and oligria. It is combined with Huashi (*Talcum*), Baimaogen (*Rhizoma Imperatae*), and Shengdihuang (*Radix Rehmanniae*), etc..

2. 用于心火炽盛,移热于小肠,症见口舌生疮,小便不利,水肿尿少。可与滑石、白茅根、生地黄等同用。

Usage and Dosage 6 - 9 g is used in decoction for oral use.

【用法用量】 水煎服,6～9 克。

Juemingzi *Semen Cassiae*

决明子

It is the ripe seed of *Cassia obtusifolia* L. or *C. tora*., family Leguminosae. Its producing areas are mainly in the provinces of Jiangsu, Anhui, Guangxi, and Sichuan, etc. the medicinal material is collected in autumn, dried in the sun, the crude or the stir-baked one can be used as medication.

为豆科植物决明或小决明的成熟种子。主产于江苏、安徽、广西、四川等地。秋季采收。晒干,打下种子。生用或炒用。

Medicinal Properties Sweet and bitter in flavor, slightly cold in nature and attributive to the liver and large intestine meridians.

【药性】 味甘、苦,性微寒。归肝、大肠经。

Actions Clear away liver-fire to improve eyesight, moisten the intestines to relax the bowels.

【功效】 清肝明目,润肠通便。

Application

1. It is used for liver-heat or wind-heat syndrome with redness, swelling and pain of the eyes. It can also clear away and purge liver-fire, accompanied with replenishing kidney-yin, and improve eyesight, therefore asthenic or sthenic syndromes of eye disease can all be treated with it. For liver-heat syndrome with redness, swelling and pain of the eyes, and tears running, it is often combined with Xiakucao (*Spica Prunellae*), Zhizi (*Fructus Gardeniae*) and others that can clear away liver-fire. For syndrome of the deficiency of liver-yin and kidney-yin with blurred vision, often used together with Gouqizi (*Fructus Lycii*) and Juhua (*Flos Chrysanthemi*) to nourish the liver and improve eyesight.

【临床应用】

1. 用于目赤肿痛。能清泻肝火,兼益肾阴,明目,因此虚实目疾均能应用。肝热目赤肿痛、流泪,多与夏枯草、栀子等清肝之品同用。如为肝肾阴虚,目暗不明,常与枸杞子、菊花等同用,以养肝明目。

2. It is used for liver-heat or hyperactivity of liver-yang with headache and dizziness. It is often combined with Gouteng (*Ramulus Uncariae cum Uncis*), Shijueming (*Concha Haliotidis*) and others to clear away heat and suppress liver-yang. It is now often used for hypertension due to hyperactivity of liver-yang.

2. 用于肝热或肝阳上亢头痛，眩晕。常与钩藤、石决明等同用以清热平肝。现多用于高血压病阳亢者。

3. For constipation due to dryness of the intestine, it is often used together with Huomaren (*Semen Cannabis*), Gualouren (*Semen Trichosanthis*) and others.

3. 用于肠燥便秘。常与火麻仁、瓜蒌仁等同用。

Usage and Dosage 10 -15 g is used in decoction for oral use or it is made tea for drinking.

【用法用量】 水煎服，10～15 克；或泡茶饮。

Notes It is not suitable for the patient with loose stool due to qi deficiency.

【使用注意】 气虚便溏者不宜。

2.2 Chinese medicinal herbs for eliminating heat and dampness

第二节 清热燥湿药

This kind of medicinal herbs are usually bitter in flavor, cold and dry in nature, are effective in clearing away heat and drying dampness and are usually accompanied with the action of clearing away heat and purging fire. They are indicated for damp-heat and fire-heat syndromes, such as damp-thermosis, or acute febrile disease due to summer-heat, or stagnation of damp and heat in the spleen and stomach with thoracic fullness, damp-heat of the large intestine with diarrhea and dysentery, damp-heat of the liver and gallbladder with jaundice, damp-heat leukorrhagia, pyretic stranguria, damp-heat Bi-syndrome, and eczema. They are generally bitter and cold, easily injuring the spleen and stomach, and dry in nature, usually consuming yin, so excessive usage should be avoided, and it is used with caution for the deficiency-cold of the spleen and stomach, or consumption of the body fluids or insufficiency of yin.

本类药物性味苦寒而燥，功能清热燥湿，又多兼清热泻火之功。适用于湿热证及火热证，如湿温，暑温，湿热蕴结脾胃之痞满，大肠湿热之泄泻、痢疾，肝胆湿热之黄疸，湿热带下，热淋，湿热痹证，湿疹，湿疮。本类药物苦寒易伤胃，性燥多伤阴，用量不宜过大。脾胃虚寒，津伤阴亏者慎用。

Huangqin *Radix Scutellariae*

The source is from the root of *Scutellaria baicalensis* Georgi, family Labiatae. The medicinal material is mainly produced in the provinces of Hebei, Shanxi, and inner Mongolia autonomous region, etc., digged up and collected in spring and autumn, usually cut into pieces, the crude one and the one stir-baked with wine or the carbonized one may be used.

Medicinal Properties Bitter in flavor, cold in nature and attributive to the lung, stomach, gallbladder and large intestine meridians.

Actions Clear away heat and remove dampness, purge the sthenic fire and remove toxic materials, cool blood and stop bleeding to prevent miscarriage.

Application

1. It is used for seasonal febrile diseases of dampness type, jaundice, dysentery and stranguria of damp-heat type, especially effective in clearing away damp-heat of both the middle and upper energizers. For the treatment of seasonal febrile disease of damp type with fever, perspiration, chest oppression, greasy fur, it is used together with Huashi (*Talcum*), Tongcao (*Medulla Tetrapanacis*), and Baidoukou (*Fructus Amomi Rotundus*), etc. such as Huangqin Huashi Tang (Decoction). For jaundice of damp-heat type, it is often combined with Yinchen (*Herba Artemisiae Scopariae*), Zhizi (*Fructus Gardeniae*), and Dahuang (*Radix et Rhizoma Rhei*), etc. so as to strengthen the effects of draining the gallbladder to relieve jaundice. For the treatment of dysentery of damp-heat type, it is combined with Huanglian (*Rhizoma Coptidis*) and Gegen (*Radix Puerariae*), such as Gegen Qin Lian Tang (Decoction), for the treatment of damp-heat of the bladder with dribbling and painful urination, used together with Mutong (*Radix Akebiae*),

黄　芩

为唇形科植物黄芩的根。主产于河北、山西、内蒙古等地。春秋季采挖。蒸透或开水润透切片。生用,酒炙用或炒炭用。

【药性】 味苦、性寒。归肺、胃、胆、大肠经。

【功效】 清热燥湿,泻火解毒,凉血止血,安胎。

【临床应用】

1. 用于湿温病,湿热黄疸,泻痢,淋证。本品尤善清中上二焦湿热。治湿温病发热汗出,胸闷苔腻,与滑石、通草、白豆蔻等同用,如黄芩滑石汤。治湿热黄疸,常配伍茵陈、栀子、大黄等,增强利胆退黄之功。治湿热泻痢,配黄连、葛根同用,如葛根芩连汤。治膀胱湿热,小便淋漓涩痛,与木通、滑石、车前子等清热利湿药同用。

Huashi (*Talcum*), Cheqianzi (*Semen Plantaginis*) and others that can eliminate heat and dampness.

2. It is used for sthenic-heat syndrome of qifen and cough due to lung-heat and good at clearing away lung-fire and sthenic-heat of the upper energizer. It can be used alone, namely Qingjin Wan (Pill), or combined with Sangbaipi (*Cortex Mori*), Zhimu (*Rhizoma Anemarrhenae*), and Maimendong (*Radix Ophiopogonis*) for stagnation of lung-heat and failure of the lung to depurate and descend marked with cough and thick sputum. For sthenic-heat of qifen with high fever, excessive thirst, urination with redness and constipation, it is often combined with Dahuang (*Radix et Rhizoma Rhei*), Zhizi (*Fructus Gardeniae*) and others that can purge fire and relax the bowels, such as Liangge San (Powder); for shaoyang syndrome with alternating episodes of chills and fever, used with Chaihu (*Radix Bupleuri*), such as Xiao Chaihu Tang (Decoction), to regulate the function of shaoyang.

2. 用于气分实热，肺热咳嗽。本品善清肺火及上焦实热。若肺热壅盛，肺失清降，咳嗽痰稠，可单用，即清金丸，也可配伍桑白皮、知母、麦门冬等同用。如气分实热，壮热烦渴，溲赤便秘，多配伍大黄、栀子等药同用以泻火通便，如凉膈散。用于少阳证寒热往来，与柴胡同用和解少阳，如小柴胡汤。

3. For exterior sores, abscess of internal organs and other heat-toxin syndromes of internal medicine, surgery and five sensory organs, it is used together with Huanglian (*Rhizoma Coptidis*), Lianqiao (*Fructus Forsythiae*), and Pugongying (*Herba Taraxaci*), etc..

3. 用于外疡内痈及其他内科、外科、五官科热毒证，可与黄连、连翘、蒲公英等配伍。

4. For hemopyretic bleeding manifested as hematemesis, hemoptysis, hematochezia, hemafecia, and metrorrhagia, it can be used alone, or combined with Sanqi (*Radix Notoginseng*), Huaihua (*Flos Sophorae*), and Baimaogen (*Rhizoma Imperatae*), etc..

4. 用于邪热迫血妄行之吐血、咳血、尿血、便血、崩漏等。可单用，或与三七、槐花、白茅根等同用。

5. For excessive fetal movement and gravid vaginal bleeding due to heat-syndrome in pregnancy, it can be used together with Baizhu (*Rhizoma Atractylodis Macrocephalae*), Danggui (*Radix Angelicae Sinensis*), and others, such as Danggui San (Powder).

5. 用于胎热所致胎动不安，胎漏下血，可与白术、当归等药物同用，方如当归散。

Usage and Dosage 3 - 9 g is used in decoction for

【用法用量】 水煎服，

oral use, the crude one is used for clearing away heat, the stir-baked one for preventing miscarriage, the carbonized one for relieving bleeding, the stir-baked with wine for clearing away heat of the upper energizer.

3～9 克。清热多生用，安胎多炒用，止血多炒炭用。清上焦热多酒炒使药力上行。

Notes It is bitter and cold and easy to injure the stomach, so it is contraindicated for deficiency and cold of the spleen and stomach.

【使用注意】 本品苦寒伤胃，脾胃虚寒者不宜用。

Huanglian *Rhizoma Coptidis*

黄　连

The source is from Rhizome of *Coptis chinensis* Franch. and *C. deltoidea* C. Y. Cheng et Hsiao or *Coptis teetoides* C. Y. Cheng, family Ranunculaceae. The producing areas are mainly in the provinces of Sichuan and Yunnan. The medicinal material is dug and collected in autumn and dried. The crude or stir-baked one can be used.

为毛茛科植物黄连、三角叶黄连或云连的根茎。主产于四川、云南。秋季采挖，干燥。生用或炒用。

Medicinal Properties Bitter in flavor, cold in nature and attributive to the heart, liver, stomach and large intestine meridians.

【药性】 味苦，性寒。归心、肝、胃、大肠经。

Actions Clear away heat and remove dampness, purge the sthenic fire and eliminate toxic materials.

【功效】 清热燥湿，泻火解毒。

Application

【临床应用】

1. It is used for dysentery and vomiting of dampness-heat type. It has a strong action of clearing away heat and eliminating dampness and is especially good at removing heat and dampness from the middle energizer, and serves as an essential medicinal herb for treatment of diarrhea and dysentery of damp-heat type. In the case accompanied with abdominal pain due to qi stagnation, it can be combined with Muxiang (*Radix Aucklandiae*) that can circulate qi and arrest pain, such as Xianglian Wan (Pill); in the case with general fever, combined with Gegen (*Radix Puerariae*) and Huangqin (*Radix Scutellariae*), such as Gegen Qin Lian Tang (Decoction); for dysentery with pus and blood, combined with Danggui (*Radix Angelicae Sinensis*), Rougui (*Cortex Cinnamomi*),

1. 用于湿热泻痢，呕吐。本品清热燥湿之力强，尤长于清中焦湿热，为治湿热泄泻、痢疾之要药。兼气滞腹痛较甚者，可与行气止痛之木香配伍，如香连丸；如见身热，可与葛根、黄芩同用，如葛根芩连汤；若下利脓血，可配伍当归、肉桂、白芍药等同用，如芍药汤；如湿热中阻，气机不畅，脘腹痞满，恶心呕吐，常与黄芩、干姜、半夏等同用，如半夏泻心汤。

Baishaoyao (*Radix Paeoniae Alba*), etc., such as Shaoyao Tang (Decoction); for damp-heat stagnation in the middle energizer and disorder of qi activity with fullness in the epigastric abdomen with nausea and vomiting, usually used together with Huangqin (*Radix Scutellariae*), Ganjiang (*Rhizoma Zingiberis*), and Banxia (*Rhizoma Pinelliae*), etc., such as Banxia Xiexin Tang (Decoction).

2. It is used for high fever and restlessness due to excessive heat and fire. It is good at clearing away sthenic-heat of heart meridian. It can be used for febrile disease with excessive fire and heat marked by high fever and restlessness and is usually combined with Zhizi (*Fructus Gardeniae*) and Huangqin (*Radix Scutellariae*), such as Huanglian Jiedu Tang (Decoction); for sthenic heart-fire and insufficiency of yin and blood manifested as dysphoria and insomnia, it can be used together with Ejiao (*Colla Corii Asini*) and Baishaoyao (*Radix Paeoniae Alba*), such as Huanglian Ejiao Tang (Decoction); for excessive heart-fire flaming up with aphthae, it can be used alone or together with the same dosage of Xixin (*Herba Asari*), which are ground into powder for use in mouth; for hemopyretic bleeding due to excessive heart-fire with hemafecia or epistaxis, used together with Dahuang (*Radix et Rhizoma Rhei*) and Huangqin (*Radix Scutellariae*), such as Xiexin Tang (Decoction).

2. 用于火热炽盛,高热烦躁。长于清心经实火。可用于温热病邪热炽盛,高热心烦,常配伍栀子、黄芩同用,如黄连解毒汤;心火亢盛,阴血不足之心烦不眠,可与阿胶、白芍药同用,如黄连阿胶汤;心火上炎,口舌生疮,可单用内服,或与细辛等分研末,掺入口腔;若心火偏亢,迫血妄行,吐血、衄血,可与大黄、黄芩同用,如泻心汤。

3. It is used for toothache due to stomach-fire and vomiting due to stomach-heat. For the former, it is used together with Shengdihuang (*Radix Rehmanniae*), Shengma (*Rhizoma Cimicifugae*), and Baizhi (*Radix Angelicae Dahuricae*), etc. so as to clear away stomach-fire and expel stagnated fire, such as Qingwei San (Powder); for the latter with uncomfortable feelings in the epigastric region, combined with Banxia (*Rhizoma Pinelliae*),

3. 用于胃火牙痛,胃热呕吐。治胃火牙痛,可与生地黄、升麻、白芷等同用,以清胃热,散郁火,如清胃散;用于胃热呕吐,脘痞不舒,可与半夏、竹茹止呕之品等同用,为治胃热呕吐常用药;如为肝火犯胃之呕吐吞酸,可与吴茱萸同

Zhuru (*Caulis Bambusae in Taeniam*) and others that can relieve vomiting, so it is a common medicinal herb for treatment of vomiting due to stomach heat; it can be also used together with Wuzhuyu (*Fructus Evodiae*), such as Zuojin Wan (Pill) to treat vomiting with acid regurgitation due to liver-fire attacking the stomach, and combined with Tianhuafen (*Radix Trichosanthis*), Dihuang (*Radix Rehmanniae*) and others that can clear away heat and promote the production of the body fluids to treat syndrome of excessive stomach-fire with polyorexia and diabetes manifested as excessive thirst and frequent drinking.

用，如左金丸。胃火炽盛，消谷善饥，烦渴多饮之消渴，可配伍天花粉、地黄等清热生津。

4. It is used for carbuncle and swelling and sore of dampness type due to heat-toxin and especially good at treatment of furunculosis since it can clear away heat and eliminate dampness, and purge fire for removing toxin. Orally it can be combined with Huangqin (*Radix Scutellariae*), Dahuang (*Radix et Rhizoma Rhei*), and Lianqiao (*Fructus Forsythiae*) and others that can clear away heat and eliminate toxic materials and also combined with other herbs for external use.

4. 用于热毒痈肿，湿疮。本品清热燥湿，泻火解毒，尤善疗疔毒。内服可与黄芩、大黄、连翘等清热解毒药同用，也可配伍其他药物外用。

Usage and Dosage 2 -5 g is used in decoction for oral use and 0.5 -1 g of the powder is swallowed and just right amount for external use. The one stir-baked with wine can clear away fire from the upper energizer and the one stir-baked with ginger juice and Wuzhuyu (*Fructus Evodiae*) can moderate the bitter and cold property so as to strengthen the action of relieving vomiting and with pork bile can purge sthenic-fire of the liver and gallbladder.

【用法用量】 水煎服，2～5 克；研末吞服，0.5～1 克。外用，适量。黄连酒炒，清上焦火；姜汁及吴茱萸炒，缓和苦寒之性，增强降逆止呕作用；猪胆汁炒，泻肝胆实火。

Notes Being extremely bitter and cold, it is easy to injure yang-qi of the spleen and stomach and contraindicated for deficiency and cold of the spleen and stomach and with caution for consumption of yin due to its bitter and

【使用注意】 本品大苦大寒，易伤脾胃阳气，脾胃虚寒者忌用。苦燥伤阴，阴虚津伤者慎用。

dry property and of body fluids due to yin deficiency.

Huangbai *Cortex Phellodendri*

The source is from the bark of a deciduous arbor, *Phellodendrou amurense* Rupr. or *P. chinense* Schneid, family Rutaceae. The medicinal material is mainly produced in the provinces of Liaoning, Jilin, and Hebei, etc. *P. chinense* Schneid in Sichuan, Guizhou, Hubei, and Yunnan, etc.. During April and May, the trees are barked and the rough skin is scraped, the left bark being dried in the sun. Usually the crude one is cut into pieces or thin pieces or further stir-baked with salt solution or with wine for medication.

Medicinal Properties Bitter in flavor, cold in nature and attributive to the kidney, bladder and large intestine meridians.

Actions Clear away heat and remove dampness, purge the sthenic fire and eliminate toxic materials, reduce asthenia-heat and bone steaming.

Application

1. It is used for syndromes of dampness-heat type in the lower energizer and very effective in clearing away dampness and heat from the lower energizer. For yellow and thick leukorrhea due to damp-heat, it is usually combined with Shanyao (*Rhizoma Dioscoreae*), Qianshi (*Semen Euryales*), and Cheqianzi (*Semen Plantaginis*), etc., such as Yihuang Tang (Decoction). For dampness and heat of the bladder marked by dripping discharge of urine with pain, it is usually combined with Cheqianzi (*Semen Plantaginis*), Huashi (*Talcum*), Mutong (*Caulis Akebiae*) and others that can clear away heat, promote urination and treat stranguria. It is combined with Cangzhu (*Rhizoma Atractylodis*), Niuxi (*Radix Achyranthis Bidentatae*), such as Sanmiao Wan (Pill) to treat beriberi and swelling and pain of foot and knees due

黄 柏

为芸香科植物黄檗(关黄柏)和黄皮树(川黄柏)除去栓皮的树皮。关黄柏主产于辽宁、吉林、河北等地,川黄柏主产于四川、贵州、湖北、云南等地。4～5月剥取树皮,刮去粗皮,晒干,润透切片或切丝。生用或盐水炙、酒炙、炒炭用。

【药性】 味苦,性寒。归肾、膀胱、大肠经。

【功效】 清热燥湿,泻火解毒,退热除蒸。

【临床应用】

1. 用于下焦湿热诸证。长于清下焦湿热。用于湿热带下,黄浊秽臭,常与山药、芡实、车前子等同用,如易黄汤。用治膀胱湿热,小便淋漓涩痛,多配伍车前子、滑石、木通等清热利尿通淋之品同用。与苍术、牛膝配伍,又用治湿热下注之脚气痿躄,足膝肿痛,如三妙丸。用于湿热泻痢,可配白头翁、黄连、秦皮等清热燥湿解毒之品同用,如白头翁汤。治湿热黄疸尿赤,常与栀子、茵陈等同用,如栀子柏皮汤。

to damp invasion of the lower energizer. For dysentery of damp-heat type, combined with Baitouweng (*Radix Pulsatillae*), Huanglian (*Rhizoma Coptidis*), Qinpi (*Cortex Fraxini*) and others that can clear away heat, eliminate dampness and toxin, such as Baitouweng Tang (Decoction); for jaundice and brownish urine due to dampness and heat, often combined with Zhizi (*Fructus Gardeniae*), Yinchen (*Herba Artemisiae Scopariae*), etc., such as Zhizi Baipi Tang (Decoction).

2. For insufficiency of kidney yin and excessive kidney-fire manifested as hectic fever, night sweat, and emission, it is often combined with Zhimu (*Rhizoma Anemarrhenae*), Shudihuang (*Radix Rehmanniae Praeparata*), Shanyurou (*Fructus Corni*), etc., such as prescription of Zhi Bai Dihuang Wan (Pill).

2．用于肾阴不足，肾火偏亢之骨蒸潮热，盗汗，遗精。常与知母相须为用，并配熟地黄、山萸肉等同用，方如知柏地黄丸。

3. It is used for pyocutaneous disease of heat type, carbuncle, furuncle, erysipelas, and burn, etc.. It is often used orally by combining it with Huanglian (*Rhizoma Coptidis*), Zhizi (*Fructus Gardeniae*) and others that can clear away heat and relieve toxin, and externally used by covering its powder on the wounded area, or decocted for external washing.

3．用于热毒疮疡，痈肿、疔疮、丹毒、烧伤等。内服常与黄连、栀子等清热解毒药同用。外用，研末外敷，或煎汤外洗。

Usage and Dosage 2-12 g is used in decoction for oral use, or in pill or powder form. Just right amount is for external use. The crude one is usually used for clearing away heat, eliminating dampness and relieving toxin, the one stir-baked with salt solution is usually used for purging fire and expelling hectic fever, and the carbonized one for arresting bleeding.

【用法用量】 水煎服，2～12克，或入丸、散。外用适量。清热燥湿解毒多生用，泻火除蒸退热多盐水炙用，止血多炒炭用。

Notes Being bitter in flavor and cold in nature, it easily injures stomach-qi, so it is contraindicated in a case with deficiency and cold of the spleen and stomach.

【使用注意】 本品苦寒，易伤胃气，脾胃虚寒者忌用。

Explanation Huanglian (*Rhizoma Coptidis*), Huangqin (*Radix Scutellariae*) and Huangbai (*Cortex*

【说明】 黄连、黄芩、黄柏，均性味苦寒，具清热燥湿、

Phellodendri) are all bitter in flavor and cold in nature, all have the actions of clearing away heat, eliminating dampness, purging fire and relieving toxin, but Huanglian (*Rhizoma Coptidis*) is good at clearing away heart or stomach fire, and more effective in relieving toxin; Huangqin (*Radix Scutellariae*) is good at clearing away lung-fire, and arresting bleeding and preventing miscarriage; Huangbai (*Cortex Phellodendri*) dominates to clear away kidney-fire and dampness-heat of the lower energizer. Therefore, there has been a saying that Huangqin (*Radix Scutellariae*) clears the fire of the upper-energizer, Huanglian (*Rhizoma Coptidis*), the fire of the middle-energizer and Huangbai (*Cortex Phellodendri*), the fire of the lower-energizer.

泻火、解毒作用。黄连善清心、胃之火，解毒之功较甚；黄芩长于清肺火，能止血、安胎；黄柏偏于清肾火及下焦湿热，故有黄芩清上焦火、黄连清中焦火、黄柏清下焦火之说。

Longdan *Radix Gentianae*

龙 胆

The source is from the root and rhizome of a perennial plant, *Gentiana scabra* Bye. or *G. triflora* Pall., family Gentianaceae. The medicinal material is produced in all parts of China, mostly in Northeast China, collected in autumn, dried in the sun. Usually the crude one is cut into segments for medication.

为龙胆科植物龙胆、三花龙胆或条叶龙胆的根。产于中国各地，以东北产量最大。秋季采挖，晒干、切段。生用。

Medicinal Properties Bitter in flavor, cold in nature, and attributive to the liver, gallbladder and bladder meridians.

【药性】 味苦，性寒。归肝、胆、膀胱经。

Actions Clear away heat and dry dampness and purge sthenic-fire from the liver and gallbladder.

【功效】 清热燥湿，泻肝胆实火。

Application

【临床应用】

1. It is indicated for all syndromes due to dampness-heat of the lower energizer and especially good at damp-heat invasion of the lower energizer manifested as jaundice, brownish urine, pudendal swelling, pruritus vuluae, leukorrhea, and eczema, etc.. In treatment of jaundice, it is usually used together with Yinchen (*Herba Artemisiae Scopariae*) and Zhizi (*Fructus Gardeniae*); in treat-

1. 用于下焦湿热诸证。尤善治肝胆湿热下注所致之黄疸、尿赤、阴肿、阴痒、带下、湿疹等证。治黄疸常与茵陈、栀子同用；治阴肿阴痒，女子带下黄稠，男子阴囊肿痛，湿疹瘙痒，常配黄柏、苦参、苍术

ment of pudendal swelling and pruritus vuluae, yellow and thick leukorrhea, swelling and painful scrotum and eczema with itching, usually combined with Huangbai (*Cortex Phellodendri*), Kushen (*Radix Sophorae Flavescentis*), and Cangzhu (*Rhizoma Atractylodis*), etc..

等同用。

2. For headache of liver-fire type marked by conjunctivitis, deafness, hypochondriac pain and bitter taste in the mouth, it is usually used together with Chaihu (*Radix Bupleuri*), Huangqin (*Radix Scutellariae*), and Mutong (*Caulis Akebiae*), etc., such as Longdan Xiegan Tang (Decoction).

2. 用于肝火头痛，目赤耳聋，胁痛口苦。多与柴胡、黄芩、木通等同用，如龙胆泻肝汤。

3. For wind-syndrome due to the domination of liver meridian-heat with high fever and infantile convulsion, and convulsion of feet and hands, it is usually used together with Gouteng (*Ramulus Uncariae cum Uncis*), Niuhuang (*Calculus Bovis*), and Huanglian (*Rhizoma Coptidis*), etc. to clear away liver-fire to stop wind.

3. 用于肝经热盛动风，高热惊厥，手足抽搐。多与钩藤、牛黄、黄连等同用，以清肝熄风。

Usage and Dosage 3 -6 g is used in decoction for oral use or used externally with proper dosage.

【用法用量】 水煎服，3～6 克。外用，适量。

Notes Being extreme bitter and cold and easily injuring stomach-qi, it is not suitable to be used excessively or for a long time, and with caution for syndrome of deficiency and cold of the spleen and stomach and consumption of the body fluids due to yin deficiency.

【使用注意】 本品苦寒之性强，容易损伤胃气，故不可多用、久用。脾胃虚寒及阴虚津伤者慎用。

Kushen *Radix Sophorae Flavescentis*

苦 参

The source is from the root of the *Sophora flavescens* Ait., family Leguminosae. The medicinal material is produced in all parts of China, collected in spring or autumn, cut into pieces, dried in the sun and the raw is used.

为豆科植物苦参的根。产于中国各地。春秋两季采收，切片，晒干。生用。

Medicinal Properties Bitter in flavor, cold in nature and attributive to the liver, stomach, large intestine and bladder meridians.

【药性】 味苦，性寒。归心、肝、胃、大肠、膀胱经。

Actions Clear away heat and dry dampness,

【功效】 清热燥湿，利尿

promote diuresis and kill worms.

杀虫。

Application

【临床应用】

1. It is suitable for dysentery of dampness-heat type and jaundice with brownish urine. It can be used alone or combined with Muxiang (*Radix Aucklandiae*) and Gancao (*Radix Glycyrrhizae*), such as Xiang Shen Wan (Pill) to treat the former syndrome; it is usually combined with Zhizi (*Fructus Gardeniae*), Yinchen (*Herba Artemisiae Scopariae*) and Longdan (*Radix Gentianae*), etc. so as to remove dampness to cure jaundice in the treatment of jaundice; combined with Cheqianzi (*Semen Plantaginis*), Zexie (*Rhizoma Alismatis*) and others that promote diuresis in the treatment of stranguria of dampness-heat type and dysuria.

1.用于湿热泻痢,黄疸尿赤。治湿热泻痢,可单用,或配伍木香、甘草同用,如香参丸;治黄疸,常配伍栀子、茵陈、龙胆等以利湿退黄;治湿热淋证,小便不利,常与车前子、泽泻等利水药同用。

2. It is used in the treatment of pruritus vuluae, eczema, and scabies. It can kill worms and arrest itching as well as clear away heat and eliminate dampness, so it is a common medicine to treat the above skin diseases, and can be used orally or externally. It is usually combined with Huangbai (*Cortex Phellodendri*), Shechuangzi (*Fructus Cnidii*), etc..

2.用于阴痒,湿疹,疥癣。既能清热燥湿,又能杀虫止痒,为治上述皮肤病的常用药。内服外用均可,常配伍黄柏、蛇床子等同用。

Usage and Dosage 3 -10 g is used in decoction and just the right amount is used externally.

【用法用量】 水煎服,3~10克。外用,适量。

Notes Contraindicated for deficiency and cold of the spleen and stomach since it is more bitter and colder in property, and it's incompatible with Lilu (*Rhizoma et Radix Veratri*).

【使用注意】 苦寒之性较甚,脾胃虚寒者忌用。反藜芦。

2.3 Heat clearing and blood cooling Chinese medicinal herbs

第三节 清热凉血药

This kind of herbs are mostly sweet and bitter in flavor and cold in nature, and attributive to xuefen, so they can clear away heat from xuefen. They are indicated for

本类药物多为味甘、苦,性寒之品,入血分,能清血分之热。适用于温热病邪入营

seasonal febrile disease involving yingfen and xuefen manifested as constantly high fever, crimson tongue, unconsciousness and delirum, macules with bleeding and internal injury diseases such as hematemesis, epistaxis caused by blood heat. Since some of the medicinal herbs are sweet in flavor, cold and moist in nature and accompanied with the action of nourishing yin, they can be used for yin-deficient syndromes.

血，高热不退，舌绛，神昏谵语，发斑出血，以及内伤杂病血热妄行之吐血、衄血等。其中部分药物甘寒质润，兼能养阴，可用于阴虚证。

Shengdihuang *Radix Rehmanniae*

生地黄

The source is from the root of *Rehmannia glutinosa* Libosch, family Scrophulariaceae. The medicinal material is mainly produced in the provinces of Henan, Hebei, Inner Mongolia Autonomous Region and the Northeast China, collected in autumn, fresh or dry crude one cut into pieces can be used.

为玄参科植物地黄的根。主产于河南、河北、内蒙古及东北。全国大部分地区有栽培。秋季采挖，鲜用或干燥切片生用。

Medicinal Properties Sweet and bitter in flavor, cold in nature and attributive to the heart, liver and kidney meridians.

【药性】 味甘、苦，性寒。归心、肝、肾经。

Actions Clear away heat and cool the blood, nourish yin and promote the production of the body fluids.

【功效】 清热凉血，养阴生津。

Application

【临床应用】

1. It is indicated for seasonal febrile disease involving yingfen and xuefen. It is effective in clearing away heat in xuefen and can nourish yin and promote the production of the body fluids as well. It is usually combined with Xuanshen (*Radix Scrophulariae*), Maimendong (*Radix Ophiopogonis*) and others that can clear away heat, promote the production of the body fluids and cool the blood, such as Qingying Tang (Decoction) for seasonal febrile diseases involving yingfen and xuefen, which are manifested as fever being more severe at night, restlessness, macules and crimson tongue.

1. 用于温热病热入营血。善清血分之热，又能滋阴生津。用于温热病热入营血，身热夜甚，烦躁谵语，发斑，舌质红绛，配伍玄参、麦门冬等清热生津凉血之品同用，如清营汤。

2. For bleeding due to blood-heat manifested as hematemesis, epistaxis, hemafecia, and hematuria, etc., it is

2. 用于血热妄行之吐血、衄血、便血、尿血等，常与侧柏

usually used together with Cebaiye (*Cacumen Biotae*), Shenheye (*Folium Nelumbinis*, unprepared), Sheng'aiye (*Folium Artemisiae Argyi*), etc., such as Sisheng Wan (Pill); for macules due to blood-heat, it is used together with Mudanpi (*Cortex Moutan Radicis*), Chishaoyao (*Radix Paeoniae Rubra*).

叶、生荷叶、生艾叶等同用，如四生丸。用于血热发斑，可与牡丹皮、赤芍药等同用。

3. It is used for syndrome of consumption of the body fluids due to yin-deficiency. For febrile disease consuming yin manifested as red tongue and oral dryness, it is combined with Shashen (*Radix Adenophorae*), Maimendong (*Radix Ophiopogonis*), and Yuzhu (*Rhizoma Polygonati Odorati*), etc.; for diabetes due to internal heat, used together with Huangqi (*Radix Astragali*), Gegen (*Radix Puerariae*), and Tianhuafen (*Radix Trichosanthis*), etc.; for febrile diseases with consumption of the body fluids manifested as constipation due to dryness of intestine, it is usually used together with Xuanshen (*Radix Scrophulariae*) and Maimendong (*Radix Ophiopogonis*), such as Zengye Tang (Decoction).

3. 用于阴虚津伤证。热病伤阴，舌红口干，可伍用沙参、麦门冬、玉竹等。内热消渴，可与黄芪、葛根、天花粉等配伍；治热伤津液而肠燥便秘，常与玄参、麦门冬同用，如增液汤。

Usage and Dosage 9–15 g is used in decoction for oral use, the fresh amount being doubled or the fresh being pounded into juice that is put in decoction. The fresh is very cold and with plenty of juice, it can clear away heat and promote the production of the body fluids, and has effect of cooling blood and arresting bleeding, so the fresh is suitable for seasonal febrile diseases and bleeding due to blood-heat; the cold nature of the dry is slightly weak while its action of nourishing yin is better, so the dry is especially suitable for yin deficiency with interior heat.

【用法用量】 水煎服，9～15克。鲜品用量加倍，或以鲜品捣汁入药。鲜品大寒多汁，清热生津，凉血止血之力较强，温热病及血热出血用之较宜；干品寒性略减，而滋阴之力较好，尤适宜于阴虚内热之证。

Notes Contraindicated for spleen deficiency with dampness and epigastric fullness with diarrhea since the medicinal herb is cold, cool and moist in nature.

【使用注意】 本品寒凉滋腻，脾虚有湿及腹满便溏者忌用。

Xuanshen *Radix Scrophulariae*

The source is from the root of *Scrophalaria ningpoensis* Hemsl, family Scrophulariaceae. The medicinal material is mainly produced in the reaches of Yangtze River and provinces of Shaanxi, Fujian, and so on. Besides, many plants are cultivated in Zhejiang province, and their roots are dug and collected in early stage of winter, piled up in the sun until the interior of the roots becomes black, and then are dried in the sun, cut into pieces and the crude form can be used.

Medicinal Properties Bitter, sweet and salty in flavor, cold in nature and attributive to the lung, stomach and kidney meridians.

Actions Clear away heat and cool the blood, nourish yin and promote the production of the body fluids, relieve toxin and benefit the throat.

Application

1. For seasonal febrile diseases involving yingfen and xuefen, consuming yin and causing blood-heat, which are manifested as fever, maculae, oral dryness, and red and crimson tongue, etc., it is usually combined with Shengdihuang (*Radix Rehmanniae*), Lianqiao (*Fructus Forsythiae*), and Jinyinhua (*Flos Lonicerae*), etc., such as Qingying Tang (Decoction); for febrile diseases causing pyrosyndrome involving both qifen and xuefen, macules and skin rash, it can also be combined with Shigao (*Gypsum Fibrosum*), Zhimu (*Rhizoma Anemarrhenae*), Daqingye (*Folium Isatidis*), etc., so as to strengthen the action of clearing away heat and purging fire, relieving toxin, or letting out the skin eruptions and resolving macules.

2. It is used for carbuncle of heat type, scrofula and subcutaneous nodule. For carbuncle and pyocutaneous disease, it is usually combined with Jinyinhua (*Flos*

玄　参

为玄参科植物玄参的根。主产于长江流域及陕西、福建等省，浙江有大量栽培。立冬前后采挖，反复堆晒至内部色黑，晒干。切片，生用。

【药性】 味苦、甘、咸，性寒。归肺、胃、肾经。

【功效】 清热凉血，滋阴生津，解毒利咽。

【临床应用】

1. 用于温热病热入营血，阴伤血热，症见身热，发斑，口干，舌质红绛者，常与生地黄、连翘、金银花等同用，如清营汤；温病气血两燔，发斑发疹，也可与石膏、知母、大青叶等同用，以加强清热泻火，解毒透疹化斑之力。

2. 用于热毒痈肿，瘰疬痰核。治痈肿疮疡，常配金银花、连翘等清热解毒药同用。

Lonicerae), Lianqiao (*Fructus Forsythiae*) and others that can clear away heat and relieve toxin; for scrofula and subcutaneous nodule, combined with Muli (*Concha Ostreae*), Beimu (*Bulbus Fritillariae Thunbergii*), etc. which can together clear away heat, relieve toxin and disperse the stagnated mass.

治瘰疬痰核，可配伍牡蛎、贝母等，共奏清热、解毒、散结之功。

3. It is used for yin-deficiency leading to hyperactivity of fire. For deficiency of lung and kidney yin manifested as cough, dryness of throat, hectic fever, night sweet and hemoptysis, it is combined with Shengdihuang (*Radix Rehmanniae*), Maimendong (*Radix Ophiopogonis*), Beimu (*Bulbus Fritillariae Thunbergii*) and others that can nourish yin and resolve phlegm; for bone steaming and consumptive fever, combined with Digupi (*Cortex Lycii Radicis*), Mudanpi (*Cortex Moutan Radicis*), etc; for diabetes of heat type, used together with Maimendong (*Radix Ophiopogonis*) and Wuweizi (*Fructus Schisandrae*).

3. 用于阴虚火旺证。肺肾阴虚，咳嗽咽燥，潮热盗汗，咯血者，可配生地黄、麦门冬、贝母等养阴化痰之品；治骨蒸劳热，配地骨皮、牡丹皮等同用。治内热消渴，则常与麦门冬、五味子配伍。

4. It is used for swollen and sore throat. Being a common medicinal herb to treat swollen and sore throat, it can always be combined with according to syndrome, whether sore throat is caused by exogenous wind and heat, or by sthenic-heat of lung meridian or by hyperactivity of fire due to yin deficiency; for that caused by exogenous wind and heat, usually combined with Niubangzi (*Fructus Arctii*) and Bohe (*Herba Menthae*); for that caused by hyperactivity of fire due to yin deficiency, usually combined with Maimendong (*Radix Ophiopogonis*), Jiegeng (*Radix Platycodi*) and Gancao (*Radix Glycyrrhizae*), such as Xuan Mai Gan Jie Tang (Decoction).

4. 用于咽喉肿痛。为治疗咽喉肿痛的常用药，无论外感风热、肺经实热、阴虚火旺之咽痛，均可随证配伍。如属外感风热者，常与牛蒡子、薄荷同用；属阴虚火旺者，常与麦门冬、桔梗、甘草配伍，即玄麦甘桔汤。

Usage and Dosage 10 –15 g is used in decoction for oral use.

【用法用量】 水煎服，10～15 克。

Notes Being cold and stagnated in nature, it is contraindicated in the case with deficiency and cold of the

【使用注意】 本品性寒而滞，脾胃虚寒、食少便溏者

spleen and stomach marked by loss of appetite and loose stool. It is incompatible with Lilu (*Rhizoma et Radix Veratri*).

不宜服用。反藜芦。

Mudanpi *Cortex Moutan Radicis*

牡丹皮

The source is from cortex of *Paeonia suffruticoas* Andr, family Ramunculaceae. The medicinal material is mainly produced in the provinces of Anhui, Shandong, etc., collected in autumn and dried in the sun. The crude or stir-baked one can be used.

为毛茛科植物牡丹的根皮。主产于安徽、山东等地。秋季采收，晒干。生用或炒用。

Medicinal Properties Bitter and pungent in flavor and slightly cold in nature, and attributive to the heart, liver and kidney meridians.

【药性】 味苦、辛，性微寒。归心、肝、肾经。

Actions Clear away heat, cool and circulate the blood to remove blood stasis.

【功效】 清热凉血，活血散瘀。

Application

【临床应用】

1. It is used for blood heat syndrome manifested as maculae and papules, haematemesis and epistaxis and has the actions of cooling blood and arresting bleeding and can clear away heat from yingfen and xuefen as well. For haematemesis, epistaxis and maculae and papules due to hemopyretic bleeding, it is usually combined with Shengdihuang (*Radix Rehmanniae*), Chishaoyao (*Radix Paeoniae Rubra*) and others that can cool blood and arrest bleeding.

1. 用于血热斑疹吐衄。能清营血分之热，又有凉血止血之功。治血热妄行之吐血、衄血、斑疹等，常与生地黄、赤芍药及其他凉血止血药同用。

2. It is used for febrile diseases injuring yin and fever due to yin deficiency. It can clear away latent pyrexia from yinfen, so it is often used in treatment of the syndrome of residual heat and consumption of the body fluids of seasonal febrile disease at the late stage manifested as fever at night and cool in the early morning, fever and bone steaming, fever bringing down with anhidrosis, and usually combined with Biejia (*Carapax Trionycis*), Shengdihuang (*Radix Rehmanniae*), Zhimu (*Rhizoma Anemarrhenae*), etc., such as Qinghao Biejia Tang

2. 用于热病伤阴，阴虚发热。能清透阴分之伏热，多用于治疗温病后期，余热未尽，阴津已伤，夜热早凉，发热骨蒸，热退无汗，常与鳖甲、生地黄、知母等同用，如青蒿鳖甲汤；如治疗温热病热入营血，见发热夜甚、发斑、舌质红绛等，常配生地黄、玄参、连翘等同用。

(Decoction); for seasonal febrile disease with heat involving yingfen and xuefen marked by fever being severe at night, macules, and crimson tongue, etc., it is usually combined with Shengdihuang (*Radix Rehmanniae*), Xuanshen (*Radix Scrophulariae*), and Lianqiao (*Fructus Forsythiae*), etc..

3. It is used for blood-stasis syndrome, and is especially suitable for stagnation of heat and stasis of blood. For amenorrhea due to stagnation of blood, dysmenorrhea, abdominal mass or traumatic injury, it is usually combined with Danggui (*Radix Angelicae Sinensis*), Taoren (*Semen Persicae*), and Dahuang (*Radix et Rhizoma Rhei*), etc..

3. 用于血瘀证,对热结血瘀者尤为适宜。治血滞经闭、痛经、癥瘕及跌打损伤等,常与当归、桃仁、大黄等配伍。

4. It is used for carbuncle, pyocutaneous disease and swelling; for overabundance of heat with carbuncle and sore toxin, it can be combined with Jinyinhua (*Flos Lonicerae*), and Lianqiao (*Fructus Forsythiae*), and Pugongying (*Herba Taraxaci*), etc.; for early stage of intestinal abscess, usually used together with Dahuang (*Radix et Rhizoma Rhei*), Taoren (*Semen Persicae*), and Mangxiao (*Natrii Sulfas*), etc., such as Dahuang Mudanpi Tang (Decoction).

4. 用于痈疡肿毒。治热毒炽盛,痈肿疮毒,可与金银花、连翘、蒲公英等同用;治肠痈初起,多配伍大黄、桃仁、芒硝等同用,如大黄牡丹皮汤。

Usage and Dosage 6-12 g is used in decoction for oral use, the crude one is used for clearing away heat and cooling blood, the carbonized for arresting bleeding, the stir-baked one with wine for dispersing blood stasis.

【用法用量】 水煎服,6～12 克。清热凉血生用,止血可炒炭用,散瘀可酒炒用。

Notes It is not suitable for blood deficiency with cold, pregnant women and a woman with excessive menstruation.

【使用注意】 血虚有寒,孕妇及月经过多者不宜用。

Chishaoyao *Radix Paeoniae Rubra*

赤芍药

The source is from root of *Paeonia lactiflora* Pall, or several other species of the same genus, family Ranunculaceae. The medicinal material is mainly produced in Inner Mongolia Autonomous Region, Sichuan, Northeast

为毛茛科植物芍药或川赤芍的根。主产于内蒙古、四川、东北等地。春、秋两季采挖,晒干,切片。生用或炒用。

China, etc., dug and collected in spring and autumn, dried in the sun and cut into pieces. The crude or the stir-baked can be used.

Medicinal Properties Bitter in flavor, slightly cold in nature and attributive to the liver meridian.

【药性】 味苦,性微寒。归肝经。

Actions Clear away heat and cool blood, remove blood stasis and relieve pain.

【功效】 清热凉血,散瘀止痛。

Application

【临床应用】

1. For seasonal febrile diseases involving yingfen and xuefen with fever that is severe at night, purplish dark eruptions and macules, crimson tongue and blood-heat syndrome with haematemesis or epistaxis, it is usually combined with Shengdihuang (*Radix Rehmanniae*), Mudanpi (*Cortex Moutan Radicis*), etc..

1. 用于温病热入营血,发热夜甚,斑疹紫暗,舌红绛,以及血热吐衄,常配生地黄、牡丹皮同用。

2. It is used for blood stasis syndrome manifested as amenorrhea, dysmenorrhea, abdominal masses and trauma, and especially suitable for heat stagnation and blood stasis or abdominal pain due to stagnation of blood. For stagnation of blood-heat with amenorrhea or dysmenorrhea, it is usually combined with Yimucao (*Herba Leonuri*), Danshen (*Radix Salviae Miltiorrhizae*) and Zelan (*Herba Lycopi*); for blood stasis with abdominal masses, used together with Mudanpi (*Cortex Moutan Radicis*), Taoren (*Semen Persicae*), etc.; for trauma and stagnated swelling and pain, usually used with Ruxiang (*Olibanum*), Moyao (*Myrrha*), Xuejie (*Resina Draconis*) and others that can circulate blood and treat injury.

2. 用于血瘀经闭、痛经、癥瘕及跌打损伤。对热结血瘀或血滞疼痛者尤为适宜。治血热瘀滞,闭经痛经,常与益母草、丹参、泽兰同用。治血瘀癥瘕,可与牡丹皮、桃仁等同用。治跌打损伤,瘀肿疼痛,多与乳香、没药、血竭等活血疗伤药同用。

In addition, it can also be used for liver-heat with red, swollen and painful eyes, and has certain action of clearing away liver-fire, it is usually combined with Juhua (*Flos Chrysanthemi*), Xiakucao (*Spica Prunellae*), etc..

此外,还可用于肝热目赤肿痛,有一定清肝火作用,常与菊花、夏枯草等同用。

Usage and Dosage 6 -12 g is used in decoction for

【用法用量】 水煎服,

oral use.

6～12 克。

Notes It is not suitable for blood-cold syndrome with amenorrhea, and incompatible with Lilu (*Rhizoma et Radix Veratri*).

【使用注意】 血寒经闭者不宜用。反藜芦。

Shuiniujiao *Cornu Bubali*

水牛角

The source is from the horn of *Bubalus bubalis* L., family Bovidae. The medicinal material is mainly produced in the areas of South and East China. The buffalo horn is soaked in warm water, dredged up, cut into pieces and then dried in the sun.

为牛科动物水牛的角。主产于华南、华东地区。劈开，用热水浸泡，捞出，镑片，晒干。

Medicinal Properties Salty in flavor, cold in nature and attributive to the heart, liver and stomach meridians.

【药性】 味咸，性寒。归心、肝、胃经。

Actions Clear away heat and relieve toxin, and cool the blood.

【功效】 清热，凉血，解毒。

Application

【临床应用】

1. For seasonal febrile diseases involving yingfen and Xuefen with fever, restlessness, coma, delirium, crimson tongue or with eruptions and macules, it is usually combined with Shengdihuang (*Radix Rehmanniae*), Xuanshen (*Radix Scrophulariae*), Jinyinhua (*Flos Lonicerae*), and Lianqiao (*Fructus Forsythiae*), etc.; for seasonal febrile diseases with high fever and convulsion, used together with Lingyangjiao (*Cornu Saigae Tataricae*), Gouteng (*Ramulms Uncariae cum Uncis*), etc. to clear away heat to stop wind.

1. 用于温热病热入营血，身热烦躁，神昏谵语，舌质红绛，或见斑疹。常配生地黄、玄参、金银花、连翘等同用；高热惊厥抽搐，可与羚羊角、钩藤等同用，以清热熄风。

2. For blood-heat syndrome with bleeding, it is usually used together with Shengdihuang (*Radix Rehmanniae*), Mudanpi (*Cortex Moutan Radicis*), Chishaoyao (*Radix Paeoniae Rubra*), etc..

2. 用于血热出血。常配生地黄、牡丹皮、赤芍药等同用。

Usage and Dosage 15-30 g is used in decoction for oral use, pounded into pieces and then decocted first, or pounded into powder for taking after it is mixed with water.

【用法用量】 水煎服，15～30 克。锉碎先煎，或锉末冲服。

2.4 Chinese medicinal herbs for eliminating heat and toxin

第四节 清热解毒药

Chinese medicinal herbs in this category can clear away heat, purge fire and is more effective in detoxifying, including clearing away heat or fire-toxin. They are mainly indicated for carbuncle, abscesses, furuncle, erysipelas, pestilent maculae, mumps, sore throat, and dysentery of heat type, snake poisoning, and scald, etc..

本类药物于清热泻火之中更长于解毒,能清解热毒或火毒。主要用于痈肿疔疮、丹毒、瘟毒发斑、痄腮、咽喉肿痛、热毒下痢、虫蛇咬伤、水火烫伤等证。

Jinyinhua *Flos Lonicerae*

金银花

The source is from the flower bud of *Lonicera japonica* Thunb., *L. hypoglauca* Miq. and *L. confusa* DC., family Caprifoliaceae. The medicinal material is produced in all parts of China and collected in summer and dried in shade. The crude, the carbonized one or distillation form can be used.

为忍冬科植物红腺忍冬、山银花或毛花柱忍冬的花蕾。产于中国各地。夏季花含苞未放时采收,阴干。生用,炒炭或蒸馏制露用。

Medicinal Properties Sweet in flavor, cold in nature and attributive to the lung, heart and stomach meridians.

【药性】 味甘,性寒。归肺、心、胃经。

Actions Clear away heat and relieve toxin, disperse wind and heat, eliminate summer-heat by cooling.

【功效】 清热解毒,疏散风热,清热解暑。

Application

【临床应用】

1. It can be used for seasonal febrile diseases or exterior syndrome of exogenous wind-heat type, no matter whether the heat of seasonal febile diseases is in weifen, qifen, or involving yingfen and xuefen. For early stage of seasonal febrile diseases, pathogenic factors being in weifen, or exterior syndrome of exogenous wind-heat type with fever and light aversion to cold, it is usually combined with Jingjie (*Herba Schizonepetae*), Bohe (*Herba Menthae*), Niubangzi (*Fructus Arctii*), etc., such as Yin Qiao San (Powder); for heat in qifen with high fever and excessive thirst, combined with Shigao (*Gypsum Fi-*

1. 用于温热病及外感风热表证。温热病无论邪在卫分、气分,或入营血均可应用。温病初起,邪在卫分,或外感风热表证,发热微恶寒者,常与荆芥、薄荷、牛蒡子等同用,如银翘散;若热在气分壮热烦渴,可与石膏、知母等同用。热入营血,斑疹隐隐,舌绛而干,则须配伍生地黄、牡丹皮等。

brosum), Zhimu (*Rhizoma Anemarrhenae*), etc.; for heat in yingfen and xuefen with eruptions, crimson and dry tongue, combined with Shengdihuang (*Radix Rehmanniae*) and Mudanpi (*Cortex Moutan Radicis*), etc..

2. It is used for carbuncle and pyocutaneous disease, and most suitable for yang syndrome of heat-toxin type, whether the carbuncle is ripe or not or the beginning of rupture. It can be used orally or the fresh is pounded for external application, or combined with Pugongying (*Herba Taxaxaci*), Yejuhua (*Flos Chrysanthemi Indici*), and Zihuadiding (*Herba Violae*), etc.; for intestinal abscess, combined with Yiyiren (*Semen Coicis*), Huangqin (*Radix Scutellariae*), Danggui (*Radix Angelicae Sinensis*), etc; for lung abscess, combined with Yuxingcao (*Herba Houttuyniae*), Lugen (*Rhizoma Phragmitis*), and Taoren (*Semen Persicae*), etc. to clear away toxic heat and remove pus.

2. 用于痈肿疮疡。热毒阳证最适宜。痈肿未成者可消,已成者可溃,初溃热毒未消者也可用。内服或鲜品捣烂外敷。或配伍蒲公英、野菊花、紫花地丁等。治肠痈,可配薏苡仁、黄芩、当归等同用;治肺痈,可与鱼腥草、芦根、桃仁等同用,以解毒排脓。

3. For blood dysentery of heat type or purulent hematochezia, it can be decocted alone into thick decoction or used together with Huangqin (*Radix Scutellariae*), Huanglian (*Rhizoma Coptidis*), Baitouweng (*Radix Pulsatillae*), etc. to strengthen the action of relieving dysentery.

3. 用于热毒血痢,便脓血,可单味生品浓煎;亦可与黄芩、黄连、白头翁等药同用,以增强止痢效果。

4. For summer-heat syndrome with excessive thirst, sore throat, summer carbuncle, and heat rash, etc., it can be steamed with water into Jinyinhua Lu (Fluid) for oral or external use.

4. 用于暑热烦渴、咽喉肿痛、热疮、痱子等。可加水蒸馏制成金银花露,供内服、外用。

Usage and Dosage 6-15 g is used in decoction for oral use, or prepared into Jinyinhua Lu (Fluid) by steaming, just right amount is used externally. Generally the crude is used, the fresh is better and the carbonized one is used for dysentery.

【用法用量】 水煎服,6～15 克。或蒸馏法制成金银花露用。外用,适量。一般生用,鲜品效好。治痢疾可炒炭用。

Explanation Rendongteng (*Caulis Lonicerae*): Its source is from the stems and leaves of *Lonicera*

【说明】 忍冬藤:为忍冬的茎叶。性味功效与金银花

japonica Thunb., family Caprifoliaceae. Its nature, flavor and actions are similar to Jinyinhua (*Flos Lonicerae*), its actions of clearing heat and relieving toxin are not so strong as Jinyinhua (*Flos Lonicerae*) but it has the actions of activating meridians and collaterals, dispersing wind-heat from meridians and collterals to arrest pain. It is usually used for wind-damp-heat Bi-syndrome marked by red-swollen-painful joints with difficult flexion and extension.

相似，清热解毒之力不及金银花，但本品又有通经络的作用，可消除经络的风热而止痛。常用于风湿热痹，关节红肿热痛，屈伸不利。

Lianqiao *Fructus Forsythiae*

连 翘

The source is from the fruit of *Forsythia Suspensa* (Thunb.) Vahl., family Oleaceae. The medicinal material is mainly produced in Northeast China, North China and Northwest China and the reaches of Yangtze River. In autumn when the fruits are ripe at the early stage, Lianqiao (*Fructus Forsythiae*) collected is known as Qingqiao, when the fruit is completely ripe, the one collected as Huangqiao and the seed as Lianqiaoxin. The crude is used.

为木犀科植物连翘的果实。主产于东北、华北、西北及长江流域。秋季果实初熟时采收为青翘，采熟透果实为黄翘，用种子为连翘心。生用。

Medicinal Properties Bitter in flavor, slightly cold in nature and attributive to the lung, heart and gallbladder meridians.

【药性】 味苦，性微寒。归肺、心、胆经。

Actions Clear away heat and relieve toxin, treat carbuncle, disperse lumps and stagnation, expel wind and heat.

【功效】 清热解毒，消痈散结，疏散风热。

Application

【临床应用】

1. It is indicated for seasonal febrile diseases and exterior syndrome of exogenous wind-heat type. Its actions are similar to those of Jinyinhua (*Flos Lonicerae*), that is, it can also clear away heat and toxin, and is accompanied with expelling wind and heat as well, so it is usually used for heat syndrome due to exogenous attack. For the beginning of seasonal febrile diseases the pathogenic factor of which is in weifen and superficial syndrome of exogenious wind-heat type, it is combined with Jinyinhua

1. 用于温热病及外感风热表证。功效与金银花相似，能清热解毒，又兼发散风热作用，为外感热病所常用。温热病初起邪在卫分，及外感风热表证，可与金银花相须为用，同入辛凉解表剂中，如银翘散；又善清心火，热病邪陷心包，烦热神昏谵语，常用连翘

(*Flos Lonicerae*), with which Lianqiao (*Fructus Forsythiae*) is added to the diaphoretic prescriptions with pungent and cool property, such as Yin Qiao San (Powder); since it is good at clearing away heart-fire, it can also be used for febrile disease involving the pericardium with restless fever, coma or delirium. Lianqiaoxin is usually used together with Maimendong (*Radix Ophiopogonis*), Zhuyexin (*Folium Phyllostachydis Henonis*), Lianzixin (*Plumula Nelumbinis*). It is also used for oral ulcer due to uprising of cardiac fire.

心,配伍麦门冬、竹叶心、莲子心等。心火上炎之口舌生疮亦可应用。

2. Lianqiao (*Fructus Forsythiae*) is a common medicine that treats surgical pyocutaneous diseases, can not only clear away heat and relieve toxin but also disperse stagnation. It is used for carbuncle of heat type and pyocutaneous disease or scrofula, etc. whether the carbuncle is ripe or not. It is usually used together with Tianhuafen (*Radix Trichosanthis*), Zihuadiding (*Herba Violae*), and Jinyinhua (*Flos Lonicerae*), etc.. For scrofula and subcutaneous nodes, it can be combined with Xiakucao (*Spica Prunellae*), Beimu (*Bulbus Fritillariae Thunbergii*), and Xuanshen (*Radix Scrophulariae*), etc..

2. 用于热毒痈肿、疮疡、瘰疬等。为治外科疮疡的常用药,不仅能清热解毒,并能散郁结,痈肿已溃未溃均可使用。常与天花粉、紫花地丁、金银花等同用。治瘰疬结核可配夏枯草、贝母、玄参等同用。

In addition, it is also used for dysuria or dribbling urination with pain, combined with Mutong (*Caulis Akebiae*), Baimaogen (*Rhizoma Imperatae*), etc..

此外,还可用于小便不利,淋沥涩痛,可配木通、白茅根等同用。

Usage and Dosage 6 -15 g is used in decotion for oral use .

【用法用量】 水煎服,6~15克。

Notes It is not suitable for deficiency and cold of the spleen and stomach and qi deficiency with thin pus.

【使用注意】 脾胃虚寒及气虚脓清者不宜用。

Zihuadiding *Herba Violae*

紫花地丁

The source is from the herb of *Viola yedoensis* Makino, family Violaceae. The medicinal material is mainly produced in the lower reaches of the Yangtze River and to its south provinces, collected in spring and au-

为堇菜科植物紫花地丁的带根全草。产于中国长江下游至南部各省。春、秋两季采收,洗净鲜用或晒干,切段。

tumn, after cleaned, the fresh form is used or dried in the sun, cut into segments and the crude form is used for medication.

生用。

Medicinal Properties Bitter and pungent in flavor, cold in nature and attributive to the heart and liver meridians.

【药性】 味苦、辛，性寒。归心、肝经。

Actions Clear away heat and remove toxin, resolve carbuncle and disperse stagnation.

【功效】 清热解毒，消痈散结。

Application

【临床应用】

1. It is used for carbuncle, furuncle, erysipelas, scrofula and all kinds of swelling toxin due to overabundance of heat, especially used for treatment of rooted furuncle. It can be decocted singly or the fresh is ground into juice for drinking and the dregs are covered on the affected place, and it is also combined with Pugongying (*Herba Taraxaci*), Jinyinhua (*Flos Lonicerae*), and Yejuhua (*Flos Chrysanthemi Indici*), etc. such as Wuwei Xiaodu Yin (Decoction).

1. 用于痈肿，疔疮，丹毒，瘰疬及一切肿毒属于热毒炽盛者，尤常用于治疗疔疮。可单味煎服，或用鲜草捣汁饮并外敷，亦可与蒲公英、金银花、野菊花等同用，如五味消毒饮。

2. For snake poisoning, the large amount of the fresh one can be ground into juice for oral use, or used with Banbianlian (*Herba Lobeliae Radicantis*).

2. 用于毒蛇咬伤。可单用鲜品大量捣汁内服，或配半边莲同用。

Usage and Dosage 15 - 30 g is used in decoction for oral use, the amount of the fresh can be doubled, ground into juice for drinking; just right amount is used externally.

【用法用量】 水煎服，15～30 克；鲜品加倍，捣汁饮。外用，适量。

Notes It is used with caution in the case with deficiency and cold of the spleen and stomach.

【使用注意】 脾胃虚寒者慎用。

Banlangen *Radix Isatidis*

板蓝根

The source is from the root of *Isatis tinctoria* L., family Cruciferae. The root is dug and collected in autumn, from which silt is removed, dried in the sun and the crude is used.

为十字花科植物菘蓝的根。秋季采挖，除去泥沙，晒干。生用。

Medicinal Properties Bitter in flavor, cold in nature and attributive to the heart and stomach meridians.

【药性】 味苦，性寒。归心、胃经。

Actions Clear away heat and remove toxin, cool the blood and benefit the throat.

【功效】 清热解毒,凉血利咽。

Application

【临床应用】

It is indicated for seasonal febrile diseases with fever, sore throat, maculae and papules, swollen head due to infection, carbuncle, and sore toxin, etc.. Since its action is stronger in clearing away heat and removing toxin, it is usually used for overabundance of heat and good at removing toxn and benefiting throat as well. For exogenous wind and heat with fever, headache or onset of seasonal febrile diseases with the above syndromes, it is usually combined with Jinyinhua (*Flos Lonicerae*), Lianqiao (*Fructus Forsythiae*), and Jingjie (*Herba Schizonepetae*), etc.; for the treatment of swollen head due to infection with red and swollen face and head, unsmooth throat, usually combined with Xuanshen (*Radix Scrophulariae*), Lianqiao (*Fructus Forsythiae*), and Niubangzi (*Fructus Arctii*), etc., such as Puji Xiaodu Yin (Decoction).

用于温热病发热、咽痛、斑疹、大头瘟、痈肿疮毒等。清热解毒之力较强,多用于热毒壅盛之证,又以解毒利咽散结见长。如外感风热发热头痛或温病初起有上述证候者,常与金银花、连翘、荆芥等同用;治大头瘟毒,头面红肿,咽喉不利者,常配伍玄参、连翘、牛蒡子等,如普济消毒饮。

It is now often used for infectious diseases of pathogenic factors, such as encephalitis B, hepatitis, and epidemic parotitis, etc..

现多用于病毒感染性疾病,如乙型脑炎、肝炎、流行性腮腺炎等。

Usage and Dosage 10 -15 g is used in decoction for oral use .

【用法用量】 水煎服,10～15克。

Notes Contraindicated for deficiency and cold of the spleen and stomach.

【使用注意】 脾胃虚寒者忌用。

Qingdai *Indigo Naturalis*

青 黛

The source is from the branch and leaf of *Baphicacanthus cusia* (Nees) Bremek, or *Polygonum tinctorium* Ait. or *Isatis tinctoria* L., family Acanthaceae, Polygonaceae or Cruciferae. The fallen leaves are collected in autumn, and soaked in water until they are rotten, dredged up from water and then just right amount of lime white is put in the rotten leaves, which is fully stirred un-

为十字花科菘蓝、爵床科植物马蓝、蓼科植物蓼蓝等叶中的色素。秋季采收以上植物的落叶,加水浸泡,至叶腐烂,捞去落叶,加适量石灰乳,充分搅拌至浸液由乌绿色转为深红色时,捞取液面泡沫,

til maceration extract becomes dark red from dark green, at last the foam on the solution is dredged up, which is dried in the sun for being used.

晒干用。

Medicinal Properties Salty in flavor, cold in nature and attributive to the liver meridian.

【药性】 味咸,性寒。归肝经。

Actions Clear away heat and liver-fire, and relieve toxin, cool blood and disperse maculae, and stop convulsion.

【功效】 清热解毒,凉血消斑,清肝泻火,定惊。

Application

【临床应用】

1. It is indicated for overabundance of pathogenic heat manifested as fever, excessive thirst, or maculae and papules, and especially suitable for syndrome of heat involving yingfen and xuefen manifested as maculae, it is usually combined with Shigao (*Gypsum Fibrosum*), Shengdihuang (*Radix Rehmanniae*), and Zhizi (*Fructus Gardeniae*), etc..

1. 用于邪热炽盛,发热,烦渴,或见斑疹。对热入营血,见发斑者尤为适宜。常配石膏、生地黄、栀子等同用。

2. For bleeding due to blood-heat manifested as haematemesis and epistaxis, it's used together with Shengdihuang (*Radix Rehmanniae*), Mudanpi (*Cortex Moutan Radicis*), Baimaogen (*Rhizoma Imperatae*) and others that can clear away heat and cool blood. Since it can clear away liver-fire and phlegm-heat, for liver-fire attacking the lung resulting in hemoptysis or bloody sputum, the single Qingdai (*Indigo Naturalis*) is effective but also combined with the powder of Haigeke (*Concha Meretricis seu Cyclinae*), that is, Dai Ge San (Powder).

2. 用于血热妄行之吐血、衄血。常与生地黄、牡丹皮、白茅根等清热凉血之品同用。因其能清肝火、痰热,故肝火犯肺,络伤血溢之咯血或痰中带血多用,单用有效,也常配海蛤壳研末同用,即黛蛤散。

3. It is generally used for mumps, laryngalgia and pyocutaneous diseases. For mumps and laryngalgia, it can be mixed with small amount of Bingpian (*Borneolum Syntheticum*) for external application, or used together with Huangqin (*Radix Scutellariae*), Banlangen (*Radix Isatidis*) and Xuanshen (*Radix Scrophulariae*) for oral use. For pyocutaneous disease of fire type, it can be combined with Pugongying (*Herba Taraxaci*), Zihuadiding

3. 用于痄腮,喉痹,疮疡。用于痄腮,喉痹,可单用与冰片少许调敷,或与黄芩、板蓝根、玄参同用内服。治火毒疮疡,可配蒲公英、紫花地丁、金银花等解毒消疮药同用。

(*Herba Violae*), Jinyinhua (*Flos Lonicerae*), and others that can relieve toxic materials and treat skin diseases.

4. It is used for convulsive epilepsy due to summer-heat and convulsion or infantile convulsion; for the former, usually combined with Gancao (*Radix Glycyrrhizae*) and Huashi (*Talcum*), such as Biyu San (Powder); for the latter, usually combined with Gouteng (*Ramulus Uncariae cum Uncis*) and Niuhuang (*Calculus Bovis*), etc..

4. 用于暑热惊痫，惊风抽搐，小儿惊风。治暑热惊痫，常与甘草、滑石同用，如碧玉散；治小儿惊风抽搐，多与钩藤、牛黄等同用。

Usage and Dosage 1.5-3 g is ground into powder that is added to pill or the powder form for oral use. It is generally not used in decoction since it is difficult to dissolve in water. Just right amount is used externally.

【用法用量】 研末入丸、散服，1.5～3克。本品难溶于水，一般不入煎剂。外用，适量。

Notes It is used with caution for deficiency and cold of the spleen and stomach.

【使用注意】 脾胃虚寒者慎用。

Chuanxinlian *Herba Andrographitis*

穿心莲

The source is from the herb of *Andrographis paniculata* (Bum. f.) Nees., family Acanthaceae. The plants are cultivated in the areas of South, East and Northwest China, at the early stage of autumn when the flower blossoms, the medicinal material is collected and dried in the sun. The crude or the fresh is used.

为爵床科植物穿心莲的全草。华南、华东、西南地区均有栽培。秋初开花时采收，晒干。生用，或鲜用。

Medicinal Properties Bitter in flavor, cold in nature and attributive to the lung, stomach, large and small intestine meridians.

【药性】 味苦，性寒。归肺、胃、大肠、小肠经。

Actions Clear away heat, eliminate toxin, dry dampness and relieve swelling.

【功效】 清热解毒，燥湿，消肿。

Application

【临床应用】

1. It is generally indicated for seasonal febrile diseases, cough due to lung-heat and pulmonary abscess. For the beginning of seasonal febrile diseases with fever and sore throat, it can be combined with Jinyinhua (*Flos Lonicerae*), Lianqiao (*Fructus Forsythiae*), and Bohe (*Herba Menthae*), etc.; for cough due to lung-heat,

1. 用于温热病及肺热咳喘，肺痈。治温热病初起，发热咽痛者，可配金银花、连翘、薄荷等同用；治肺热咳喘，配黄芩、桑白皮等清肺泄热之品；治肺痈咳吐脓痰，多与鱼

combined with Huangqin (*Radix Scutellariae*), Sangbaipi (*Cortex Mori Radicis*) and others that clear away lung-heat; for pulmonary abscess with thick sputum, mostly combined with Yuxingcao (*Herba Houttuyniae*), Jiegeng (*Radix Platycodi*), etc. to clear away lung-heat and resolve pus. It is now widely used for upper respiratory tract infection and other infectious diseases.

腥草、桔梗等配伍清肺排脓。现广泛用于上呼吸道感染及其他感染性疾病。

2. It is generally indicated for dysentery due to damp-heat and stranguria due to heat. For dysentery due to damp-heat, it can be used alone or combined with Machixian (*Herba Portulacae*), Huanglian (*Rhizoma Coptidis*), etc.; for stranguria due to heat with dribbling urination with pain, mostly combined with Cheqianzi (*Semen Plantaginis*), Baimaogen (*Rhizoma Imperatae*), and Huangbai (*Cortex Phellodendri*), etc..

2. 用于湿热泻痢，热淋。治湿热泻痢，可单用或与马齿苋、黄连等同用；治热淋涩痛，多与车前子、白茅根、黄柏等同用。

3. For carbuncle, pyogenic infection and snake-bite poisoning, the fresh can be ground into pieces for external application, or combined with Jinyinhua (*Flos Lonicerae*), Zaoxiu (*Rhizoma Paridis*), and Yejuhua (*Flos Chrysanthemi Indici*), etc. for being used internally.

3. 用于痈肿疮毒，毒蛇咬伤。可用鲜品捣烂外敷，或与金银花、蚤休、野菊花等内服。

Usage and Dosage 6 -9 g is used in decoction for oral use. Or added to pill, powder or tablet, or prepared into injection. Just right amount is used externally.

【用法用量】 水煎服，6～9克。或入丸、散、片剂，或制成注射剂。外用，适量。

Notes It is not suitble for deficiency and cold of the spleen and stomach.

【使用注意】 脾胃虚寒者不宜用。

Banbianlian *Herba Lobeliae Chinensis*

半边莲

The source is from the whole plant of *Lobelia chinensis* Lour., family Campanulaceae. The medicinal material is produced in all parts of China but more in the reaches of the Yangtze River and the south provinces of China, collected in summer, dried in the sun or in shade. The crude or the fresh can be used.

为桔梗科植物半边莲的全草。产于中国各地，以长江流域及南方各省较多。夏季采收，晒干或阴干。生用或用鲜品。

Medicinal Properties Bitter in flavor, cold in nature and attributive to the heart, small intestine and lung

【药性】 味苦，性寒。归心、小肠、肺经。

meridians.

Actions Clear away heat and eliminate toxin, promote diuresis to relieve edema.

【功效】 清热解毒,利水消肿。

Application

【临床应用】

1. It is indicated for snake-bite poisoning, bee or scorpion injuries and carbuncle of heat type, especially for snake-bite poisoning and it is a common Chinese medicine to treat snake-bite poisoning. It is used internally or externally, or the fresh is ground for external application.

1. 用于毒蛇咬伤,蜂蝎刺螫,热毒痈肿。尤善于解蛇毒,为救治毒蛇咬伤常用之品。亦可用于蜂、蝎及蜈蚣螫咬,及其他热毒痈肿,内服外用均可,或以鲜品捣烂外敷。

2. It is indicated for ascites, edema and dysuria. It has remarkable and constant actions in promoting diuresis, can be used singly or together with Cheqianzi (*Semen Plantaginis*), Zexie (*Rhizoma Alismatis*) and others that promote diuresis.

2. 用于水肿,腹水,小便不利。有显著而持久的利水作用,可单用,或配车前子、泽泻等利水药同用。

Usage and Dosage 10 -15 g is used in decoction for oral use; 30 -60 g of the fresh is used; just right amount is used externally.

【用法用量】 水煎服,10～15克;鲜品30～60克。外用,适量。

Notes Contraindicated for deficiency syndrome with edema.

【使用注意】 虚证水肿忌用。

Guanzhong *Rhizoma Dryopteris Crassirhizomae* 贯 众

The source is from rhizome with petiole base of *Dryopteris crassirhizoma* Nakai, family Dryopteridaceae and *Blechnum orientale* L., family Blechnaceae. The medicinal material is mainly produced in the provinces of Liaoning, Jilin, and Heilongjiang, etc., collected in autumn, dried in the sun. The crude is cut into pieces for being used or the carbonized one is used.

为鳞毛蕨科植物粗茎鳞毛蕨的根茎及叶柄残基。主产于辽宁、吉林、黑龙江等地。秋季采挖,晒干。切片生用或炒炭用。

Medicinal Properties Bitter in flavor, slightly cold in nature, small toxic and attributive to the liver and spleen meridians.

【药性】 味苦,性微寒。有小毒。归肝、脾经。

Actions Clear away heat and eliminate toxin, kill worms, cool the blood and arrest bleeding.

【功效】 清热解毒,杀虫,凉血止血。

Application

1. It is indicated for cold due to wind-heat, seasonal febrile diseases with maculae and papules, carbuncle of heat type and mumps. It is usually combined with Jinyinhua (*Flos Lonicerae*), Lianqiao (*Fruclus Forsythiae*), Daqingye (*Folium Isatidis*), and Pugongying (*Herba Taraxaci*), etc.. It is now used for influenza, measles, mumps, and encephalitis B. etc..

2. It is indicated for many kinds of intestinal parasitosis such as tapeworm, hook worm and roundworm. For killing typeworm and hook worm, it is usually combined with Binglang (*Semen Arecae*); for treatment of roundworms with abdominal pain, usually combined with Shijunzi (*Fructus Quisqualis*), Kuliangenpi (*Cortex Meliae Radicis*), etc.; for pinworm, it can be decocted alone for washing the round of anus before sleeping.

3. It is indicated for bleeding such as haematemesis, epistaxis, hemafecia, metrorrhagia, and especially for profuse uterine bleeding, being more effective in treatment of blood-heat syndrome. It can be used alone and also combined with Cebaiye (*Cacumen Biotae*), Baimaogen (*Rhizoma Imperatae*) and others that can cool the blood and arrest bleeding.

Usage and Dosage 10 -15 g is used in decoction for oral use, the crude is suitable for killing worms and clearing away heat and eliminate toxin and the charred one for arresting bleeding.

【临床应用】

1. 用于风热感冒，温热斑疹，热毒痈肿，痄腮。常配金银花、连翘、大青叶、蒲公英等同用。现多用于治流行性感冒、麻疹、流行性腮腺炎、乙型脑炎等。

2. 用于绦虫、钩虫、蛔虫等多种肠寄生虫。驱杀绦虫、钩虫，常与槟榔同用；治蛔虫虫积腹痛，常配使君子、苦楝根皮等同用；治蛲虫，可单以本品煎汁，临睡前洗肛门周围。

3. 用于吐血、衄血、便血、崩漏等，尤善治崩漏下血，对血热证更宜。可单用，也可配伍侧柏叶、白茅根等其他凉血止血药同用。

【用法用量】 水煎服，10～15 克。杀虫及清热解毒宜生用，止血炒炭用。

Baitouweng *Radix Pulsatillae*

The source is from the root of *Pulsatilla chinensis* (Bunge) kegel, family Ranunculaceae. The medicinal material is produced in the areas of Northeast China, Inner Mongolia Autonomous Region and North China. It is dug and collected in spring and autumn, its leaves, flower stems and fibrous roots being removed and its root stock

白头翁

为毛茛科植物白头翁的根。分布于东北、内蒙古及华北等地。春、秋季采挖，除去叶及残留的花茎和须根，保留根头白绒毛，晒干。生用。

enlarged and covered with white hairs being kept, and dried in the sun. The crude can be used.

Medicinal Properties　Bitter in flavor, cold in nature, and attributive to the large intestine meridian.

【药性】味苦,性寒。归大肠经。

Actions　Clear away heat and eliminate toxin, cool the blood and treat dysentery.

【功效】清热解毒,凉血止痢。

Application

【临床应用】

1. It is indicated for dysentery of heat type and an essential medicine to treat dysentery and especially suitable for dysentery of serious heat with the fresh blood. It can be used alone or combined with Huanglian (*Rhizoma Coptidis*), Huangbai (*Cortex Phellodendri*), and Qinpi (*Cortex Fraxini*), etc., such as Baitouweng Tang (Decoction). It is also effective to treat bacillary and amebic dysentery.

1. 用于热毒痢疾。为治痢疾要药,以热毒甚,痢下鲜血者尤为适宜。可单用,或配伍黄连、黄柏、秦皮同用,如白头翁汤。用于治疗细菌性痢疾及阿米巴痢疾有效。

2. For scrofula, carbuncle and scaby head, it can be used internally or externally. For damp-heat in the lower part with pudendal itching, and leukorrhea, it can be combined with Kushen (*Radix Sophorae Flavescentis*), which are decocted for externally washing.

2. 用于瘰疬,痈肿,秃疮。可内服或外用。用于治下部湿热,阴痒,白带。可与苦参配伍,煎汤外洗。

Usage and Dosage　9 -15 g is used in decoction for oral use. Just right amount is used externally.

【用法用量】水煎服,9～15 克。外用,适量。

Notes　Contraindicated for dysentery due to deficiency and cold.

【使用注意】虚寒泄痢患者忌服。

Yuxingcao　*Herba Houttuyniae*

鱼腥草

The source is from herb of *Houttuynia cordata* Thunb., family Saururaceae. The medicinal material is mainly produced in all provinces of the south to the reaches of the Yangtze River, collected in summer, dried in the sun and the crude form is used.

为三白草科植物蕺菜的全草。主产于长江流域以南各省。夏秋间采集,晒干。生用。

Medicinal Properties　Pungent in flavor, cold in nature and attributive to the lung meridian.

【药性】味辛,性寒。归肺经。

Actions　Clear away heat and eliminate toxin, treat carbuncle and promote pus drainage, promote diuresis for

【功效】清热解毒,消痈排脓,利尿通淋。

treating stranguria.

Application

1. It is indicated for cough due to lung-heat, pulmonary abscess, and an essential medicine to treat pulmonary abscess. For pulmonary abscess marked by cough with bloody purulent sputum, it is usually combined with Jiegeng (*Radix Platycodi*), Lugen (*Rhizoma Phragmitis*), and Gualou (*Fructus Trichosanthis*), etc.. For cough due to lung-heat with yellow and thick sputum, it is usually used together with Huangqin (*Radix Scutellariae*), Beimu (*Bulbus Fritillariae Thunbergii*), and Zhimu (*Rhizoma Anemarrhenae*) and others that can clear away heat and resolve phlegm.

2. For pyocutaneous diseases of heat type, it is usually combined with Jinyinhua (*Flos Lonicerae*), Pugongying (*Herba Taraxaci*), Yejuhua (*Flos Chrysanthemi Indici*) and others that can clear away heat and eliminate toxin, the fresh being ground into pieces for external application.

3. For stranguria of damp-heat type and edema, it can combined with Cheqianzi (*Semen Plantaginis*) and Haijinsha (*Spora Lygodii*) to play a role together in inducing diuresis for treating stranguria.

Usage and Dosage 15 -30 g is used in decoction for oral use, just right amount for external use. But it is not suitable to be decocted for a long time since it includes volatile oil.

【临床应用】

1. 用于肺热咳嗽,肺痈。为治肺痈要药。治肺痈咳唾脓血,常与桔梗、芦根、瓜蒌等同用。治肺热咳嗽,痰黄稠,多与黄芩、贝母、知母等清热化痰之品同用。

2. 用于热毒疮疡。常与金银花、蒲公英、野菊花等清热解毒之品共用,亦可单用鲜品捣烂外敷。

3. 用于湿热淋证,水肿。可配车前子、海金沙等药同用共奏利尿通淋之功。

【用法用量】 水煎服,15～30 克。外用,适量。本品含挥发油,不宜久煎。

Jinqiaomai *Rhizoma Fagopyri Cymosi*

The source is from rhizome of *Fagopyrum cymosum* (Trev.) Meisn., family Polygonaceae. The medicinal material is produced in the provinces of Shaanxi, Jiangsu, Jiangxi, and Zhejiang, etc., dug and collected in autumn, dried in the sun, cut into segments or small pieces for being used.

金荞麦

为蓼科植物野荞麦的根茎及块根。产于陕西、江苏、江西、浙江等地。秋季采挖,晒干。切成段或小块用。

Medicinal Properties Bitter in flavor, neutral in nature and attributive to the lung, spleen and stomach meridians.

【药性】 味苦,性平。归肺、脾、胃经。

Actions Clear away heat and eliminate toxin, clear the lung to resolve phlegm.

【功效】 清热解毒,清肺化痰。

Application

【临床应用】

1. It is indicated for cough due to lung-heat, pulmonary abscess with vomiting of pus and blood. It can clear away lung-heat and eliminate toxin and is as a common medicinal herb like Yuxingcao (*Herba Houttuyniae*) to treat cough due to lung-heat and pulmonary abscess. The both medicinal herbs can be combined with each other or with others that clear away lung-heat and resolve phlegm.

1. 用于肺热咳嗽,肺痈吐脓血。本品能清肺热,解毒,与鱼腥草同为治肺热咳嗽及肺痈的常用药。两者可相须为用,或配伍其他清肺化痰之品同用。

2. It is used for carbuncle of heat type, erisipelas, snake-bite poisoning. It can be used internally or externally. It is effective for the fresh leaves to be ground singly into pieces for external application, or they can be used together with others that clear away heat and eliminate toxin.

2. 用于热毒痈肿、丹毒、毒蛇咬伤。内服或外用均可。单用鲜叶捣烂外敷有效,亦可与其他清热解毒之品同用。

Usage and Dosage 15–25 g is used in decoction for oral use. For pulmonary abscess, it should be stewed with water in a separated container.

【用法用量】 水煎服,15～25克。治肺痈,金荞麦加水置于容器内,隔水蒸服效好。

Hongteng *Caulis Sargentodoxae*

红 藤

The source is from the stem of a deciduous woody vine, *Sargentodoxa cuneata* Rehd. et Wits., family Lardizabalaceae. The medicinal material is mainly produced in provinces of Jiangxi, Hubei, Hunan, and Jiangsu, etc. and collected in autumn and summer, cut into segments when fresh and dried in the sun for use.

为大血藤科植物大血藤的藤茎。主产于江西、湖北、湖南、江苏等地。夏、秋季采收,除去枝叶,砍成短节,趁鲜切片,晒干。生用。

Medicinal Properties Bitter in flavor, slightly cold in nature and attributive to the large intestine and liver meridians.

【药性】 味苦,性微寒。归大肠、肝经。

Actions Clear away heat and eliminate toxin, circulate the blood to remove blood stasis.

【功效】 清热解毒,活血祛瘀。

Application

1. It is indicated for periappendicular abscess with abdominal pain and an essential medicine to treat periappendicular abscess. It can be used together with Dahuang (*Radix et Rhizoma Rhei*), Mudanpi (*Cortex Moutan Radicis*), Jinyinhua (*Flos Lonicerae*) and others that can clear away heat, eliminate toxin and cool the blood so as to strengthen the action of eliminating toxic materials and dissipating abscess.

2. For trauma and irregular menstruation due to blood stasis. It can be used alone or together with Danggui (*Radix Angelicae Sinensis*), Chuanxiong (*Rhizoma Chuanxiong*), and Chishaoyao (*Radix Paeoniae Rubra*), etc..

Usage and Dosage 15 - 30 g is used in decoction for oral use, just right amount is used externally.

Notes Contraindicated in pregnant women.

【临床应用】

1. 用于肠痈腹痛。为治肠痈要药。可与大黄、牡丹皮、金银花等清热、解毒、凉血药同用,以加强解毒消痈之力。

2. 用于跌打损伤、月经不调等瘀血证。可单用,或与当归、川芎、赤芍药等同用。

【用法用量】 水煎服,15～30 克。外用,适量。

【使用注意】 孕妇不宜多服。

Baijiangcao *Herba Patriniae*

The source is from the root and stem of *Patrinia Scabiosaefolia* Fisch, family Valerianaceae. The medicinal material is mainly produced in the provinces of middle and lower reaches of the Yangtze River, collected in autumn, washed, dried in shade and cut into segments and the crude one is used.

Medicinal Properties Pungent and bitter in flavor, slightly cold in nature and attributive to the large intestine and liver meridians.

Actions Clear away heat and eliminate toxin, relieve abscess and promote pus drainage, remove blood stasis and alleviate pain.

Application

1. It is indicated for carbuncle due to heat, for both carbuncle over the body surface and abscess of internal

败酱草

为败酱科植物黄花败酱的根茎。主产于长江流域中下游各省。秋季采收,洗净。阴干,切段。生用。

【药性】 味辛、苦,性微寒。归大肠、肝经。

【功效】 清热解毒,消痈排脓,祛瘀止痛。

【临床应用】

1. 用于热毒痈肿。外痈内痈均可用,尤善治肠痈。若

organs, especially effective for periappendicular abscess. For periappendicular abscess with pus, it is usually combined with Yiyiren (*Semen Coicis*) and Fuzi (*Radix Aconiti Praeparata*), such as Yiyi Fuzi Baijiang San (Powder). For the early stage of that, it is usually combined with Jinyinhua (*Flos Lonicerae*), Pugongying (*Herba Taraxaci*), and Mudanpi (*Cortex Moutan Radicis*), etc. so as to clear away heat and eliminate toxic materials to dissipate abscess. For pulmonary abscess, used together with Yuxingcao (*Herba Houttuyniae*), Lugen (*Rhizoma Phragmitis*), and Jiegeng (*Radix Platycodi*), etc.. For carbuncle and skin infection, usually used together with Jinyinhua (*Flos Lonicerae*) and Lianqiao (*Fructus Forsythiae*), etc. which can be used externally or orally.

肠痈脓成,常与薏苡仁、附子同用,如薏苡附子败酱散。若初起未化脓者,常与金银花、蒲公英、牡丹皮等同用,清热解毒促其消散。治肺痈,可与鱼腥草、芦根、桔梗等同用。治痈肿疮毒,常与金银花、连翘等药同用,外敷内服均可。

2. For postpartum abdominal pain and dysmenorrhea due to blood stasis, it can be decocted alone for oral use or used together with Danggui (*Radix Angelicae Sinensis*) and Chuanxiong (*Rhizoma Chuanxiong*), etc..

2. 用于产后瘀滞腹痛、痛经。可单用煎服,或配当归、川芎等同用。

Usage and Dosage 6 -15 g is used in decoction for oral use . Just right amount is for external use.

【用法用量】 水煎服,6~15克。外用,适量。

Notes Contraindicated in a case with deficiency of the spleen and stomach manifested as poor appetite and diarrhea.

【使用注意】 脾胃虚弱,食少泄泻者忌服。

2.5 Asthenic-heat clearing Chinese medicinal herbs

第五节 清虚热药

This kind of medicinal herbs are mainly effective in clearing away asthenic-heat and reduce hectic fever due to yin deficiency, and indicated for syndromes due to yin-asthenia generating interior heat, such as hectic fever, low fever in the afternoon, feverish palms and soles, restlessness and insomnia, night sweat, red tongue with little

本类药物以清虚热、退骨蒸为主要功效,适用于阴虚内热之骨蒸潮热,午后发热,手足心热,虚烦不寐,盗汗,舌红少苔,脉细数。亦可用于温热病后期,邪热未尽,已伤阴液,

coating, rapid and thready pulse. They are also used for the late stage of seasonal febrile diseases manifested as residual heat and consumption of yin-fluids resulting in fever at night subsiding in the morning, fever being gone but anhidrosis, and crimson tongue, etc..

而致夜热早凉、热退无汗、舌质红绛等。

Qinghao *Herba Artemisiae Annuae*

青蒿

The source is from the herb of *Artemisia annua* L., family Compositae. The medicinal material is produced in all parts of China, collected in autumn that the flowers are vigorious. The fresh can be used or dried in shade and cut into segments for being used.

为菊科植物黄花蒿的地上部分。产于中国各地。秋季花盛开时采割。鲜用或阴干,切段生用。

Medicinal Properties Bitter and purgent in flavor, cold in nature and attributive to the liver, gallbladder and kidney meridians.

【药性】 味苦、辛,性寒。归肝、胆、肾经。

Actions Clear away asthenic-heat and summer-heat and prevent recurrence of malaria.

【功效】 清虚热,解暑热,截疟。

Application

【临床应用】

1. It is indicated for fever and hectic fever due to yin deficiency. Since it attributes to yinfen and clear away asthenic-heat, and is accompanied with relieving and dispering action, especially effective in hectic fever due to yin deficiency with anhidrosis. It is usually combined with Yinchaihu (*Radix Stellariae*), Huhuanglian (*Rhizoma Picrorrhizae*), Zhimu (*Rhizoma Anemarrhenae*), and Biejia (*Carapax Trionycis*), etc., such as Qinggu San (Powder); for the late stage of seasonal febrile diseases with residual heat, fever at night subsiding in the morning, fever being gone but anhidrosis, or prolonged low fever after febrile disease, it is usually used together with Biejia (*Carapax Trionycis*), Mudanpi (*Cortex Moutan Radicis*), and Shengdihuang (*Radix Rehmanniae*), etc., such as Qinghao Biejia Tang (Decoction).

1. 用于阴虚发热,骨蒸劳热。本品入阴分清虚热,兼有透散之功,尤宜于骨蒸无汗者。常与银柴胡、胡黄连、知母、鳖甲等同用,如清骨散;温热病后期,余热未清,夜热早凉,热退无汗,或热病后低热不退等。常与鳖甲、牡丹皮、生地黄等同用,如青蒿鳖甲汤。

2. It is indicated for summer-heat syndrome or the syndrome with dampness and damp-warm disease with

2. 用于暑热证,暑热挟湿及湿温病湿热交蒸者。治暑

alternating steaming of damp and warm. For summer-heat with fever and perspiration, it can be used together with Xiguacuiyi (*Pericarpium Citrulli*), Jinyinhua (*Flos Lonicerae*), Heye (*Folium Nelumbinis*) and others that clear away summer-heat. For summer-heat syndrome with dampness or damp-warm syndrome, fever with unsmooth sweating, dizziness, headache and heavy feelings of body, combined with Huoxiang (*Herba Agastache seu Pogostemonis*), Peilan (*Herba Eupatorii*), Huashi (*Talcum*) and others that resolve and remove dampness.

热发热汗出，可与西瓜翠衣、金银花、荷叶等清解暑热之品同用。如治暑热挟湿或湿温证，发热汗出不畅，头昏痛，肢体沉重，可配藿香、佩兰、滑石等化湿、利湿之品。

3. It is used for malaria with alternating episodes of chills and fever, can prevent recurrence of malaria and can be used alone or combined with Huangqin (*Radix Scutellariae*), Huashi (*Talcum*), and Qingdai (*Indigo Naturalis*), etc. according to syndrome. Arteannuin is now extracted from the herb and prepared into tablet, injection, etc. for being used so as to improve therapeutic effects further.

3. 用于疟疾寒热。本品为治疟疾常用之品。可单用，或随证配伍黄芩、滑石、青黛等同用。现代从其中提取青蒿素，制成片剂、注射剂等应用，进一步提高疗效。

Usage and Dosage 6-12 g is used in decoction for oral use. It is not suitable to be decocted for a long time, or the fresh can be pounded into juice for medication.

【用法用量】 水煎服，6～12克。不宜久煎；或鲜用绞汁饮。

Digupi *Cortex Lycii Radicis*

地骨皮

The source is from the root cortex of *Lycium chinensis* Mill, and *L. barbarum* L., family Solanaceae. The medicinal herb is produced in all parts of China, and *Lycium barbarum* L. in the provinces of Ningxia, Gansu, etc.. It is dug and collected in the early stage of spring or after autumn, dried in the sun for medication.

为茄科植物枸杞或宁夏枸杞的根皮。产于中国各地，宁夏枸杞产宁夏、甘肃等地。春初或秋后采挖，剥取根皮，晒干。生用。

Medicinal Properties Sweet and bland in flavor, cold in nature and attributive to the lung, liver and kidney meridians.

【药性】 味甘、淡，性寒。归肺、肝、肾经。

Actions Cool the blood and reduce bone steaming, clear the lung to lower lung-fire.

【功效】 凉血退蒸，清肺降火。

Application

1. It is used for fever due to yin-deficiency, hectic fever due to yin deficiency with night sweating, and as an essential herb to treat fever due to yin deficiency. It is usually combined with Zhimu (*Rhizoma Anemarrhenae*), Biejia (*Carapax Trionycis*), Yinchaihu (*Radix Stellariae*), etc..

2. It is used for cough and dyspnea due to lung-heat. It can clear away both asthenia and sthenia heat and is especially effective in clearing and purging lung-heat and fire hiding in the lung, usually combined with Sangbaipi (*Cortex Mori*), Gancao (*Radix Glycyrrhizae*), etc., such as Xiebai San (*Powder*).

3. For bleeding due to blood-heat manifested as haematemesis, epistaxis and hematuria, It can be used alone or together with Baimaogen (*Rhizoma Imperatae*), Cebaiye (*Cacumen Biotae*), etc..

4. For diabetes due to internal heat, it can be used together with Shengdihuang (*Radix Rehmanniae*), Tianhuafen (*Radix Trichosanthis*), Wuweizi (*Fructus Schisandrae*) and others that promote the production of the body fluids to relieve thirst.

Usage and Dosage 6.-15 g is used in decoction for oral use.

【临床应用】

1. 用于阴虚发热，骨蒸盗汗。为治阴虚发热常用药。常与知母、鳖甲、银柴胡等配伍同用。

2. 用于肺热咳喘。虚热、实热均可清，尤擅清泄肺热，除肺中伏火。常与桑白皮、甘草等同用，如泻白散。

3. 用于血热妄行之吐血、衄血、尿血。可单用，或配白茅根、侧柏叶等凉血止血药同用。

4. 用于内热消渴。可与生地黄、天花粉、五味子等生津止渴药同用。

【用法用量】 水煎服，6～15 克。

Baiwei *Radix Cynanchi Atrati*

The source is from the root and rhizome of *Cynanchum atratum* Bunge or *C. versicolor* Bunge, family Asclepiadaceae. The medicinal material is produced in all parts of China, dug and collected in autumn, dried in the sun and used alone.

Medicinal Properties Bitter and salty in flavor and cold in nature and attributive to the lung, liver and stomach meridians.

Actions Clear away heat, cool the blood, promote

白 薇

为萝藦科植物白薇和蔓生白薇的根及根茎。产于中国各地。秋季采挖，晒干。生用。

【药性】 味苦、咸，性寒。归肺、肝、胃经。

【功效】 清热凉血，利尿

diuresis and relieve stranguria, eliminate toxin to treat sore.

通淋,解毒疗疮。

Application

【临床应用】

1. It is indicated for the late stage of seasonal febrile diseases with the pathogenic factors involving yingfen and xuefen with prolonged fever and fever due to yin-deficiency. It can clear away both sthenia and asthenia heat. For seasonal febrile diseases involving yingfen and xuefen, fever being severe at night or maculae and papules, it can be used together with Shengdihuang (*Radix Rehmanniae*), Mudanpi (*Cortex Moutan Radicis*), etc.; for prolonged fever or fever due to yin deficiency, and hectic fever due to yin deficiency, usually combined with Shengdihuang (*Radix Rehmanniae*), Zhimu (*Rhizoma Anemarrhenae*), and Qinghao (*Herba Artemisiae Annuae*), etc..

1. 用于温热病后期邪入营血、余热未尽、阴虚内热等。既能清实热,又能退虚热。用于温病邪入营血,发热夜甚,身发斑疹。可配生地黄、牡丹皮等。治余热未尽,阴虚发热,骨蒸潮热,常与生地黄、知母、青蒿等同用。

2. For stranguria of heat type and stranguria complicated by hematuria, it is usually combined with Mutong (*Caulis Akebiae*), Huashi (*Talcum*), and Cheqianzi (*Semen Plantaginis*), etc..

2. 用于热淋、血淋。常配伍木通、滑石、车前子等同用。

3. For overabundance of toxin due to blood-heat manifested as swollen and painful carbuncle, swollen-sore throat, snake-bite poisoning, used both internally and externally or together with other herbs that clear away heat and eliminate toxic materials.

3. 用于血热毒盛的疮痈肿痛,咽喉肿痛,毒蛇咬伤。内服外敷均可,也可配伍其他清热解毒药同用。

In addition, it can also be used for cough due to lung-heat or exogenous fever due to yin-deficiency.

此外,还可用于肺热咳嗽,阴虚外感发热。

Usage and Dosage 4-9 g is used in decoction for oral use.

【用法用量】 水煎服,4~9克。

Notes Contraindicated for deficiency and cold of the spleen and stomach with poor appetite and loose stool.

【使用注意】 脾胃虚寒,食少便溏者不宜服用。

Huhuanglian *Rhizoma Picrorrhizae*

胡黄连

The source is from the rhizome of *Picrorhizae scrophulariflora* Pennell, family Scrophulariaceae. The medicinal

为玄参科植物胡黄连的根茎。主产于云南、西藏。秋

material is mainly produced in the areas of Yunnan and Tibet of China, collected in autumn, dried in the sun, cut into pieces and the crude form is used.

季采挖,晒干,切片。生用。

Medicinal Properties Bitter in flavor, cold in nature and attributive to the heart, liver, stomach and large intestine meridians.

【药性】 味苦,性寒。归心、肝、胃、大肠经。

Actions Clear away asthenia heat, and reduce fever of infantile malnutrition, and eliminate dampness-heat.

【功效】 清虚热,除疳热,清湿热。

Application

【临床应用】

1. For fever due to yin deficiency and hectic fever due to yin deficiency, it is usually combined with Yinchaihu (*Radix Stellariae*), Digupi (*Cortex Lycii Radicis*), etc. such as Qinggu San (Powder).

1. 用于阴虚发热,骨蒸潮热。常与银柴胡、地骨皮等同用,如清骨散。

2. For infantile malnutrition with fever, indigestion, abdominal distention and weight-loss, and prolonged low fever, it is usually used together with Dangshen (*Radix Codonopsis*), Baizhu (*Rhizoma Atractylodis Macrocephalae*), Shanzha (*Fructus Crataegi*) and others that can tonify qi and digest food, such as Fei'er Wan (Pill).

2. 用于小儿疳积发热,消化不良,腹胀体瘦,低热不退。常与党参、白术、山楂等益气、消食之品配伍,如肥儿丸。

3. It is used for dysentery of dampness-heat type and hemorrhoids. Compared with Huanglian (*Rhizoma Coptidis*), it has the weaker action to clear away heat, dry dampness and eliminate toxin, and is good at clearing away dampness-heat of the stomach and intestine. For dysentery of dampness-heat, it can be combined with Huangqin (*Radix Scutellariae*), Huangbai (*Cortex Phellodendri*), and Baitouweng (*Radix Pulsatillae*), etc.; for hemorrhoids with swelling and pain, used together with Diyu (*Radix Sanguisorbae*), Huaihua (*Flos Sophorae*), etc..

3. 用于湿热泻痢,痔疮。有类似黄连而较弱的清热燥湿、解毒作用,善除胃肠湿热。治湿热下痢,可与黄芩、黄柏、白头翁等同用。治痔疮肿痛,可与地榆、槐花等同用。

Usage and Dosage 5 –10 g is used in decoction for oral use .

【用法用量】 水煎服,5~10 克。

Notes Used with caution for deficiency and cold of

【使用注意】 脾胃虚寒

the spleen and stomach.

者慎用。

Yinchaihu　*Radix Stellariae*

银柴胡

The source is from the root of *Stellaria dichotoma* L. var. *lanceolata* Bunge, family Caryophyllaceae. The medicinal herb is mainly produced in the areas of Ningxia, Inner Mongolia autonomous region, Gansu, and Shaanxi, etc., collected after autumn, dried in the sun, cut into pieces and the crude form is used.

为石竹科植物银柴胡的根。主产于宁夏、内蒙古、甘肃、陕西等地。秋后采挖，晒干，切片。生用。

Medicinal Properties　Sweet in flavor and slightly cold in nature and attributive to the liver and stomach meridians.

【药性】　味甘，性微寒。归肝、胃经。

Actions　Clear away asthenia-heat, and reduce fever of infantile malnutrition.

【功效】　清虚热，除疳热。

Application

【临床应用】

1. For yin-deficiency with fever, bone steaming and hectic fever, and night sweat, it is usually used together with Digupi (*Cortex Lycii Radicis*), Qinghao (*Herba Artemisiae Annuae*), and Biejia (*Carapax Trionycis*), etc., such as Qinggu San (Powder).

1. 用于阴虚发热，骨蒸劳热盗汗。多与地骨皮、青蒿、鳖甲同用，如清骨散。

2. For infantile malnutrition with fever, abdominal enlargement, emaciation, it is usually used together with Dangshen (*Radix Codonopsis*), Huhuanglian (*Rhizoma Picrorrhizae*), and Jineijin (*Endothelium Corneum Gigeriae Galli*), etc. to play a role in reducing accumulation and clearing away fever of infantile malnutrition.

2. 用于小儿疳积发热，腹大，消瘦。可与党参、胡黄连、鸡内金等同用，共奏消积除疳之功。

Usage and Dosage　3 -10 g is used in decoction for oral use.

【用法用量】　水煎服，3～10克。

Notes　Contraindicated for wind-cold syndrome due to exogenous attack and blood-deficiency without fever.

【使用注意】　外感风寒，血虚无热者忌用。

3 Cathartics

第三章 泻下药

Any medicinal herb that can cause diarrhea or lubricate the large intestine, aid in moving the bowels and relieve constipation is known as cathartics.

凡能引起腹泻，或润滑大肠，促使排便的药物称泻下药。

They have the actions of aiding in moving the bowels, clearing away pathogenic heat and purging the retention of water. Therefore, they are mainly indicated to treat constipation, various interior excess syndromes due to food and water retention, and interior excess syndrome due to invasion by heat, etc..

泻下药有通利大便、清泄热邪、攻逐水饮的作用。主要适用于大便秘结、实积停滞、水饮滞留，以及实热壅滞等证。

In the light of the difference of the cathartic actions and adaptive conditions, this kind of herbs are classified into three subcategories, that is, purgatives, moistening purgatives and drastic purgatives, of which purgatives and drastic purgatives have the potent actions, especially the latter, while moistening purgatives have moderate actions of lubricating intestines.

根据泻下作用强弱及适应范围的不同，本章药物可分为攻下、润下、峻下逐水三类。其中攻下药和峻下逐水药作用峻猛，尤以后者为甚，润下药润滑肠道，作用缓和。

Therefore purgatives and drastic purgatives should be used with caution or contraindicated in cases of chronic disease with asthenia of healthy qi, pregnancy, menstruation, postpartum, and old and weak patients. So long as the disease is cured, their administration must be stopped and the overdosage must be avoided. For a case of interior sthenia and deficiency of healthy qi, they should be used together with tonics.

攻下药与逐水药，对久病正虚，年老体弱，以及妇女月经期、妊娠、产后，均应慎用或忌用。中病即止，不可过量。里实而正虚者，当与补益药同用。

3.1 Purgatives

第一节 攻下药

Medicinal herbs in this category are bitter in flavor

本类药物药性多苦寒，既

and cold in nature, have descending and cooling properties, and remarkable action of removing stagnation by purgation. They are mainly indicated for syndromes such as constipation due to heat stagnation and seasonal febrile disease with interior stasis of heat, fever having not come down due to obstruction of fuqi or flaring of fire.

能泻下,又能泄热,有泻下攻积作用。主要用于热结便秘及温热病邪热内结,腑气不通以致热势不退或火热上炎诸证。

Purgatives are usually used together with the qi-circulating medicinal herbs so as to strengthen the effects in removing stagnation by purgation. For constipation due to heat stagnation, they are combined with heat clearing and fire purging medicinal herbs; for constipation due to cold stagnation, combined with the interior warming herbs; for constipation due to interior-sthenia but deficiency of healthy qi, combined with tonics.

应用攻下药,常配伍行气药,加强泻下攻积效果。热结便秘者,配清热泻火药;寒积便秘者,配温里药;里实便秘而正虚者配补益药。

Dahuang *Radix et Rhizoma Rhei*

大 黄

The source is from the root and rhizome of *Rheum palmatum* L., *R. tanguticum* Maxim. ex Balf. or *R. officinale* Baill., family Polygonaceae. *Rheum palmatum* L., and *R. tanguticum* Maxim. ex Balf. are also called north *Radix et Rhizoma Rhei*, which is mainly produced at the provinces of Qinghai, Gansu, etc.; *R. officinale* Baill is called South *Radix et Rhizoma Rhei*, which is mainly produced in Sichuan Province. They are collected in the end of autumn or the next spring before the plants will sprout, the hair and coat being removed, cut into pieces or lumps and then dried in the sun. The crude, or the one steamed or stir-baked with wine, or the one charred can be used for medication.

为蓼科植物掌叶大黄、唐古特大黄或药用大黄的根及根茎。掌叶大黄和唐古特大黄称为北大黄,主产于青海、甘肃等地;药用大黄称南大黄,主产于四川。秋末茎叶枯萎或次年春发芽前采挖。除去须根,刮去外皮,切块,干燥。生用,或酒炒,酒蒸,炒炭用。

Medicinal Properties Bitter in flavor, cold in nature and attributive to the spleen, stomach, large intestine, liver and heart meridians.

【药性】 味苦,性寒。归脾、胃、大肠、肝、心经。

Actions Remove stagnation by purgation, clear away heat and purge fire, cool the blood and stop bleeding, remove toxin and promote blood circulation to remove

【功效】 泻下攻积,清热泻火,凉血止血,解毒,活血祛瘀。

blood stasis.

Application

1. It is used for stagnation in the passway of the intestine and obstruction of the bowels, an essential medicinal herb to treat the syndrome of stagnation with constipation and especially effective in treatment of constipation due to stagnation of heat. For constipation due to stagnation of sthenic-heat and abdominal pain against pressing, it is usually used together with Mangxiao (*Natrii Sulfas*), Zhishi (*Fructus Aurantii Immaturus*) and Houpo (*Cortex Magnoliae Officinalis*), such as Da Chengqi Tang (Decoction); if the constipation is accompanied with deficiency of qi and blood, Renshen (*Radix Ginseng*), Danggui (*Radix Angelicae Sinensis*), etc. are added to the above prescription again to support healthy qi and attack pathogenic factors, such as Huanglong Tang (Decoction); for yin deficiency due to stagnation of heat, Shengdihuang (*Radix Rehmanniae*) and Maimendong (*Radix Ophiopogonis*), etc. are combined with, such as Zengye Chengqi Tang (Decoction); for constipation due to insufficiency of spleen yang and stagnation of cold, Fuzi (*Radix Aconiti Lateralis Praeparata*), Ganjiang (*Rhizoma Zingiberis*), etc. can be also combined with, such as Wenpi Tang (Decoction).

2. It is used for dysentery due to stagnation. For early stage of dysentery of dampness-heat type with abdominal pain and tenesmus, it is usually combined with Huanglian (*Rhizoma Coptidis*), Muxiang (*Radix Aucklandiae*), etc. such as Shaoyao Tang (Decoction); for abdominal pain due to food retention and unsmooth dysentery, combined with Qingpi (*Pericarpium Citri Reticulatae Viride*), Muxiang (*Radix Aucklandiae*), etc..

3. For headache, redness of eye, sore throat and swollen painful gums, and oral ulcer, etc. caused by

【临床应用】

1. 用于胃肠积滞,大便秘结。为治疗积滞便秘要药,尤宜于热结便秘。治实热内结便秘,腹痛拒按者,常与芒硝、枳实、厚朴同用,如大承气汤;如兼见气血虚者,再配人参、当归等,以扶正攻邪,如黄龙汤;热结阴伤者,配生地黄、麦门冬等药,如增液承气汤;至于脾阳不足,冷积便秘,也可以配附子、干姜等同用,如温脾汤。

2. 用于积滞泻痢。治湿热痢疾初起,腹痛里急后重,常与黄连、木香等同用,如芍药汤;治食积腹痛,泻痢不畅,可与青皮、木香等同用。

3. 用于火热上炎之头痛、目赤、咽痛、齿龈肿痛、口舌生

flaring of fire, it can be used whether there is constipation or not., usually combined with Huanglian (*Rhizoma Coptidis*), Huangqin (*Radix Scutellariae*), and Niuhuang (*Calculus Bovis*), etc. such as Xiexin Tang (Decoction).

疮等,无论有无便秘均可应用。常与黄连、黄芩、牛黄等配伍,如泻心汤。

4. It is used for bleeding due to blood-heat manifested as haematemesis and epistaxis or bleeding due to blood stasis causing blood not to attribute to channels, since it can promote blood circulation as well as purge fire and stop bleeding without blood stasis. It can be used alone or together with other medicinal herbs for cooling blood and stopping bleeding.

4. 用于血热出血。既能泻火止血,又兼活血作用,止血而不留瘀。凡血热妄行之吐血、衄血,或瘀血血不归经所致的出血均可应用。可单用,或与其他清热凉血止血药同用。

5. Oral or external use is for pyocutaneous disease due to toxic heat, burn and scald. For carbuncle due to toxic heat, it is usually combined with Jinyinhua (*Flos Lonicerae*), Pugongying (*Herba Taraxaci*) and Lianqiao (*Fructus Forsythiae*), etc.; for intestinal abscess, usually combined with Mudanpi (*Cortex Moutan Radicis*), Taoren (*Semen Persicae*), etc., such as Dahuang Mudanpi Tang (Decoction); for burn and scald, can be used alone in powder form, or combined with Diyu (*Radix Sanguisorbae*) powder, being mixed with sesame oil for external application.

5. 用于热毒疮疡,烧烫伤。既可内服,又能外用。治热毒痈肿,常与金银花、蒲公英、连翘等同用;治疗肠痈,常与牡丹皮、桃仁等同用,如大黄牡丹皮汤;治烧烫伤,可单用研粉,或配地榆粉、麻油调敷患处。

6. It is used for postpartum abdominal pain due to blood stasis, abdominal mass, trauma and syndrome of blood retention. For postpartum abdominal pain due to blood stasis, it can be used together with Taoren (*Semen Persicae*), etc., such as Xiayuxue Tang (Decoction), for trauma and blood stasis with swelling and pain, used together with Taoren (*Semen Persicae*), Honghua (*Flos Carthami*), etc., such as Fuyuan Huoxue Tang (Decoction).

6. 用于产后瘀血腹痛,癥瘕积聚,跌打损伤及蓄血证。治妇女产后血瘀腹痛,可与桃仁等同用,如下瘀血汤。治跌打损伤,瘀血肿痛,可与桃仁、红花等同用,如复元活血汤。

In addition, it can also clear away dampness-heat, so it is indicated for jaundice of dampness-heat type and

此外,本品亦能清湿热,用于湿热黄疸及淋证。治黄

stranguria. For jaundice, it is usually combined with Yinchen (*Herba Artemisiae Scopariae*), Zhizi (*Fructus Gardeniae*), and Huangqin (*Radix Scutellariae*), etc., such as Yinchenhao Tang (Decoction); for stranguria due to dampness-heat in the lower energizer, it is usually combined with Mutong (*Caulis Akebiae*), Cheqianzi (*Semen Plantaginis*), and Zhizi (*Fructus Gardeniae*), etc., such as Bazheng San (Powder).

疸,常配茵陈、栀子、黄芩等同用,如茵陈蒿汤;治下焦湿热淋证,常配木通、车前子、栀子等同用,如八正散。

Usage and Dosage 5 -30 g is used in decoction for oral use, just right amount for external use, and the crude one with stronger purgative action is used for downward discharging. It is later added to decoction or soaked in boiling water for oral use, and is not decocted for a long time. That prepared with wine is suitable for blood stasis because of its better action of circulating blood. The carbonized form is usually used for bleeding syndrome.

【用法用量】 水煎服,5～30 克。外用,适量。生用泻下作用较强,欲攻下者生用,入煎剂后下或开水泡服,不宜久煎。酒制大黄泻下力减弱,活血作用较好,宜用于瘀血证。大黄炭多用于出血证。

Notes Used carefully or contraindicated during pregnancy, menstruation or in a case with deficiency of the spleen and stomach, and used with caution during lactation since Dahuang (*Radix et Rhizoma Rhei*) may induce a infant to have diarrhea.

【使用注意】 妇女月经期,孕妇及脾胃虚弱者忌用或慎用。妇女哺乳期服大黄,会引起婴儿腹泻,当慎用。

Mangxiao *Natrii Sulfas*

芒 硝

The Chinese medicine is the refined crystalline sodium sulphate, usually made from natural sources, natrii sulfas as its chief component. The medicinal material is mainly produced in the provinces of Hebei, Henan, Shandong, and Jiangsu, etc.. The mineral substance containing Natrii sulfas is decocted in hot water with pieces of turnips, and the upper part of the decocton is taken out and treated by cooling, the refined sodium sulphate can be crystallized out, which is called Mangxiao (*Natrii Sulfas*). The dehydrated white powder of Mirabilite is called Xuanmingfen (*Natrii Sulfus Exsiccatus*).

为硫酸盐类矿物芒硝族芒硝经加工精制而成的结晶体。主要成分为含水硫酸钠。主产于河北、河南、山东、江苏等省。天然产品用热水与萝卜共煮后取上层液,冷却后析出的结晶即芒硝。芒硝经风化失去结晶水而成的白色粉末称玄明粉。

Medicinal Properties Salty and Bitter in flavor,

【药性】 味咸、苦,性寒。

cold in nature and attributive to the stomach and large intestine meridians.

归胃、大肠经。

Actions Soften dried feces to induce downward discharging, clear away heat.

【功效】 泻下，软坚，清热。

Application

【临床应用】

1. For constipation caused by accumulation of sthenic-heat in the stomach and intestine, it is especially suitable for constipation due to dry feces with difficulty in defecation, usually combined with Dahuang (*Radix et Rhizoma Rhei*), such as Da Chengqi Tang (Decoction).

1. 用于胃肠实热积滞便秘，大便燥结难解者最为适宜。常与大黄相须为用，如大承气汤。

2. For sore throat and aphthae, it is usually combined with Pengsha (*Borax*), Zhusha (*Cinnabaris*) and Bingpian (*Borneolum Syntheticum*) that are pounded into powder for external use, that is, Bingpeng San (Powder). Also put in watermelon, and prepared into Xigua Shuang (*Pulvis Pericarpii Citrulli Preparatus*) for external use. The solution form of Xuanmingfen (*Natrii Sulfus Exsiccatus*) can be used for eye drops to treat bloodshot eyes.

2. 用于咽痛，口疮，目赤。治咽痛口疮，常与硼砂、朱砂、冰片为散外用，即冰硼散。亦可置于西瓜中制成西瓜霜外用。玄明粉化水，可以滴眼，治目赤肿痛。

3. It is generally indicated for the swelling and sores of carbuncles. It can be wrapped with gauze or dissolved in water for external application to treat the early stage of mastitis. It is also combined with Dahuang (*Radix et Rhizoma Rhei*) and garlic (*Bulbus Allii*), which are ground into pieces for external use to treat the early stage of intestinal abscess.

3. 用于痈疮肿痛。治乳痈初起，可用之化水或用纱布包裹外敷。治肠痈初起，可与大黄、大蒜同用，捣烂外敷。

Usage and Dosage 10 -18 g is used in decotion for oral use, dissolved in decoction or in boiling water for oral use. Just right amount is for external use. Xuanmingfen (*Natrii Sulfas Exsiccatus*) is usually used in oral and eye department.

【用法用量】 内服，10～18克，冲入药汁或开水溶化后服。外用，适量。口腔、眼科外用时多用玄明粉。

Notes Contraindicated during prenancy and lactation.

【使用注意】 孕妇及哺乳期妇女忌用。

Luhui *Aloe*

The source is from the juice of the base of the leaf of a perennial evergreen plant, *Aloe ferox* Mill, Berger, family Liliaceae, and the juice is further concentrated and made into a kind of dried extract. The medicinal material is mainly produced in Africa and cultivated in the areas of Guangdong, Guangxi, and Fujian, etc. of China. All year round the juice out of the cut leaves is collected, put in a pot and decocted into thick extract that is poured into a container and cooled, added in pill or powder for being used.

Medicinal Properties Bitter in flavor, cold in nature and attributive to the liver and large intestine meridians.

Actions Purge the bowels, clear away fire from the liver and kill worms.

Application

1. It is used for constipation due to heat stagnation, especially suitable for constipation due to sthenic-heat accompanied with the flaring of heart-fire and liver-fire with restlessness and insomnia since it can clear liver-fire. It is usually combined with Zhusha (*Cinnabaris*), such as Gengyi Wan (Pill).

2. For overabundance of fire in the liver meridian manifested as constipation, bloody urine, dizziness, hypochondriac pain and convulsion, it is usually used together with Longdan (*Radix Gentianae*), Huanglian (*Rhizoma Coptidis*), and Qingdai (*Indigo Naturalis*), etc., such as Danggui Long Hui Wan (Pill).

3. For infantile malnutrition and accumulation of worms with abdominal pain, usually combined with paraciticides, Dangshen (*Radix Codonopsis*), Baizhu (*Rhizoma Atractylodis Macrocephalae*) and others that can tonify the spleen.

芦 荟

为百合科植物库拉索芦荟及好望角芦荟的叶汁浓缩后的干燥物。主产于非洲，中国广东、广西、福建等地有栽培。全年可采，割取植物的叶片，收集其流出的液汁，置锅内熬成稠膏，倾入容器，冷却凝固。入丸、散用。

【药性】 味苦，性寒。归肝、大肠经。

【功效】 泻下，清肝，杀虫。

【临床应用】

1. 用于热结便秘。因能清肝火，故实热便秘兼心肝火旺，烦躁失眠者用之尤宜，常与朱砂配用，如更衣丸。

2. 用于肝经火盛，症见便秘溲赤，眩晕，胁痛，惊痫。常与龙胆、黄连、青黛等同用，如当归龙荟丸。

3. 用于小儿疳积，虫积腹痛。常配驱虫药同用，并加党参、白术等补益健脾药。

In addition, it is used externally for chronic eczema, sore and fistula.

此外，外用可治顽癣，疮瘘。

Usage and Dosage 2－5 g is added to pill or powder for oral use; just right amount for external use.

【用法用量】 入丸散服，2～5克。外用，适量。

Notes Contraindicated in a case with deficiency of the spleen and stomach with poor appetite and loose stool, and pregnant women since it is extremely bitter in flavor.

【使用注意】 味极苦，脾胃虚弱，食少便溏及孕妇忌用。

Fanxieye　*Folium Sennae*

番泻叶

The source is from the leaflet of *Cassia angustifolia* Vahl and *C. acutifolia* Delile, family Leguminosae. The former is mainly produced in India, Egypt and Sudan, and the latter in Egypt, and also cultivated in Guangdong, Guangxi and Yunnan of China. After September, the medicinal material is collected, dried in the sun and the crude form is used.

为豆科植物狭叶番泻和尖叶番泻的叶。前者主产于印度、埃及和苏丹。后者主产于埃及，中国广东、广西、云南有栽培。通常9月采收，晒干。生用。

Medicinal Properties Sweet and bitter in flavor, cold in nature and attributive to the large intestine meridian.

【药性】 味甘、苦，性寒。归大肠经。

Actions Purge and relax the bowels.

【功效】 泻下导滞。

Application

【临床应用】

For constipation due to stagnation of heat, or chronic habitual constipation, it is usually soaked alone in boiling warter for oral use or combined with Zhishi (*Fructus Aurantii Immaturus*), Houpo (*Cortex Magnoliae Officinalis*), etc., it is now used as intestine clearing agent before GI fluoroscopy.

用于热结便秘，也可用于慢性习惯性便秘。多单味泡服，亦可与枳实、厚朴等同用。

现常用于胃肠检查前的肠道清洁剂。

Usage and Dosage 1.5－3 g is soaked in warm boiled water for oral use; 5－9 g is used in decoction and added to later.

【用法用量】 温开水泡服，1.5～3克；水煎服，5～9克，宜后下。

Notes Contraindicated during pregnancy, lactation and menstruation. Overdosage should be avoided because it can cause side effects such as nausea, vomiting and abdominal pain.

【使用注意】 妇女哺乳期、月经期及孕妇忌用。剂量过大，有恶心、呕吐、腹痛等副作用。

3.2 Moistening purgatives

第二节 润下药

They are mostly sweet in flavor and moist in property, include oil and mostly belong to fruits and seeds of the plants. They can lubricate the large intestine to promote bowels to be discharged but not to induce violent diarrhea. They are commonly used in constipation and dry stool due to the elderly and weak that are deficient in the blood and body fluids. They can be combined with the medicinal herbs that can circulate qi, and those that can tonify blood or nourish yin according to syndromes.

大多味甘质润，富含油脂，以植物的种仁为多。能润滑大肠，促使排便而不致峻泻。适用于年老、体弱、血少津枯所致的肠燥便秘。使用时可配伍行气药，并随证配伍补血药或养阴药。

Huomaren *Fructus Cannabis*

火麻仁

The source is from the fruits of *Cannabis sativa* L., family Moraceae. The medicinal material is produced in all parts of China, collected in autumn when the fruits are ripe, dried in the sun and broken. The crude form is used for medication.

为桑科植物大麻的成熟种子。产于中国各地。秋季果实成熟时采收，晒干，打碎。生用。

Medicinal Properties Sweet in flavor, bland in nature and attributive to the spleen, large and small intestine meridians.

【药性】 味甘，性平。归脾、大肠经。

Actions Moisten the intestine to relieve constipation.

【功效】 润肠通便。

Application

【临床应用】

For constipation due to dryness of intestine. For the elderly or pregnant women that are weak or deficient in the body fluids and blood, it can be combined with Danggui (*Radix Angelicae Sinensis*) and Shudihuang (*Radix Rehmanniae Praeparata*). For constipation due to pathogenic heat injuring yin or constitutional yin deficiency, it can be combined with Dahuang (*Radix et Rhizoma Rhei*) and Houpo (*Cortex Magnoliae Officinalis*), such as Maziren Wan (Pill).

用于肠燥便秘。老人、产妇及体弱津血不足而致的便秘，可与当归、熟地黄等同用。热邪伤阴或素体阴虚，大便秘结，可与大黄、厚朴配伍，如麻子仁丸。

Usage and Dosage 10 -30 g is used in decoction

【用法用量】 水煎服，

for oral use, broken and then added to decoction.

10～30 克,打碎入煎。

Yuliren *Semen Pruni*

郁李仁

The source is from the seeds of *Prumus humilis* Bunge or *P. japonica* Thunb., family Rosaceass. The medicinal material is mainly produced in the areas of Hebei, Liaoning, and Inner Mongolia autonomgus region, etc., collected in autumn when the fruits are ripe, dried in the sun and the crude form is used.

为蔷薇科植物欧李、郁李或长柄扁桃的成熟种子。主产于河北、辽宁、内蒙古等地。秋季果实成熟时采摘。除去果肉,去壳取仁,晒干。生用。

Medicinal Properties Pungent, bitter and sweet in flavor, bland in nature and attributive to the spleen, large and small intestine meridians.

【药性】 味辛、苦、甘,性平。归脾、大肠、小肠经。

Actions Moisten the intestine to relieve constipation, promote diuresis and relieve edema.

【功效】 润肠通便,利水消肿。

Application

【临床应用】

1. For constipation due to dryness of intestine, it is usually combined with Huomaren (*Fructus Cannabis*), Baiziren (*Semen Biotae*), and Xingren (*Semen Armeniacae Amarum*), such as Wuren Wan (Pill).

1. 用于肠燥便秘。多与火麻仁、柏子仁、杏仁同用,如五仁丸。

2. For edema, abdominal fullness, beriberi and dysuria, it is usually used together with Sangbaipi (*Cortex Mori Radicis*), Chixiaodou (*Semen Phaseoli*), etc. such as Yuliren Tang (Decoction).

2. 用于水肿腹满,脚气浮肿,小便不利。常与桑白皮、赤小豆等同用,如郁李仁汤。

Usage and Dosage 3 - 9 g is used in decoction for oral use, broken and then added to decoction.

【用法用量】 水煎服,3～9 克,打碎入煎。

Notes used in pregnant women with caution.

【使用注意】 孕妇慎用。

3.3 Drastic purgatives

第三节 峻下逐水药

They are mostly bitter, cold and toxic and will elicit the body's response to excrete water, sometimes in a violent manner and can cause diarrhea, and some are accompanied with inducing diuresis to reduce swelling and distension. They are indicated for general edema, abdominal

本类药物多苦寒有毒,药力峻猛,能引起剧烈腹泻,有的兼能利尿,使体内水饮从二便排出,消除肿胀。适用于全身水肿,大腹胀满,以及体内

fullness and water retention but the healthy qi is not weakened. Since they have violent effect in purging water and severe side effects, when used, they are usually combined with tonics to protect healthy qi. Preparing, dosage, administration and contraindication, etc. must be seriously controlled so as to ensure the safety of medicinal application.

停饮而正气未衰之证。逐水药攻伐力强，副作用大，易伤正气，使用时常配伍补益药以保护正气。对炮制、用量、用法、禁忌等均须严格控制，以保证用药安全。

Gansui *Radix Euphorbiae Kansui*

甘 遂

The source is from the root tuber of *Euphorbia Kansui* T.N. liou ex T. P. Wang, family Euphorbiaceae. The medicinal material is mainly produced in the areas of Shanxi, Shanxi, and Henan, etc. dug and collected in the end of autumn or at the early stage of spring, skined, then dried in the sun and prepared with vinegar for being used.

为大戟科植物甘遂的块根。主产于陕西、山西、河南等地。秋末或春初采挖，除去外皮，晒干。醋制用。

Medicinal Properties Bitter and sweet in flavor and cold in nature, toxic and attributive to the lung, kidney and large intestine meridians.

【药性】 味苦、甘，性寒。有毒。归肺、肾、大肠经。

Actions Purge the bowels to eliminate the retention of phlegm, induce diuresis to relieve edema.

【功效】 泻下逐饮，利水消肿。

Application

【临床应用】

1. It can be used for edema, tympanites and localized fluids in the chest and hypochondrium but the healthy qi is not weakened since it has violent effect in purging and eliminating the retention of phlegm. It can be powdered singly for oral use or used together with Daji (*Radix Euporbiae Pekinensis*), Yuanhua (*Flos Genkwa*), etc., such as Shizao Tang (Decoction); for the syndrome resulting from water retention and heat accumulating in the thorax, it is used together with Dahuang (*Radix et Rhizoma Rhei*) and Mangxiao (*Natrii Sulfas*), such as Da Xianxiong Tang (Decoction). Now it is mostly used for ascites due to cirrhosis, exudative pleurisy and intestinal obstruction, etc..

1. 用于水肿，鼓胀，胸胁停饮。本品泻水逐饮之力峻，前证正气未衰者，均可用之。可单用研末服，或与大戟、芫花等同用，如十枣汤；若水饮与热邪结聚而致的结胸证，可与大黄、芒硝同用，如大陷胸汤。现多用于肝硬化腹水、渗出性胸膜炎、肠梗阻等。

2. For epilepsy of wind-phlegm type, it can be poun-

2. 用于风痰癫痫。可研

ded into powder that is added to a pork heart to be stewed, and then it is prepared with Zhusha (*Cinnabaris*) into pills for oral use, such as Suixin Dan (Pill).

末入猪心煨后,与朱砂为丸服,如遂心丹。

3. For pyocutaneous disease, the powder is mixed with water for external application.

3. 用于疮疡肿毒。可用甘遂末水调外敷。

Usage and Dosage 0.5－1.5 g is added to pill or powder form for oral use, just right amount of the raw is for external use and it must be prepared with vinegar for oral use so as to decrease the toxicity.

【用法用量】 入丸散服,0.5～1.5克。外用,适量,生用。内服须醋制以减低毒性。

Notes Contraindicated in pregnant women or the weak, it is incompatible with Gancao (*Radix Glycyrrhizae*).

【使用注意】 孕妇及体虚者忌用。反甘草。

Daji *Radix Euphorbiae Pekinensis*

大 戟

The source is from the root of *Euphorbia pekinensis* Rupr., family Euphorbiaceae. The medicinal material is maily produced in Jiangsu, Sichuan, Jiangxi and Guangxi provinces, dug and collected in the end of autumn or the early stage of spring. The roots without fibrous stems and hair are dried in the sun and prepared with vinegar to be used.

为大戟科植物大戟的根。主产于江苏、四川、江西、广西等地。秋末或春初采挖。除去残茎及须根,晒干。醋制过用。

Medicinal Properties Bitter and pungent in flavor, cold in nature, toxic and attributive to the lung, kidney and large intestine meridians.

【药性】 味苦、辛,性寒。有毒。归肺、肾、大肠经。

Actions Purge the bowels to eliminate the retention of phlegm, relieve swelling and dissipate the masses.

【功效】 泻下逐水,消肿散结。

Application

【临床应用】

1. It is used for edema, tympanites and localized fluids in the chest and hypochondrium. It has violent effects in purging and eliminating the retention of phlegm. It can be used alone, or used together with Gansui (*Radix Euphorbiae Kansui*) and Yuanhua (*Flos Genkwa*), such as Shizao Tang (Decoction) to treat edema and tympanites without exhaustion of the healthy qi; For retention of phlegm and dampness in the chest and hypochondrium

1. 用于水肿,鼓胀,胸胁停饮。本品泻水逐饮作用峻猛。治水肿、鼓胀,正气未衰者,可单用,或与甘遂、芫花同用,如十枣汤。治痰湿水饮停于胸膈而致胸胁隐痛,痰涎黏稠者,可与甘遂、白芥子等同用,以祛痰逐饮。

manifested as pain in the chest and hypochondrium, sticky and thick sputum, it can be used together with Gansui (*Radix Euphorbiae Kansui*) and Baijiezi (*Semen Sinapis Albae*), etc. to resolve phlegm and eliminate the retention of phlegm.

2. For carbuncle, sore, scrofula and subcutaneous nodule, it can be used orally or by external application.

Usage and Dosage 1.5 - 3 g is used in decoction for oral use; 1 g is added to pill or powder form and just right amount for external use. If taken orally, it must be prepared with vinegar to decrease the toxicity.

Notes Contraindicated in pregnant women and the weak. It is incompatible with Gancao (*Radix Glycyrrhizae*).

2. 用于痈肿疮毒,瘰疬痰核。内服或外敷均可。

【用法用量】 水煎服,1.5～3 克;入丸散,1 克。外用,适量。内服须醋制以减低毒性。

【使用注意】 孕妇及体虚者忌用。反甘草。

Yuanhua *Flos Genkwa*

The source is from the flower bud of *Daphne genkwa* sieb. et Zucc, family Thymelaeaceae. The medicinal material is mainly produced in Anhui, Jiangsu, Zhejiang and Sichuan provinces, collected in spring before the flower blossoms, dried in the sun or by fire, the crude one or the one prepared with vinegar is used for medication.

Medicinal Properties Pungent and bitter in flavor, cold in nature, toxic and attributive to the lung, kidney and large intestine meridians.

Actions Purge the bowels to eliminate the retention of phlegm, resolve phlegm to relieve cough, kill worms and treat sore.

Application

1. It is used for retention of phlegm in the chest and hypochondrium, edema and tympanites. As it has similar action of purging and eliminating the retention of phlegm to Gansui (*Radix Euphorbiae Kansui*) and Daji (*Radix Euphorbiae Pekinensis*), the three kinds are often combined with each other, such as Shizao Tang (Decoction)

芫 花

为瑞香科植物芫花的花蕾。主产于安徽、江苏、浙江、四川等地。春季花未开放前采摘,晒干或烘干。生用或醋制用。

【药性】 味辛、苦,性温。有毒。归肺、肾、大肠经。

【功效】 泻水逐饮,祛痰止咳,杀虫疗疮。

【临床应用】

1. 用于胸胁停饮,水肿,鼓胀。泻水逐饮功似甘遂、大戟,三者常同用,如十枣汤、舟车丸。

and Zhouche Wan (Pill).

2. For cough and dyspnea due to phlegm, it can be used alone or together with others that resolve phlegm, relieve cough and dyspnea. Recently, it is also used for chronic bronchitis.

2. 用于咳嗽痰喘。可单用或配其他化痰止咳平喘药同用。现可用于治疗慢性支气管炎。

3. For eczema on the head, tinea tonsure and hard tinea, it can be used alone or together with Xionghuang (*Realgar*), which are pounded together into powder that are mixed with pork fat for exteranl application.

3. 用于头疮、白秃、顽癣等。可单用或与雄黄共研末，猪脂调外敷。

Usage and Dosage 1.5－3 g is used in decoction for oral use; 0.6－1 g is added to powder form; just right amount for external use; if taken orally, it must be prepared with vinegar to decrease its toxicity.

【用法用量】 水煎服，1.5～3克；入散剂0.6～1克。外用，适量。内服须醋制减毒。

Notes Contraindicated in the weak and pregnant women. It is incompatible with Gancao (*Radix Glycyrrhizae*).

【使用注意】 虚弱者及孕妇忌用。反甘草。

Qianniuzi *Semen Pharbitidis*

牵牛子

The source is from the seed of *Pharbitis nil* (L.) Choisy or *P. purpurea* (L.) voight, family Convolvulaceae. Spermoderm grey-dark or yellow-white is separately called Heichou or Baichou. The medicinal material is produced in all parts of China, cut in autumn when the fruits are ripe and the fruit shell does not split open, and dried in the sun. The seeds are gathered without impurity and then dried in the sun. The crude or stir-baked one can be used.

为旋花科植物裂叶牵牛或圆叶牵牛的成熟种子。表面灰黑色者称黑丑，淡黄色者称白丑。产于中国各地。秋季果实成熟，果壳未裂开时将全株割下，晒干，打下种子，除去杂质，晒干。生用或炒用。

Medicinal Properties Bitter and pungent in flavor, cold in nature, toxic and attributive to the lung, kidney and large intestine meridians.

【药性】 味苦、辛，性寒。有毒。归肺、肾、大肠经。

Actions Purge the bowels, promote diuresis, eliminate stagnated accumulation and kill worms.

【功效】 泻下，利水，消积，杀虫。

Application

【临床应用】

1. It is used in a case with edema or tympanites but with healthy qi, it can be used alone or combined with

1. 用于水肿、鼓胀。适用于正气未衰者。可单用，或配

Gansui (*Radix Euphorbiae Kansui*), Daji (*Radix Euphorbiae Pekinensis*), etc. such as Zhouche Wan (Pill).

甘遂、大戟等同用，如舟车丸。

2. For dyspnea and cough due to phlegm retention, it can be used together with Tinglizi (*Semen Lepidii seu Descurainiae*), Xingren (*Semen Armeniacae Amarum*), etc..

2. 用于痰饮喘咳。可与葶苈子、杏仁等同用。

3. For stagnation of dampness-heat with constipation, stagnation of dampness-heat in the stomach and intestine with constipation and abdominal distention or dysentery with tenesmus, it is used together with Muxiang (*Radix Aucklandiae*), Binglang (*Semen Arecae*), and Zhishi (*Fructus Aurantii Immaturus*), etc.; for constipation, it is also used together with Taoren (*Semen Persicae*), which are pounded into powder and prepared into pill for administration.

3. 用于湿热积滞，大便秘结。治肠胃湿热积滞，便秘腹胀，或痢疾里急后重者，可与木香、槟榔、枳实等同用。治大便秘结，还可与桃仁同用，研末和蜜丸服。

4. For abdominal pain due to accumulation of worms, and for abdominal pain and indigestion due to ascariasis and taeniasis, etc., it is used together with Binglang (*Semen Arecae*), Shijunzi (*Fructus Quiqualis*), etc..

4. 用于虫积腹痛。凡蛔虫、绦虫等肠道寄生虫引起的腹痛，消化不良，可与槟榔、使君子等同用。

Usage and Dosage 3 - 6 g is used in decoction for oral use; 1.5 - 3 g is added to pill or powder form. The fried one can make the medicinal property moderate.

【用法用量】 水煎服，3～6 克。入丸散服，1.5～3 克。炒后可使药性缓和。

Notes Contraindicated in pregnant women and a case with edema due to spleen-deficiency.

【使用注意】 孕妇及脾虚水肿者忌用。

4 Dampness Removing Chinese Medicinal Herbs

第四章 祛湿药

Any medicines that remove dampness from the body and treat syndromes caused by dampness are considered as dampness removing Chinese medicinal herbs. Of them, those that take removing wind-dampness and relieving pains due to arthralgia as their main actions are considered as antirheumatic Chinese medicinal herbs; those that display aromatic properties and have the action to dissolve dampness and to strengthen the function of the spleen fall into dampness resolving aromatic herbs; those that mainly promote the removal of water and permeate the dampness are considered as medicinal herbs for promoting diuresis and resolving dampness.

凡能祛除体内之湿邪,治疗湿邪所致诸证的药物,称为祛湿药。其中以祛除风湿,解除痹痛为主要作用的药物称祛风湿药。气味芳香,具化湿健脾作用的药物称芳香化湿药。有通利水道,渗泄水湿作用的药物称利水渗湿药。

They are indicated for wind-cold-damp Bi-syndrome, edema, stranguria, jaundice and syndrome of dampness obstruction in the middle energizer, etc..

本类药物适用于风寒湿痹、水肿、淋证、黄疸及湿阻中焦证等。

Some of them are warm and dry in nature or their permeating and purging properties are violent, and easily consume yin and blood, therefore, they are used with caution in a case with insufficiency of yin, deficiency of blood or consumption of the body fluids.

某些药物性温燥,或渗泄之性强,易耗伤阴血,故阴亏血虚、津伤者慎用。

4.1 Antirheumatic Chinese medicinal herbs

第一节 祛风湿药

They can remove pathogenic wind-damp from the muscles, channels and collaterals, tendons and bones, and joints. Some of them also separately have the actions of

本类药物能祛除肌肉、经络、筋骨、关节间的风湿之邪,其中有些还分别具有止痛、舒

relieving pain, relaxing and activating the tendons, invigorating the liver and kidney and strengthening tendons and bones. They are indicated for wind-damp Bi-syndrome, painful tendons and bones, stiffness of tendons and muscles, soreness and flaccidity of lumbus and knees, flaccidity and weakness of lower limbs, numbness or hemiplegia, etc..

筋、通络及补肝肾、强筋骨等作用。适用于风湿痹证、筋骨疼痛、筋脉拘急、屈伸不利、腰膝酸软、下肢痿弱、麻木不仁或半身不遂等证。

Bi-syndrome is distinctive in overabundance of wind, damp, cold or heat, affected location or the course of disease, therefore, when they are used, they should be selected and combined with other relative medicinal herbs according to different symptoms and signs so as to achieve responding effects. If the syndromes are accompied with superficial syndrome, diaphoretics must be combined; if blood stasis is in the body, blood activating ones should be combined; if the wind and dampness are predominant, channels warming ones must be combined; if the heat is predominant, heat clearing ones must be combined; if the syndromes are with deficiency of qi and blood, qi and blood tonifying ones should be combined.

痹证有风胜、湿胜、寒胜、热胜的区别,以及痹痛部位的不同和病程长短的差异,故使用时应有所选择,并配伍有关药物,才能收到应有的效果。如兼有表证,与解表药同用;有瘀血者,配伍活血化瘀药;寒湿偏胜者,配伍温经药;热象较显者,配伍清热药;气血亏虚者,配伍补益气血药。

If Bi-syndrome lasts a long period, a formula prepared into medicinal wine or pill would be more suitable.

痹证病程较长,可制成酒剂或丸剂以便于服用。

Duhuo *Radix Angelicae Pubescentis*

独 活

The source is from the root of *Angelica pubescens* Maxim. f. biserrata shan. et Yuan, family Umbelliferae. The medicinal material is mainly produced in Sichuan, Hubei, Anhui provinces, etc., dug and collected in the end of autumn and early stage of spring, dried in the sun, cut into pieces and the crude form is used.

为伞形科植物重齿毛当归的根。主产于四川、湖北、安徽等地。秋末或春初采挖,晒干,切片。生用。

Medicinal Properties Pungent and bitter in flavor, warm in nature and attributive to the liver and bladder meridians.

【药性】 味辛、苦,性温。归肝、膀胱经。

Actions Expel wind and dampness, stop pain of Bi-syndrome and relieve exogenous pathogenic factors.

【功效】 祛风湿,止痹痛,解表。

Application

1. It is used for Bi-syndrome of wind-cold-dampness type with pain, especially in the back and the lower half of the body with soreness and pain due to dampness. For general arthritis, it is combined with Qianghuo (*Rhizoma et Radix Notopterygii*) and Qinjiao (*Radix Gentianae Macrophyllae*); for prolonged Bi-syndrome accompanied with insufficiency of the liver and kidney, and deficiency of qi and blood, combined with Sangjisheng (*Ramulus Taxilli*), Duzhong (*Cortex Eucommiae*), Niuxi (*Radix Achyranthis Bidentatae*) and others that tonify the liver and kidney, such as Duhuo Jisheng Tang (Decoction).

2. For superficial syndrome of wind-cold type with dampness-syndrome, which is manifested as aversion to cold and fever, headache, general heavy sensation of body, sore and painful lumbus and legs, combined with Qianghuo (*Rhizoma et Radix Notopterygii*), Fangfeng (*Radix Saposhnikoviae*) and Jingjie (*Herba Schizonepetae*).

Usage and Dosage 3 - 10 g is used in decoction for oral use.

Explanation Duhuo (*Radix Angelicae Pubescentis*) and Qianghuo (*Rhizoma et Radix Notopterygii*) can all expel wind, dampness and cold, and relieve pain, treat rheumatic arthralgia with pain and superficial syndrome of wind-cold-damp type. But Qianghuo (*Rhizoma et Radix Notopterygii*) tends to treat superficial syndrome and has strong action of promoting sweating to expel cold, so it is often used to expel wind and dampness and treat Bi-syndrome of the upper part of the body; Duhuo (*Radix Angelicae Pubescentis*) has weaker action of eliminating exogenous pathogenic factors and works on the side of expelling wind and dampness, and of relieving pain of Bi-syn-

【临床应用】

1. 用于风寒湿痹证。对湿邪偏重,腰背和下半身酸重疼痛者,尤为适宜。若治全身性关节痹痛,可配羌活、秦艽一起使用;痹证日久,肝肾不足,气血亏虚者,配桑寄生、杜仲、牛膝等补肝肾之品,如独活寄生汤。

2. 用于风寒表证挟湿,症见恶寒发热,头痛,身重,腰腿酸痛。可配羌活、防风、荆芥使用。

【用法用量】 煎服,3～10 g。

【使用说明】 独活与羌活均有祛风湿、散寒止痛作用,都可以治疗风湿痹痛,风寒湿表证。但羌活偏于解表,发汗散寒力量强,用于祛风湿,多治上半身痹痛;而独活解表力较弱,偏于祛风湿,除痹痛,并偏治下半身痹痛。对于全身关节疼痛,两药配伍同用,效果更好。

drome, so it is more on the side of treating pain of Bi-syndrome in the lower part of the body. Both Duhuo (*Radix Angelicae Pubescentis*) and Qianghuo (*Rhizoma et Radix Notopterygii*) can combine together to treat general joint pain so that better effect will be achieved.

Weilingxian *Radix Clematidis*

威灵仙

The source is from the root and rhizome of the perennial trailing shrub, *Clematis chinensis* Osbeck. or *C. hexapetala* Pall. or *C. manshurica* Rupr., family Ranunculaceae. The medicinal material is mainly produced in Jiangsu, Anhui and Zhejiang provinces, etc., dug and collected in autumn, cleaned, dried in the sun and the crude one may be used.

为毛茛科植物威灵仙、棉团铁线莲或东北铁线莲的根及根茎。主产于江苏、安徽、浙江等省。秋季采挖,除去泥沙,晒干。生用。

Medicinal Properties Pungent and salty in flavor, warm in nature and attributive to the bladder meridian.

【药性】 味辛、咸,性温。归膀胱经。

Actions Expel wind and dampness, dredge the channel and remove fishbone stuck in the throat.

【功效】 祛风湿,通经络,消骨鲠。

Application

【临床应用】

1. It is indicated for pain of Bi-syndrome of wind-dampness type, especially migratory Bi-syndrome due to preponderant wind, which is manifested as soreness and pains of general joints, tendons and bones which are wandering, it is powdered alone and then mixed with wine for being used or combined with Danggui (*Radix Angelicae Sinensis*), Guizhi (*Ramulus Cinnamomi*), Fangfeng (*Radix Saposhnikoviae*), Chuanxiong (*Rhizoma Chuanxiong*), and Jianghuang (*Rhizoma Curcume Longae*), etc..

1. 主治风湿痹痛,尤宜于风邪偏胜之行痹,症见全身上下关节、筋骨酸痛,呈游走性。单用为末,温酒调服有效;也可配当归、桂枝、防风、川芎、姜黄等同用。

2. For fishbone stuck in the throat, its decoction to which sugar and vinegar is added is slowly swallowed in several times. The decoction is also taken orally to treat sore throat.

2. 主治骨鲠喉间。煎汤加糖、醋,分次含口中缓缓咽下。煎汤内服也可以治疗咽喉疼痛。

Usage and Dosage 5 - 10 g is used in decoction for oral use and 30-50 g for fishbone stuck in the throat.

【用法用量】 煎服,5~10 g。治骨鲠可用 30~50 g。

Chuanwu *Radix Aconiti*

The source is from the root of *Aconiti*, family Ranunculaceae. The medicinal material is mainly produced in Sichuan, Yunnan, Shaanxi and Hunan provinces, etc., dug and collected in summer and autumn, dried in the sun, the crude or prepared one being used.

Medicinal Properties Pungent and bitter in flavor, warm in nature, extremely toxic and attributive to the heart, spleen, liver and kidney meridians.

Actions Expel wind and cold, and eliminate dampness to relieve pain.

Application

1. It is used for Bi-syndrome of wind-cold-dampness type; for headache, general pain, swollen and painful joints with stiffness due to cold and dampness, it is usually combined with Mahuang (*Herba Ephedrae*), Baishaoyao (*Radix Paeoniae Alba*), and Huangqi (*Radix Astragali*), etc., such as Wutou Tang (Decoction); for apoplexy with numbness and muscular spasm, usually combined with Ruxiang (*Olibanum*), Moyao (*Myrrha*), etc., such as Xiao Huoluo Dan (Pill).

2. It is indicated for all kinds of pains. It is well effective in relieving pains and can be used for pains due to cold. It is boiled alone into thick decoction to which honey is added for oral use, that is, Da Wutou Jian (Decoction); for traumatic stasis and pain, usually combined with Moyao (*Myrrha*), Ruxiang (*Olibanum*), and Sanqi (*Radix Notoginseng*), etc., it can also serve as anesthesia to relieve pain.

Usage and Dosage 1.5 - 3 g is used in decoction for oral use. If it is put in powder or the agent prepared with wine, the dosage should be decreased and if put in decoction, it should be decocted first for a half to one hour to decrease its toxicity. Just right amount is for external

川 乌

为毛茛科植物乌头的母根。主产于四川、云南、陕西、湖南等地。夏、秋季采挖，晒干。生用或制后用。

【药性】 味辛、苦，性温。有大毒。归心、脾、肝、肾经。

【功效】 祛风除湿，散寒止痛。

【临床应用】

1. 用于风寒湿痹。治寒湿头痛，身痛，历节疼痛，不可屈伸者，常与麻黄、白芍药、黄芪等同用，如乌头汤；治中风手足不仁，筋脉挛痛，常与乳香、没药等同用，如小活络丹。

2. 用于各种痛证。本品止痛作用好，可用于诸寒疼痛。单用浓煎加蜜服，即大乌头煎；治外伤瘀痛，常与乳香、没药、三七等同用。亦可用于麻醉止痛。

【用法用量】 水煎服，1.5～3克。入散剂或酒剂，减少用量。入汤剂先煎0.5～1小时以减毒。外用，适量。内服制用，生品一般外用。

use. The prepared one is used orally and generally the crude one is used externally.

【使用注意】 孕妇忌用。反半夏、瓜蒌、贝母、白及、白蔹。不宜久服。

Notes It is contraindicated in pregnant women and incompatible with Banxia (*Rhizoma Pinelliae*), Gualou (*Fructus Trichosanthis*), Beimu (*Bulbus Fritillariae Thunbergii*), Baiji (*Rhizoma Bletillae*) and Bailian (*Radix Ampelopsis*). It is not taken for a long time.

【说明】 另有草乌，为毛茛科北乌头的块根。功似川乌而毒性更强。

Explanation In addition, Caowu (*Radix Aconiti Kusnezoffii*) is the root tuber of *Aconiti*, family Ranunculaceae, its action is like that of Chuanwu (*Radix Aconiti*) but its toxicity is stronger.

Fangji *Radix Stephaniae Tetrandrae*

防 己

为防己科植物粉防己(汉防己)或马兜铃科植物广防己(木防己)的根。前者主产于浙江、安徽、江西、湖北等地。后者主产于广东、广西等地。秋季采挖，晒干，切片。生用。

The source is from the tuberous root of a perennial trailing vine, *Stephania tetrandra* S. Moore, family Menispermaceae, or the tuberous root of a perennial trailing vine, *Aristolochia fangchi* Wu, family Aristolochiaceae. The former is mainly produced in Zhejiang, Anhui, Jiangxi, and Hubei provinces, etc.. The latter in Guangdong and Guangxi provinces, etc.. They are collected in autumn, dried in the sun, the crude one being cut into pieces for being used.

【药性】 味苦、辛，性寒。归膀胱、肾、脾经。

Medicinal Properties Bitter and pungent in flavor, cold in nature and attributive to the bladder, kidney and spleen meridians.

【功效】 祛风湿，止痹痛，利水消肿。

Actions Expel wind and dampness, relieve pain of Bi-syndrome, induce diuresis to relieve edema.

【临床应用】

Application

1. 用于痹证。尤宜于湿热偏胜者，症见骨节红肿疼痛，屈伸不利，常与薏苡仁、滑石等同用，如宣痹汤；治风寒湿痹，关节疼痛，常与附子、肉桂、白术等同用，如防己汤。

1. For Bi-syndrome, especially that due to preponderant damp and heat, which is manifested as red swollen and painful joints and stiffness, it is usually combined with Yiyiren (*Semen Coicis*), Huashi (*Talcum*), etc., such as Xuanbi Tang (Decoction); for that of wind-cold-dampness type with painful joints, usually used together with Fuzi (*Radix Aconiti Lateralis Praeparata*), Rougui

(*Cortex Cinnamomi*), and Baizhu (*Rhizoma Atractylodis Macrocephalae*), etc., such as Fangji Tang (Decoction).

2. It is used for edema, ascitic fluid and dysuria; for edema and abdominal fullness, and difficulty in urination and defecation, it can be combined with Jiaomu (*Semen Zanthoxyli*), Tinglizi (*Semen Lepidii seu Descurainiae*), Dahuang (*Radix et Rhizoma Rhei*), etc., such as Ji Jiao Li Huang Wan (Pill); for deficiency of yin with edema caused by wind, used together with Huangqi (*Radix Astragali*) and Baizhu (*Rhizoma Atractylodis Macrocephalae*), such as Fangji Huangqi Tang (Decoction).

2. 用于水肿,腹水,小便不利。治水肿腹满,二便不利,可与椒目、葶苈子、大黄等同用,如己椒苈黄丸;治脾虚风水水肿,可与黄芪、白术合用,如防己黄芪汤。

Usage and Dosage 5 - 10 g is used in decoction for oral use. Mufangji (*Cocculus Trilobus*) is suitable for expelling wind to relieve pain and Hanfangji (*Stephania Tetranda S. Moore*) is suitable for promoting diuresis to relieve edema.

【用法用量】 水煎服,5~10 克。祛风止痛宜木防己,利水消肿宜汉防己。

Notes Used with caution in the weak with yin deficiency and poor appetite, since the Chinese medicinal herb is very bitter and cold and easily damages stomach-qi. Fangji from a perennial trailing vine, *Aristolochia fangchi* Wu, family Aristolochiaceae contains such chief element as aristolochine, which can result in acute damage to kidney function.

【使用注意】 本品大苦大寒,易伤胃气,体弱阴虚,胃纳不佳者慎用。属马兜铃科植物的防己,因含有马兜铃酸等主要成分,可导致急性肾功能损害,应慎用。

Qinjiao *Radix Gentianae Macrophyllae*

秦 艽

The source is from the roots of a perennial herb, *Gentiana macrophylla* Pall. or *G. straminea* Maxim. or *G. crassicaulis* Duthie ex Burk., family Gentianaceae. The medicinal material is mainly produced in Shaanxi, Gansu, and Sichuan provinces and Inner Mongolia Autonomous Region, etc., dug and collected in spring and autumn, dried in the sun, the crude one being cut into pieces for being used.

为龙胆科植物秦艽、麻花秦艽、粗茎秦艽或小秦艽的根。主产于陕西、甘肃、四川、内蒙古等地。春、秋两季采挖,晒干,切片。生用。

Medicinal Properties Bitter and pungent in

【药性】 味苦、辛,性微

flavor, slightly cold in nature and attributive to the stomach, liver and gallbladder meridians.

寒。归胃、肝、胆经。

Actions Expel wind and dampness, relieve pain of Bi-syndrome and asthenia heat, clear away dampness-heat.

【功效】 祛风湿，止痹痛，退虚热，清湿热。

Application

【临床应用】

1. It is indicated for Bi-syndrome of wind-dampness type. It is cold but not dry in nature, so it is suitable for all kinds of Bi-syndrome of wind-dampness type, especially for heat-Bi-syndrome. If joints are red, swollen and painful, it is usually combined with Rendongteng (*Caulis Lonicerae*), Fangji (*Radix Stephaniae Tetrandrae*), and Huangbai (*Cortex Phellodendri*), etc.; for Bi-syndrome of wind-cold-dampness type, usually combined with Qianghuo (*Rhizoma et Radix Notopterygii*), Duhuo (*Radix Angelicae Pubescentis*), Guizhi (*Ramulus Cinnamomi*), etc..

1. 用于风湿痹痛。本品性寒不燥，各种风湿痹痛均可应用，尤以热痹为宜。关节红肿热痛，常与忍冬藤、防己、黄柏等同用；治风寒湿痹，多与羌活、独活、桂枝等同用。

2. For bone steaming and hectic fever, it is usually used together with Zhimu (*Rhizoma Anemarrhenae*), Digupi (*Cortex Lycii Radicis*), and Biejia (*Carapax Trionycis*), etc., such as Qinjiao Biejia Tang (Decoction).

2. 用于骨蒸潮热。常与知母、地骨皮、鳖甲等同用，如秦艽鳖甲汤。

3. For jaundice of dampness-heat type, it is usually combined with Yinchenhao (*Cacumen Artemisiae Scopariae*), Zhizi (*Fructus Gardeniae*), and Zhuling (*Polyporus*), etc..

3. 用于湿热黄疸。常与茵陈蒿、栀子、猪苓等配伍。

Usage and Dosage 3 - 9 g is used in decoction for oral use.

【用法用量】 水煎服，3～9克。

Qishe *Agkistrodon Acutus*

蕲 蛇

The source is from the viscerated and dried body of *Agkistrodon acutus* (Guenther), family Grotalidae. The medicinal material is mainly produced in the areas of Hubei, Jiangxi, and Zhejiang, etc. caught in summer and autumn. The viscerated and dried body is prepared with

为蝰蛇科动物五步蛇除去内脏的全体。主产于湖北、江西、浙江等地。夏、秋两季捕捉，剖开腹部，除去内脏，干燥，以黄酒润透去皮骨，切

millet wine (with skin and bone removed), being cut into pieces for being used.

段用。

Medicinal Properties Sweet and salty in flavor, warm in nature, toxic and attributive to the liver meridian.

【药性】 味甘、咸,性温。有毒。归肝经。

Actions Expel wind, dredge the channels, relieve convulsion.

【功效】 祛风通络,定惊止痉。

Application

【临床应用】

1. For obstinate Bi-syndrome of wind-dampness type manifested as numbness of the extremities and muscular spasm, it is usually combined with Fangfeng (*Radix Saposhnikoviae*), Qianghuo (*Rhizoma et Radix Notopterygii*), and Danggui (*Radix Angelicae Sinensis*), etc. so as to expel wind and promote blood circulation.

1. 用于风湿顽痹,肌肤麻木,筋脉拘挛。常配防风、羌活、当归等同用,以祛风活血。

2. For deviation of the eyes and mouth resulting from apoplexy, hemiplegia, paralysis of limbs, it can be combined with Huangqi (*Radix Astragali*), Danggui (*Radix Angelicae Sinensis*), and Guizhi (*Ramulus Cinnamomi*), etc..

2. 用于中风口眼歪斜,半身不遂,肢体瘫痪。可配伍黄芪、当归、桂枝等同用。

3. For leprosy, numbness of the extremities and itching of skin, it is usually combined with Wushaoshe (*Zaocys*), Xionghuang (*Realgar*), and Shengdahuang (*Radix et Rhizoma Rhei*), etc., such as Qufeng San (Powder).

3. 用于麻风疠毒,手足麻木,皮肤瘙痒。多与乌梢蛇、雄黄、生大黄等同用,如驱风散。

4. For acute or chronic infantile convulsion and tetanus, it is usually combined with Wushaoshe (*Zaocys*) and Wugong (*Scolopendra*) which are powdered together, the powder being mixed with wine that is boiled for being used.

4. 用于小儿急、慢惊风,破伤风。常与乌梢蛇、蜈蚣同研末,煎酒调服。

Usage and Dosage 3 - 9 g is used in decoction for oral use, 1 - 1.5 g in the powder and just right amount for external use.

【用法用量】 水煎服,3～9克;研末服,1～1.5克。外用,适量。

Sangjisheng *Ramulus Taxilli*

桑寄生

The source is from the stem and branch of *Taxillus*

为桑寄生科植物桑寄生

chinensis (DC.) Danser, family Loranthaceae. The medicinal material is mainly produced in Guangdong, Guangxi and Yunnan provinces, etc., cut and collected from winter to the next spring, cut into segments, dried in the sun or after steaming.

的带叶茎枝。主产于广东、广西、云南等地。冬季至次春采割，除去粗茎。切段，干燥，或蒸后干燥。

Medicinal Properties Bitter and sweet in flavor, bland in nature and attributive to the liver and kidney meridians.

【药性】 味苦、甘，性平。归肝、肾经。

Actions Expel wind and dampness, invigorate the liver and kidney, strengthen tendons and bones and prevent miscarriage.

【功效】 祛风湿，补肝肾，强筋骨，安胎。

Application

1. It is used for Bi-syndrome of wind-dampness type with weakness of waist and knees; especially suitable for chronic rheumatism with yin deficiency of the liver and kidney manifested as weakness of waist and knees and flaccidity of extremities, it is usually combined with Duhuo (*Radix Angelicae Pubescentis*), Qinjiao (*Radix Gentianae Macrophyllae*), and Guizhi (*Ramulus Cinnamomi*), etc., such as Duhuo Jisheng Tang (Decoction).

2. For threatened abortion with spot vaginal bleeding and habitual miscarriage due to yin deficiency of the liver and kidney, it is usually combined with Ejiao (*Colla Corii Asini*), Xuduan (*Radix Dipsaci*), and Tusizi (*Semen Cuscutae*), etc., such as Shoutai Wan (Pill).

【临床应用】

1. 用于风湿痹痛，腰膝酸痛。对于痹痛日久，肝肾亏损，腰膝酸软，筋骨无力者尤宜，常与独活、秦艽、桂枝等同用，如独活寄生汤。

2. 用于肝肾亏虚之胎漏下血，习惯性流产。常配阿胶、续断、菟丝子等同用，如寿胎丸。

Usage and Dosage 10 – 15 g is used in decoction for oral use.

【用法用量】 水煎服，10～15克。

Wujiapi *Cortex Acanthopanacis Radicis*

五加皮

The source is from the root cortex of *Acanthopanax gracilistylis* W. W. Smith, family Araliaceae, the medicinal material is mainly produced in Hubei, Henan, and Anhui provinces, etc., dug and collected in summer and autumn, dried in the sun, cut into thick pieces and the

为五加科植物细柱五加的根皮。主产于湖北、河南、安徽等地。夏、秋季采挖，剥取根皮，晒干，切厚片。生用。

crude one is used for medication.

Medicinal Properties Pungent and bitter in flavor, warm in nature and attributive to the liver and kidney meridians.

【药性】 味辛、苦,性温。归肝、肾经。

Actions Expel wind-damp, strengthen the tendons and bones, and induce diuresis.

【功效】 祛风湿,强筋骨,利尿。

Application

【临床应用】

1. For Bi-syndrome of wind-dampness type with muscular spasm and stiffness, it can be soaked alone in wine, or used together with Mugua (*Fructus Chaenomelis*), Sangjisheng (*Ramulus Taxilli*), etc..

1. 用于风湿痹痛,筋脉拘挛,屈伸不利。可单用浸酒,或与木瓜、桑寄生等同用。

2. For yin deficiency of the liver and kidney with weakness of waist and knees or retarded ambulation of children, it is usually combined with Huainiuxi (*Radix Achyranthis Bidentatae*), Duzhong (*Cortex Eucommiae*), Buguzhi (*Fructus Psoraleae*) and others that tonify the kidney and strengthen the bone.

2. 用于肝肾不足,腰膝软弱,小儿行迟。多与怀牛膝、杜仲、补骨脂等补肾壮骨药同用。

3. For swollen face and extremities and dysuria, it is usually combined with Fulingpi (*Cortex Sclerotii Poria*), Jupi (*Pericarpium Citri Tangerinae*), and Dafupi (*Pericarpium Arecae*), etc., such as Wupi Yin (Decoction).

3. 用于面目、四肢浮肿,小便不利。常与茯苓皮、橘皮、大腹皮等同用,如五皮饮。

Usage and Dosage 5 - 10 g is used in decoction for oral use.

【用法用量】 水煎服,5~10克。

Explanation In addition, Xiangjiapi (*Cortex Periplocae*) is from the root and bark of *Periploca Sepium* Bge.. It is toxic in nature, can invigorate the heart, induce diuresis and arrest pain. The function is different with Wujiapi (*Cortex Acanthopanacis Radicis*), so the both Chinese medicinal herbs should not be used confusedly.

【说明】 另有香加皮,为萝藦科植物杠柳的根皮。有毒。能强心,利尿,止痛。与本品功效不同,不可混用。

4.2 Dampness resolving Chinese medicinal herbs

第二节 芳香化湿药

Medicines in this category are pungent, bitter,

本类药物气味芳香,味多

aromatic in flavor, warm and dry in nature, and have the actions to circulate qi, dissolve and dry dampness, and to improve the spleen's transformation and transportation. They are indicated for obstruction of dampness in the middle energizer, disorder of the spleen's and stomach's transformation and transportation, which is manifested as epigastric and abdominal distention and fullness, nausea, vomiting, loss of appetite, heaviness of limbs, loose stool, turbid and greasy coating on the tongue, etc.. Some of them can also clear away summer-heat and remove turbidity so they are indicated for syndromes of dampness-warm, or summer-heat-dampness type.

苦、辛,性偏温燥。具有行气化湿,健脾助运之功。适用于湿阻中焦,脾胃运化失常之脘腹胀闷,恶心呕吐,食欲不振,肢体困重,大便溏薄,舌苔浊腻等。有些药物又能解暑辟秽,用于湿温、暑湿等证。

For a cold-damp type, the interior warming Chinese medicinal herbs should be combined; for a damp-heat type, those for clearing away heat and drying dampness should be combined; for more severe stagnation of qi, those that circulate qi should be combined with; for hamper of the spleen's transformation and transportation due to spleen deficiency, those that tonify qi and invigorate the spleen should be combined.

寒湿者,配温里药;湿热者,配清热燥湿药;气滞较甚者,配行气药;脾虚不运者,配补气健脾药。

They are a bit on warm and dry side in nature, easily consuming qi and damaging yin, therefore, they are used with caution in a case with deficiency of yin, dryness of blood and deficiency of qi, and not taken for a long time due to their aromatic flavor.

化湿药性偏温燥,易于耗气伤阴,阴虚血燥及气虚者慎用。本类药气味芳香,不宜久煎。

Huoxiang *Herba Agastachis*

藿 香

The source is from the aerial parts of a perennial herb, *Pogostemon cabin* (Blanco) Benth., family Labiatae. The medicinal material is mainly produced in Guangdong Province, cut and collected in summer and autumn, the fresh is cut into segments, or dried in shade for being used.

为唇形科植物广藿香的地上部分。主产于广东。夏、秋季采割,鲜时切段用,或阴干。生用。

Medicinal Properties Pungent in flavor, slightly warm in nature and attributive to the spleen and stomach

【药性】 味辛,性微温。归脾、胃经。

meridians.

Actions Eliminate dampness, clear away summer-heat and stop vomiting.

【功效】 化湿,解暑,止呕。

Application

【临床应用】

1. For the obstruction of dampness and stagnation of qi in the middle energizer manifested as fullness in the chest and epigastrium, loss of appetite and nausea, fatigue of the body and spirits, it is usually combined with Cangzhu (*Rhizoma Atractylodis*), Houpo (*Cortex Magnoliae Officinalis*), etc..

1. 用于中焦湿阻气滞,脘腹痞闷,食少作呕,神疲体倦,多与苍术、厚朴等同用。

2. It is indicated for the early stage of summer-heat-dampness and dampness-warm syndromes of seasonal febrile disease. For affection of exogenous wind-cold in summer and retention of dampness and cold in the interior manifested as aversion to cold, fever, headache, fullness and pain in the chest and epigastrium, vomiting and diarrhea, it is usually combined with Zisuye (*Folium Perillae*), and Houpo (*Cortex Magnoliae Officinalis*), etc., such as Houxiang Zhengqi San (Powder). For the early stage of damp-febrile disease, used together with Huangqin (*Radix Scutellariae*), Huashi (*Talcum*), and Yinchen (*Herba Artemisiae Scopariae*), etc., such as Ganlu Xiaodu Dan (Pill).

2. 用于暑湿证及湿温证初起。暑季外感风寒,内伤湿冷而致恶寒发热,头痛,脘腹胀痛,呕吐泄泻,常配伍紫苏叶、厚朴等同用,如藿香正气散。湿温病初起,湿热并重,可与黄芩、滑石、茵陈等同用,如甘露消毒丹。

3. It is used for vomiting, and is an essential medicine for the treatment of dampness-retention syndrome with vomiting. It is usually combined with Banxia (*Rhizoma Pinelliae*), to which Huanglian (*Rhizoma Coptidis*), Zhuru (*Caulis Bambusae in Taeniam*), etc. are added again for vomiting being a bit on the heat side; for that due to pregnancy, it is combined with Sharen (Fructus Amomi) and Zisugeng (*Caulis Perillae*).

3. 用于呕吐。为治湿浊呕吐要药,常与半夏配伍。偏热者,再配黄连、竹茹等;妊娠呕吐,也可配砂仁、紫苏梗同用。

Usage and Dosage 3 - 10 g is used in decoction for oral use. The amount of the fresh is doubled.

【用法用量】 水煎服,3~10克。鲜品用量加倍。

Peilan *Herba Eupatorii*

The source is from the aerial part of a perennial herb, *Eupatorium fortunei* Turcz., family Compositae. The medicinal material is mainly produced in the areas of Jiangsu, Hebei, and Shandong, etc., cut and collected in autumn and summer, the fresh being cut into segments or dried in the sun for being used.

Medicinal Properties Pungent in flavor, bland in nature and attributive to the spleen, stomach and lung meridians.

Actions Eliminate dampness due to aromatic nature, clear away summer-heat from the superficies.

Application

1. For dampness-retention syndrome involving the spleen and stomach, it is usually combined with Huoxiang (*Herba Agastachis*), or with Cangzhu (*Rhizoma Atractylodis*), Houpo (*Cortex Magnoliae Officinalis*), etc.; for dampness-heat in spleen meridian with sweetness and greasiness in the mouth, plenty of saliva, and foul breath, etc., it can be decocted alone for oral use.

2. For affection of exogenous summer-heat and dampness or the early stage of damp febrile disease with fever, fullness in the head, fullness and oppression in the chest and epigastrium, oral stickness, white-greasy or yellow-greasy coating, it is usually combined with Huoxiang (*Herba Agastachis*), Heye (*Folium Nelumbinis*), Qinghao (*Herba Artemisiae Annuae*), etc., also used together with Huashi (*Talcum*), Yiyiren (*Semen Coicis*), etc..

Usage and Dosage 3 - 9 g is used in decoction for oral use. The amount of the fresh is doubled.

佩　兰

为菊科植物佩兰的地上部分。主产于江苏、河北、山东等地。夏、秋季采割，切段鲜用或晒干生用。

【药性】 味辛，性平。归脾、胃、肺经。

【功效】 芳香化湿，发表解暑。

【临床应用】

1. 用于湿阻中焦证。常与藿香相须为用，或配伍苍术、厚朴等同用。若脾经湿热之口中甜腻、多涎、口臭等，可单味煎服。

2. 用于外感暑湿或湿温初起，见身热头胀，胸脘痞闷，口黏，舌苔白腻或黄腻。常与藿香、荷叶、青蒿等同用；也可与滑石、薏苡仁等同用。

【用法用量】 水煎服，3～9克。鲜品用量加倍。

Cangzhu *Rhizoma Atractylodis*

The source is from the rhizome of *Atractylodes lancea* (Thunb.) DC. or *A. chinensis* (DC.) koidz., family

苍　术

为菊科植物茅苍术或北苍术的根茎。前者主产于江

Compositae. The former is mainly produced in Jiangsu, Hubei, and Henan provinces, etc., that produced in Maoshan of Jiangsu Province having the best quality. The latter is mainly produced in Inner Mongolia Autonomous Region and Shanxi and Liaoning provinces, etc.. The medicinal material is dug and collected in spring and autumn, dried in the sun, steeped thoroughly in water or water in which rice has been washed and then cut into pieces. The stir-baked one is used.

苏、湖北、河南等地。以产于江苏茅山一带者质量最好。后者主产于内蒙古、山西、辽宁等地。春、秋季采挖,晒干,水或米泔水润透切片。炒用。

Medicinal Properties Pungent and bitter in flavor, warm in nature and attributive to the spleen and stomach meridians.

【药性】 味辛、苦,性温。归脾、胃经。

Actions Eliminate dampness and invigorate the spleen, expel wind, damp and cold.

【功效】 燥湿健脾,祛风湿散寒。

Application

【临床应用】

1. For dampness-retention syndrome involving the middle-energizer with distention and pain in the chest and abdomen, poor appetite, nausea and vomiting, it is usually combined with Houpo (*Cortex Magnoliae Officinalis*), and Jupi (*Pericarpium Citri Tangerinae*), such as Pingwei San (Powder).

1. 用于湿滞中焦,脘腹胀痛,食欲不振,恶心呕吐。常与厚朴、橘皮配伍,如平胃散。

2. For Bi-syndrome of wind-dampness type, especially suitable for Bi-syndrome with domination of dampness marked by general soreness, heaviness, distension and pain, it is usually combined with Duhuo (*Radix Angelicae Pubescentis*), Qinjiao (*Radix Gentianae Macrophyllae*), etc.; for Bi-syndrome of dampness-heat type, combined with Shigao (*Gypsum Fibrosum*), Zhimu (*Rhizoma Anemarrhenae*), etc., such as Baihu Jia Cangzhu Tang (Decoction).

2. 用于风湿痹证。以治痹证湿胜,头身酸重胀痛者尤宜,常配独活、秦艽等同用。若湿热痹痛,可配石膏、知母等同用,如白虎加苍术汤。

3. For flaccidity-syndrome of dampness-heat type, leukorrhea due to turbid dampness, damp ulcer, and eczema, etc., it is usually combined with Huangbai (*Cortex Phellodendri*), such as Ermiao San (Powder).

3. 用于湿热痿证、湿浊带下、湿疮、湿疹等。常与黄柏同用,如二妙散。

4. For affection of exogenous wind-cold-dampness, it is usually combined with Baizhi (*Radix Angelicae Dahuricae*), Xixin (*Herba Asari*), etc..

4. 用于外感风寒挟湿证。多与白芷、细辛等同用。

In addition, it can bright the eyes, so it can be used for night blindness.

此外,本品还能明目,可用治夜盲证。

Usage and Dosage 3 - 9 g is used in decoction for oral use.

【用法用量】 水煎服,3~9克。

Notes It is not suitable for yin deficiency generating interior heat and perspiration due to loose superficies.

【使用注意】 阴虚内热、表疏汗出者不宜用。

Houpo *Cortex Magnoliae Officinalis*

厚 朴

The source is from the dried bark and bark of branch, root of *Magnolia officinalis* Rehd. et Wils. or *M. officinalis* Rehd. et Wils. var. biloba Rehd. et Wils., family Magnoliaceae. The medicinal material is mainly produced in Sichuan, Hubei, and Anhui provinces, etc., skined during April, May and June. Bark of branch and root are directly dried in shade and the dried bark is put in boiling water for a while and then piled in the wet shade for sweating until the surface becomes purple-brown or brown color. The bark softened is rolled up, and then dried. The crude one may be used or the prepared one with ginger juice is used.

为木兰科植物厚朴或凹叶厚朴的干皮、根皮及枝皮。产于四川、湖北、安徽等地。4~6月剥取。根皮及枝皮直接阴干,干皮置沸水中微煮后堆置阴湿处,"发汗"至内表面变紫褐色或棕褐色时,蒸软取出,卷成筒状,干燥。生用或姜汁制用。

Medicinal Properties Bitter and pungent in flavor, warm in nature and attributive to the spleen, stomach, lung and large intestine meridians.

【药性】 味苦、辛,性温。归脾、胃、肺、大肠经。

Actions Activate circulation of qi, remove dampness, promote digestion and relieve dyspnea.

【功效】 行气,燥湿,消积,平喘。

Application

【临床应用】

1. For obstruction of dampness and stagnation of qi in the middle energizer manifested as epigastic and abdominal distention and pain, nausea, etc.. It is good at relieving fullness and distention and usually combined with Cangzhu (*Rhizoma Atractylodis*), Jupi (*Pericarpium*

1. 用于中焦湿阻气滞之脘腹胀痛、呕逆等证。本品尤善消除胀满,常与苍术、橘皮等同用,如平胃散。

Citri Tangerinae), etc., such as Pingwei San (Powder).

2. For accumulation of food and stagnation of qi in the stomach and intestine with constipation, it is usually combined with Zhishi (*Fructus Aurantii Immaturus*) and Dahuang (*Radix et Rhizoma Rhei*), such as Houpo Sanwu Tang (Decoction).

2. 用于肠胃积滞，大便秘结。常与枳实、大黄同用，如厚朴三物汤。

3. For stagnation of phlegm and dampness in the lung with chest distress, cough with plenty of sputum, thick and greasy tongue coating, it is usually combined with Zisuzi (*Fructus Perillae*), Xingren (*Semen Armeniacae Amarum*), etc. to resolve phlegm, lower qi and relieve dyspnea.

3. 用于痰湿阻肺，胸闷咳喘痰多，舌苔厚腻。常配伍紫苏子、杏仁等以化痰降气平喘。

Usage and Dosage 3 - 10 g is used in decoction for oral use.

【用法用量】 水煎服，3～10克。

Sharen *Fructus Amomi*

砂 仁

The source is from the ripe fruit of *Amomum villosum* lour (Yangchunsha), *A. longiligulare* T. L. Wu, family Zingiberaceae (*Hainansha or Leukesha*). Yangchunsha is mainly produced in Guangdong, Guangxi provinces, etc.; and Hainansha in Guangdong and Hainan provinces, and Lükesha in Vietnam, Thailand, and Indonesia, etc.. They are collected in summer and autumn when the fruits are ripe, dried in the sun or in low temperature, the crude one being used.

为姜科植物阳春砂、海南砂或绿壳砂的成熟果实。阳春砂主产于广东、广西等地；海南砂主产于广东、海南等地；绿壳砂产于越南、泰国、印度尼西亚等地。夏、秋季果实成熟时采收，晒干或低温干燥。生用。

Medicinal Properties Pungent in flavor, warm in nature and attributive to the spleen and stomach meridians.

【药性】 味辛，性温。归脾、胃经。

Actions Eliminate dampness and promote the circulation of qi, warm the middle energizer to stop vomiting and diarrhea, and prevent miscarriage.

【功效】 化湿行气，温中止呕，止泻，安胎。

Application

【临床应用】

1. For obstruction of dampness in the stomach and spleen and stagnation of spleen qi and stomach qi with

1. 用于脾胃湿阻气滞之脘腹胀满，不思饮食。更宜于

epigastric fullness and distention, loss of appetite, more suitable for cold-dampness syndrome, it is usually combined with Houpo (*Cortex Magnoliae Officinalis*), Jupi (*Pericarpium Citri Tangerinae*), and Zhishi (*Fructus Aurantii Immaturus*), etc.. For stagnation of qi due to deficiency of the spleen, usually combined with Dangshen (*Radix Codonopsis*), Baizhu (*Rhizoma Atractylodis Macrocephalae*), and Fuling (*Poria*), etc., such as Xiang Sha Liujunzi Tang (Decoction).

寒湿证,常与厚朴、橘皮、枳实等同用。若脾虚气滞,多配伍党参、白术、茯苓等同用,如香砂六君子汤。

2. For vomiting and diarrhea due to asthenia-cold of the spleen and stomach. It can be taken in powder form or combined with Ganjiang (*Rhizoma Zingiberis*) and Fuzi (*Radix Aconiti Lateralis Praeparata*), etc..

2. 用于脾胃虚寒吐泻。可单用研末吞服,或与干姜、附子等同用。

3. For vomiting due to pregnancy and threatened abortion due to stagnation of qi, the fried one that is powdered is taken to treat the former symptom; it is combined with Renshen (*Radix Ginseng*), Huangqi (*Radix Astragali*), and Baizhu (*Rhizoma Atractylodis Macrocephalae*), etc. to treat the latter symptom.

3. 用于气滞妊娠呕吐及胎动不安。治妊娠呕吐,可单用炒研末服;胎动不安,可配人参、黄芪、白术等同用。

Usage and Dosage 3–6 g is used in decoction for oral use, not suitable to be taken for a long time.

【用法用量】 水煎服,3~6克。不宜久煎。

4.3 Chinese medicinal herbs for promoting diuresis and resolving dampness

第三节 利水渗湿药

This kind of herbs are mostly sweet and bland in flavor and have the actions of promoting the flow of water and relieving edema, inducing diuresis to treat stranguria, removing dampness and treating jaundice. They are indicated for dysuria, edema, stranguria, jaundice, and Bi-syndrome due to dampness, etc..

本类药物味多甘淡,具有利水消肿、利尿通淋、利湿退黄等功效。适用于小便不利、水肿、淋证、黄疸、湿温、湿痹等证。

In multi-syndrome conditions such as a syndrome of the above accompanied by superficial syndrome, they

兼表证者,配解表药;脾肾阳虚者,配温补脾肾药;热

should be combined with diaphoretics; with deficiency of spleen-yang and kidney-yang, combined with medicinal herbs that warm and invigorate the spleen and kidney; with stranguria caused by heat, combined with heat clearing herbs; with stranguria complicated by hematuria, combined with heat clearing and blood cooling medicinal herbs.

淋者,配清热药;血淋者,配清热凉血药。

Fuling *Poria*

The source is from the sclerotium of *Poria cocos* (schw) Wolf, family Polyporaceae. The sclerotium mostly parasitizes on the root of Japanese red pine and *Pinus massoniana* Lamb., family Pinaceae. The medicinal material is mainly produced in the areas of Yunnan, Hubei, and Sichuan, etc., dug and collected from July to September, piled repeatedly, dried in the sun. The crude one is used.

Medicinal Properties Sweet and bland in flavor, mild in nature, and attributive to the heart, spleen and kidney meridians.

Actions Promote diuresis to resolve dampness from the lower energizer, invigorate the spleen and tranquilize the mind.

Application

1. It is used for edema and dysuria. For all kinds of edema; for that caused by hypofunction of bladder-qi, it is combined with Guizhi (*Ramulus Cinnamomi*), Zhuling (*Polyporus*), Baizhu (*Rhizoma Atractylodis Macrocephalae*), and Zexie (*Rhizoma Alismatis*), etc., such as Wuling San (Powder); for that with deficiency of qi, combined with Fangji (*Radix Stephaniae Tetrandrae*), Huangqi (*Radix Astragali*); for that with yang-deficency of the spleen and kidney, combined with Fuzi (*Radix Aconiti Praeparata*), Ganjiang (*Rhizoma Zingiberis*), etc., such as Zhenwu Tang (Decoction).

2. For all syndromes of spleen-deficiency, especially

茯 苓

为多孔菌科真菌茯苓的菌核。多寄生于松科植物赤松或马尾松等的树根上。主产于云南、湖北、四川等地。7～9月采挖,反复堆置、晒干。生用。

【药性】 味甘、淡,性平。归心、脾、肾经。

【功效】 利水渗湿,健脾安神。

【临床应用】

1. 用于水肿,小便不利。可用于各种水肿证。膀胱气化不利所致,可与桂枝、猪苓、白术、泽泻等同用,如五苓散;气虚者配防已、黄芪;脾肾阳虚者,配附子、干姜等同用,如真武汤。

2. 用于脾虚诸证。对脾

effective in spleen-deficiency with dampness, it is combined with Dangshen (*Radix Codonopsis*) and Baizhu (*Rhizoma Atractylodis Macrocephalae*), such as Sijunzi Tang (Decoction). For retention of fluid due to spleen-deficiency, combined with Guizhi (*Ramulus Cinnamomi*) and Baizhu (*Rhizoma Atractylodis Macrocephalae*), etc., such as Ling Gui Zhu Gan Tang (Decociton); for diarrhea due to spleen deficiency, combined with Shanyao (*Rhizoma Dioscoreae*), Baizhu (*Rhizoma Atractylodis Macrocephalae*), and Yiyiren (*Semen Coicis*), etc..

虚有湿者尤宜,可与党参、白术配伍,如四君子汤。若脾虚饮停,可与桂枝、白术等同用,如苓桂术甘汤;若脾虚泄泻,可与山药、白术、薏苡仁等同用。

3. For deficiency of both the heart and spleen manifested as restlessness, palpitation and insomnia, it is usually combined with Huangqi (*Radix Astragali*), Danggui (*Radix Angelicae Sinensis*) and Yuanzhi (*Radix Polygalae*), such as Guipi Tang (Decoction).

3. 用于心脾两虚之心神不宁,心悸失眠。常与黄芪、当归、远志同用,如归脾汤。

Usage and Dosage 10 - 15 g is used in decoction for oral use.

【用法用量】 水煎服,10～15克。

Zhuling *Polyporus*

猪 苓

The source is from the sclerotium of *Polyporus umbellatus* (Pers) Fries, family Polyporaceae. The sclerotium mostly parasitizes on the rotten root of birch, Chinese sweet gum, etc.. The medicinal material is mainly produced in the areas of Shaanxi, Hebei, and Yunnan, etc., dug and collected in spring and autumn, dried in the sun, cut into pieces and the crude one is used.

为多孔菌科真菌猪苓的菌核。多寄生于桦树、枫树、柞树等的腐枯根上。主产于陕西、河北、云南等地。春、秋两季采挖,晒干,切片。生用。

Medicinal Properties Sweet and bland in flavor, mild in nature and attributive to the kidney and bladder meridians.

【药性】 味甘、淡,性平。归肾、膀胱经。

Actions Promote diuresis to resolve dampness.

【功效】 利水渗湿。

Application

【临床应用】

The herb is used for dysuria, edema, diarrhea, and turbid stranguria, etc.. Its action of promoting diuresis is stronger than that of Fuling (*Poria*), but it has no action of invigorating the spleen. Therefore, to treat edema

用于小便不利、水肿、泄泻、淋浊等。利水作用强于茯苓,但无健脾作用。治脾虚水肿,须与茯苓、白术、泽泻等同

syndrome due to spleen-deficiency, it must be combined with Fuling (*Poria*), Baizhu (*Rhizoma Atractylodis Macrocephalae*), and Zexie (*Rhizoma Alismatis*), etc., such as Siling San (*Powder*). For dysuria due to yin-deficiency, combined with Zexie (*Rhizoma Alismatis*), Huashi (*Talcum*), Ejiao (*Colla Corii Asini*), etc., such as Zhuling Tang (Decoction).

用,如四苓散。若阴虚小便不利,可与泽泻、滑石、阿胶等同用,如猪苓汤。

Usage and Dosage 5－10 g is used in decoction for oral use.

【用法用量】 水煎服,5～10克。

Zexie *Rhizoma Alismatis*

泽　泻

The source is from the stem tuber of *Alisma orientale* (Sam) Juzep., family Alismataceae. The medicinal material is mainly produced in Fujian, Sichuan, and Jiangxi provinces, etc., dug and collected in winter when the tuber and leaves become yellow, dried in the sun or in the shade. The crude one or the one stir-baked with salt can be used.

为泽泻科植物泽泻的块茎。主产于福建、四川、江西等地。冬季茎叶开始枯萎时采挖,晒干或阴干。生用或盐水炒用。

Medicinal Properties Sweet and bland in flavor, cold in nature and attributive to the kindey and bladder meridians.

【药性】 味甘、淡,性寒。归肾、膀胱经。

Actions Promote diuresis to resolve dampness from the lower energizer and expel heat.

【功效】 利水渗湿,泄热。

Application For edema, dysuria, diarrhea, turbid stranguria, leucorrhagia, and dizziness due to retention of phlegm, especially effective in dampness-heat type in the lower energizer, it is usually combined with Zhuling (*Polyporus*), Fuling (*Poria*), etc.; for dizziness due to retention of phlegm, combined with Baizhu (*Rhizoma Atractylodis Macrocephalae*), such as Zexie Tang (Decoction).

【临床应用】 用于水肿、小便不利、泄泻、淋浊带下及痰饮眩晕等。下焦湿热者尤为适用。常与猪苓、茯苓等同用。若治痰饮眩晕,可与白术配伍,如泽泻汤。

Usage and Dosage 5－10 g is used in decoction for oral use.

【用法用量】 水煎服,5～10克。

Yiyiren *Semen Coicis*

薏苡仁

The source is from the dried mature seed of *Coix*

为禾本科植物薏苡的成

lacrymajobi L. var. mayuan (Roman.) stapf, family Gramineae. The medicinal material is mainly produced in the areas of Fujian, Hebei, and Liaoning, etc., collected in autumn when the fruits are ripe, shelled, dried in the sun and then peeled. The raw or the stir-baked one can be used.

熟种仁。主产于福建、河北、辽宁等地。秋季果实成熟时采割，脱粒，晒干，除去外壳及种皮。生用或炒用。

Medicinal Properties Sweet and bland in flavor, slightly cold in nature and attributive to the spleen, stomach and lung meridians.

【药性】 味甘、淡，性微寒。归脾、胃、肺经。

Actions Promote diuresis to resolve dampness and invigorate the spleen, treat Bi-syndrome and clear away heat to drain the pus.

【功效】 利水渗湿，健脾，除痹，清热排脓。

Application

【临床应用】

1. It is used for spleen-deficiency syndrome with accumulation of dampness manifested as dysuria, edema, beriberi or diarrhea due to spleen-deficiency. For edema, it is usually combined with Fuling (*Poria*), Baizhu (*Rhizoma Atractylodis Macrocephalae*), and Huangqi (*Radix Astragali*), etc.; for spleen deficiency with loss of appetite and diarrhea, it is usually used together with Dangshen (*Radix Codonopsis*) and Baizhu (*Rhizoma Atractylodis Macrocephalae*).

1. 用于脾虚湿胜之小便不利，水肿，脚气，脾虚泄泻。治水肿，多与茯苓、白术、黄芪等配伍；若治脾虚食少便溏，多与党参、白术同用。

2. For Bi-syndrome with dominant dampness manifested as bodily heaviness and soreness and rigidity of limbs, it is used together with Mugua (*Fructus Chaenomelis*) every time; for that with dominant heat, it is combined with Dilong (*Lumbricus*), Fangji (*Radix Stephaniae Tetrandrae*); for that with dominant cold, combined with Mahuang (*Herba Ephedrae*) and Guizhi (*Ramulus Cinnamomi*); for that with heavy dampness, combined with Cangzhu (*Rhizoma Atractylodis*).

2. 用于痹证湿胜，身重酸痛，肢体拘急。每与木瓜同用。偏热者配地龙、防己；偏寒者配麻黄、桂枝；湿重者配苍术同用。

3. It is used for pulmonary and intestinal abscess. For pulmonary abscess with cough and thick sputum, it is usually combined with Lugen (*Rhizoma Phragmitis*),

3. 用于肺痈，肠痈。治肺痈咳吐脓痰，常与芦根、冬瓜仁、桃仁等同用，如苇茎汤；治

Dongguaren (*Semen Benincasae*), and Taoren (*Semen Persicae*), etc., such as Weijing Tang (Decoction); for intestinal abscess, used together with Baijiangcao (*Herba Patriniae*), Mudanpi (*Cortex Moutan Radicis*), and Taoren (*Semen Persicae*), etc..

肠痈,可与败酱草、牡丹皮、桃仁等同用。

Usage and Dosage 10 - 30 g is used in decoction for oral use. The stir-baked one is used for invigorating the spleen to stop diarrhea and the raw for other syndromes.

【用法用量】 水煎服,10~30克。健脾止泻炒用,余均可生用。

Notes The medicinal herb is moderate in action, so the dosage should be large. It can be made gruel to be taken and is a good food as dietotherapy besides adding it to decoction, pill and powder.

【说明】 本品力缓,用量宜大。除入汤剂、丸散外,亦可作粥食,为食疗佳品。

Cheqianzi *Semen Plantaginis*

车前子

The source is from the mature seed of the perennial herb, *Plantago asiatica* L. or *P. depressa* Willa., family Plantaginaceae. The medicinal material is produced in all parts of China, collected in summer and autumn when the seed is ripe. The crude one or the one parched with salty water is used.

为车前科植物车前或平车前的成熟种子。产于中国各地。夏、秋两季种子成熟时采收。生用或盐水炙用。

Medicinal Properties Sweet in flavor, cold in nature and attributive to the kidney, liver and lung meridians.

【药性】 味甘,性寒。归肾、肝、肺经。

Actions Induce diuresis to treat stranguria, resolve dampness to stop diarrhea, clear away liver-fire to improve eyesight and clear away lung-heat to resolve phlegm.

【功效】 利水通淋,渗湿止泻,清肝明目,清肺化痰。

Application

1. For edema and stranguria, especially suitable for stranguria of damp and heat types manifested as oliguria with reddish urine, difficulty and pain in micturition, it is usually combined with Mutong (*Caulis Akebiae*), Huashi (*Talcum*) and Bianxu (*Herba Polygoni Avicularis*), such as Bazheng San (Powder).

【临床应用】

1. 用于水肿,淋证。尤宜于湿热淋证,小便短赤涩痛,常与木通、滑石、萹蓄同用,如八正散。

2. It is used for diarrhea due to summer-heat-dampness. It can promote diuresis to make defecation forming, so it can be used for watery diarrhea due to domination of dampness. It can be used alone or together with Baizhu (*Rhizoma Atractylodis Macrocephalae*), Fuling (*Poria*), and Zexie (*Rhizoma Alismatis*), etc..

2. 用于暑湿泄泻。本品能利小便以实大便，可用于湿胜水泻，可单用，或与白术、茯苓、泽泻等同用。

3. For conjunctivitis due to flaring up of liver-fire, it is usually combined with Juhua (*Flos Chrysanthemi*) and Juemingzi (*Semen Cassiae*); for insufficiency of liver-yin and kidney-yin manifested as dim eyesight and nebula, used together with Shudihuang (*Radix Rehmanniae Praeparata*) and Gouqizi (*Fructus Lycii*).

3. 用于目赤肿痛。肝火上炎之所致者，常与菊花、决明子同用；若肝肾阴亏，目暗昏花，翳障，可与熟地黄、枸杞子同用。

4. For cough of lung-heat type, usually combined with Gualou (*Fructus Trichosanthis*), Beimu (*Bulbus Fritillariae*), and Pipaye (*Folium Eriobotryae*), etc..

4. 用于痰热咳嗽。多与瓜蒌、贝母、枇杷叶等同用。

Usage and Dosage 10 - 15 is used in decoction for oral use. It is wrapped with gauze and then put in decoction to be decocted.

【用法用量】 水煎服，10～15克。布包入煎。

Mutong *Caulis Akebiae*

木 通

The source is from the stem of the deciduous woody lianna, *Akebia trifoliata* (Thunb.) Koidz. var *australis* (Diels) Rehd., *Akebia trifoliata* (Thunb.) Koidz., and *Akebia quinata* (Thunb.) Decne, family Akebia. The above medicinal material is mainly produced in the areas of Jiangsu, Zhejiang, Shanxi, and Hebei provinces. The source of Guanmutong (*Caulis Aristolochiae Manshuriensis*) is from the stem of *Aristolochia manshuriensis* Kom., family Aristolochiacere. Its material is mainly produced in the areas of Jilin, Liaoning, and Heilongjiang, etc., collected in autumn, dried in the sun, cut into pieces and the crude form is used.

木通科植物白木通或三叶木通、木通的木质茎。主产于江苏、浙江、山西、河北等地。关木通为马兜铃科植物东北马兜铃的藤茎。主产于吉林、辽宁、黑龙江等地。秋季采收，晒干，切片。生用。

Medicinal Properties Bitter in flavor, cold in nature and attributive to the heart, small intestine and bladder meridians.

【药性】 味苦，性寒。归心、小肠、膀胱经。

Actions Clear away heart-heat, promote diuresis, menstruation and lactation.

【功效】 清心火,利小便,通经下乳。

Application

【临床应用】

1. It is used for stranguria of heat type. For flaring up of heart-fire manifested as aphthae and heart-fire involving small intestine marked by restlessness and darkish urine, it is usually combined with Shengdihuang (*Radix Rehmanniae*), Gancao (*Radix Glycyrrhizae*), Zhuye (*Folium Phyllostachydis Nigrae*), such as Dao Chi San (Powder); for dampness-heat in the bladder with dripping discharge, difficulty and pain in micturition, usually combined with Cheqianzi (*Semen Plantaginis*), Qumai (*Herba Dianthi*), etc., such as Bazheng San (Powder).

1. 用于热淋。治心火上炎,口舌生疮,及心火移热于小肠之心烦尿赤,多与生地黄、甘草、竹叶等同用,如导赤散。治膀胱湿热,小便淋漓涩痛,常与车前子、瞿麦等配伍,如八正散。

2. It is used for amenorrhea due to blood stasis, and especially suitable for that accompanied by blood-heat, it is combined with Honghua (*Flos Carthami*), Taoren (*Semen Persicae*), and Danshen (*Radix Salviae Miltiorrhizae*), etc..

2. 用于血瘀经闭,尤以兼血热者为宜。配伍红花,桃仁、丹参等同用。

3. For shortness of lactation or galactostasis, it is combined with Wangbuliuxing (*Semen Vaccariae*), Loulu (*Radix Rhapontici seu Echinopsis*), etc., or boiled with pig feet for oral use.

3. 用于产后乳少或乳汁不下。可与王不留行、漏芦等同用,或与猪蹄炖汤服。

4. For arthralyia of dampness-heat type, it is usually combined with Qinjiao (*Radix Gentianae Macrophyllae*), Fangji (*Radix Stephaniae Tetrandrae*), and Yiyiren (*Semen Coicis*), etc..

4. 用于湿热痹痛。多配伍秦艽、防己、薏苡仁等同用。

Usage and Dosage 3-6 g is used in decoction for oral use.

【用法用量】 水煎服,3~6克。

Notes The dosage of Guanmutong (*Caulis Aristolochiae Manshuriensis*) is not suitable to be overlarge and it is contraindicated in a case with incomplete function of the heart and kidney, and used with caution in pregnant women, since Guanmutong (*Caulis Aristolochiae Manshuriensis*) contains aristolochine, whose overdosage can

【使用注意】 关木通含有马兜铃酸,过量可引起急性肾功能衰竭,心肾功能不全者忌用。孕妇慎用。

result in acute renal failure.

Haijinsha *Spora Lygodii*

海金沙

The source is from the mature spore of the perennial climbing fern, *Lygodium japonicum* (Thunb.) sw., family Lygodiaceae. The medicinal material is mainly produced in the areas of Guangdong, Zhejiang, etc., collected in autumn, dried in the sun and the crude one is used.

为海金沙科植物海金沙的成熟孢子。主产于广东、浙江等地。秋季采收，晒干。生用。

Medicinal Properties Sweet in flavor, cold in nature and attributive to the bladder and small intestine meridians.

【药性】 味甘，性寒。归膀胱、小肠经。

Action Induce diuresis to treat stranguria.

【功效】 利尿通淋。

Application

【临床应用】

1. It can be used to treat various syndromes of stranguria and especially is a main medicine for treating stranguria caused by urinary stones. For stranguria of heat type, it can be combined with Cheqianzi (*Semen Plantaginis*) and Jinqiancao (*Herba Lysimachiae*); for that complicated by hematuria, used together with Niuxi (*Radix Achyranthis Bidentatae*), Hupo (*Succinum*) and Xiaoji (*Herba Cephalanoploris*); for that caused by urinary stones, used together with Jineijin (*Endotholium Corneum Gigeriae Galli*) and Jinqiancao (*Herba Lysimachiae*).

1. 用于各种淋证。尤为治砂淋要药。治热淋，可与车前子、金钱草同用；治血淋，可与牛膝、琥珀、小蓟同用；治砂淋，与鸡内金、金钱草同用。

2. For dysuria and edema, it is usually used together with Zexie (*Rhizoma Alismatis*), Zhuling (*Polyporus*), Fangji (*Radix Stephaniae Tetrandrae*), and Mutong (*Caulis Akebiae*), etc..

2. 用于小便不利，水肿。多与泽泻、猪苓、防己、木通等同用。

Usage and Dosage 6 - 15 g is used in decoction for oral use, wrapped with gauze and then put in decoction to be decocted.

【用法用量】 水煎服，6～15克。布包入煎。

Difuzi *Fructus Kochiae*

地肤子

The source is from the mature fruit of *Kochia scoparia* (L.) Schrad., family Chenopodiaceae. The medicinal material is produced in most areas of China, cut in

为藜科植物地肤的成熟果实。中国大部分地区均产。秋季果实成熟时割取全株，晒

autumn when the fruit is ripe, dried in the sun and then the fruit is collected and can be used in the crude form.

干,打下果实。生用。

Medicinal Properties Bitter in flavor, cold in nature and attributive to the bladder meridian.

【药性】 味苦,性寒。归膀胱经。

Actions Clear away heat and eliminate dampness, and alleviate itching.

【功效】 清热利湿,止痒。

Application

【临床应用】

1. For dampness-heat in the bladder with dysuria, and difficulty and pain in urination, it is usually combined with Mutong (*Caulis Akebia*), Qumai (*Herba Dianthi*), and Dongkuizi (*Semen Abutili*), etc., such as Difuzi Tang (Decoction).

1. 用于膀胱湿热,小便不利,淋漓涩痛。常与木通、瞿麦、冬葵子等同用,如地肤子汤。

2. For skin eczema, damp sore and pruritussvuluae, it is usually combined with Shechuangzi (*Fructus Cnidii*), Chantui (*Periostracum Cicadae*), and Huangbai (*Cortex Phellodendri*), etc. which are decocted together for washing.

2. 用于皮肤湿疹,湿疮,阴痒。常与蛇床子、蝉蜕、黄柏等同用,煎汤外洗。

Usage and Dosage 10 - 15 g is used in decoction for oral use and just right amount for external use.

【用法用量】 水煎服,10~15克。外用,适量。

Bixie *Rhizoma Dioscoreae Hypoglaucae*

萆 薢

The source is from Rhizome of *Discorea hypoglauca* Polibin and several other species of the same genus, family Dioscoreaceae, or some species of *Smilax* (Liliaceae) are also used medicinally. The medicinal material is mainly produced in the areas of Zhejiang, Hubei, and Guangxi, etc., dug and collected in spring and autumn, cut into pieces, dried in the sun and the crude form is used.

为薯蓣科植物绵萆薢和粉背薯蓣的根茎。主产于浙江、湖北、广西等地。春、秋季采挖,切片,晒干。生用。

Medicinal Properties Bitter in flavor, slightly cold in nature and attributive to the liver and stomach meridians.

【药性】 味苦,性微寒。归肝、胃经。

Actions Eliminate dampness and turbidity, and expel wind.

【功效】 利湿去浊,祛风除湿。

Application

【临床应用】

1. The herb is used for chyloid stranguria and whitish

1. 用于膏淋,白浊。为治

turbid urine and is the main one for treating turbid urine or chyloid stranguria. It is usually combined with Wuyao (*Radix Linderae*). Yizhiren (*Fructus Alpiniae Oxyphyllae*), and Shichangpu (*Rhizoma Acori Graminei*), etc., such as Bixie Fen qing Yin (Decoction).

小便混浊或如米泔膏淋之要药。常与乌药、益智仁、石菖蒲同用,如萆薢分清饮。

2. For Bi-syndrome of dampness type manifested as bodily heaviness, sore and painful waist and knees, it is usually combined with Yiyiren (*Semen Coicis*), Cangzhu (*Rhizoma Atractylodis*), and Niuxi (*Radix Achyranthis Bidentatae*), etc..

2. 用于痹证湿胜,肢体重着,腰膝酸痛,常配薏苡仁、苍术、牛膝等同用。

Usage and Dosage 10 - 15 g is used in decoction for oral use.

【用法用量】 水煎服,10～15克。

Jinqiancao *Herba Lysimachiae*

金钱草

The source is from the whole plant of *Lysimachia christinae* Hance, family Primulaceae. The medicinal material is mainly produced in all provinces of the South to the Yangtze River, collected in summer and autumn, dried in the sun, cut into pieces and the crude form is used.

为报春花科植物过路黄的全草。产于江南各省。夏、秋两季采收。晒干,切段。生用。

Medicinal Properties Sweet and bland in flavor, slightly cold in nature and attributive to the liver, gallbladder, kidney and bladder meridians.

【药性】 味甘、淡,性微寒。归肝、胆、肾、膀胱经。

Actions Eliminate dampness to treat jaundice, induce diuresis to treat stranguria, eliminate toxic materials and relieve swelling.

【功效】 除湿退黄,利尿通淋,解毒消肿。

Application

【临床应用】

1. For jaundice of dampness-heat type, it is usually combined with Yinchenhao (*Herba Ariemisiae Scopariae*), Zhizi (*Fructus Gardeniae*) and Huzhang (*Rhizoma Polygoni Cuspidati*).

1. 用于湿热黄疸。常与茵陈蒿、栀子、虎杖同用。

2. For stranguria, especially suitable for stony stranguria, large dosage can be decocted alone for drinking as tea, or used together with Haijinsha (*Spora Lygodii*), Jineijin (*Endothelium Corneum Gigeriae Galli*), and

2. 用于淋证。尤宜于治石淋,可单用大剂量煎汤代茶,或与海金沙、鸡内金、滑石等同用。

Huashi (*Talcum*), etc..

3. For pyocutaneous disease with swelling and poisoning snake bite, the fresh can be ground into juice for drinking, the dregs of the juice being used as external application.

3. 用于疮疡肿毒,毒蛇咬伤。可用鲜品捣烂取汁饮,药渣外敷。

Usage and Dosage 15 - 60 g is used in decoction for oral use, the amount of the fresh should be doubled and just right amount is for external use.

【用法用量】 水煎服,15～60克。鲜品用量加倍。外用,适量。

Yinchenhao *Herba Artemisiae Scopariae*

茵陈蒿

The source is from the whole herb of *Artemisia Capillaris* Thunb., or *Artemisia scoparia* Waldst, et kit, family Compositae. The medicinal material is produced in all parts of China, collected in spring when the young plant is 10 cm high or in autumn when the bud has grown up, the root and impurity being removed. The crude is dried in the sun for use.

为菊科植物茵陈蒿或滨蒿的全草。产于中国各地。春季幼蒿苗高约 10 cm 时采收,或秋季花蕾长成时采割,除去根及杂质,晒干。生用。

Medicinal Properties Bitter in flavor, slightly cold in nature and attributive to the spleen, stomach, liver and gallbladder meridians.

【药性】 味苦,性微寒。归脾、胃、肝、胆经。

Actions Clear away heat and eliminate dampness, drain the gallbladder to relieve jaundice.

【功效】 清热利湿,利胆退黄。

Application

【临床应用】

1. It is a main medicinal herb for treating jaundice and can treat all kinds of syndromes of jaundice by the herb in combination with others. For yang-jaundice of dampness-heat type, it is usually combined with Zhizi (*Fructus Gardeniae*), Huangbai (*Cortex Phellodendri*), and Dahuang (*Radix et Rhizoma Rhei*), such as Yinchenhao Tang (Decoction); for that of dominant dampness type with heat, combined with Fuling (*Poria*), Zhuling (*Polyporus*), such as Yinchen Wuling San (Powder); for yin-jaundice of dampness-heat type, must be combined with Fuzi (*Radix Aconiti Lateralis Praeparata*), Ganjiang (*Rhizoma Zingiberis*), etc., such as

1. 用于黄疸。为治黄疸要药,经配伍可治各型黄疸病证。治湿热阳黄,多与栀子、黄柏、大黄同用,如茵陈蒿汤;湿重于热,可与茯苓、猪苓同用,如茵陈五苓散;若治寒湿阴黄,须与附子、干姜等配伍,如茵陈四逆汤。

Yinchen Sini Tang (Decoction).

2. For damp-thermosis, eczema and damp sore, it is combined with Huangbai (*Cortex Phellodendri*), Kushen (*Radix Sophorae Flavescentis*), Shechuangzi (*Fructus Cnidii*), and Difuzi (*Fructus kochiae*), etc. to be decocted for oral use or for external washing.

2. 用于湿温,湿疹,湿疮。可与黄柏、苦参、蛇床子、地肤子等同用内服,或煎汤外洗。

Usage and Dosage 10 - 30 g is used in decoction for oral use and just right amount for external use.

【用法用量】 水煎服,10～30 克。外用,适量。

Notes Contraindicated for jaundice with yellowish skin due to accumulation of blood and for that with lustreless yellow due to deficiency of the blood.

【使用注意】 蓄血发黄及血虚萎黄者忌用。

5 The Interior Warming Chinese Medicinal Herbs

第五章 温里药

Any medicinal herb that has the ability to warm up the interior and dispel cold to act on internal conditions is known as the interior warming Chinese medicinal herbs.

凡能温散里寒，治疗里寒证的药物，称为温里药。

The category of medicinal herbs are warm and heat in nature, and can expel interior cold and invigorate yang-qi. They are indicated for syndrome due to invasion of cold into the interior which affects yang-qi; or cold conditions in the interior due to yang weakness manifested as cold and pain in the chest and epigastric abdomen, vomiting, nausea, diarrhea and dysentery, chillness with cold limbs, and clear and profuse urine, etc.. Some of them can recuperate the depleted yang and rescue the patient from collapse, and are indicated for syndrome of yang exhaustion. In addition, some can warm the lung to resolve retention of phlegm, warm the liver to treat colic, lower the adverse-rising qi to relieve hiccup, and can be used for cough due to lung-cold, colic and vomiting due to stomach-cold, cold and pain in the epigastric abdomen.

本类药物性温热，能祛散里寒，振奋阳气，适用于寒邪内侵，阳气受抑；或阳气衰弱，阴寒内生之里寒证，症见脘腹冷痛、呕吐、呃逆、泄泻痢疾、畏寒肢冷、小溲清长等。部分药物能回阳救逆，适用于亡阳证。此外，有的能温肺化饮，温肝治疝，降逆止呃。可治肺寒咳喘，疝气痛及胃寒呕吐，脘腹冷痛。

They must be used in proper combination according to different syndromes. For yang deficiency with interior cold, they should be combined with yang tonifying medicinal herbs; for syndrome of yang exhaustion and collapse of qi, combined with Renshen (*Radix Ginseng*) to tonify qi and treat collapse of qi; for cold accumulation and qi stagnation, combined with qi circulating medicinal herbs; for water retention due to yang deficiency, combined with the medicinal herbs for inducing diuresis and eliminating the

使用时，还须根据不同病证，进行恰当配伍。阳虚内寒，配补阳药；亡阳气脱者，配人参以益气固脱；寒凝气滞，配行气药；阳虚水停者，配利水渗湿药。

dampness.

They are pungent, hot and dry in property and can help fire injure yin if they are used improperly, therefore they are contraindicated for heat syndrome and yin-deficiency syndrome, and used with caution in yin deficient and bleeding patients and pregnant women.

温里药辛热而燥,应用不当易助火伤阴,故热证、阴虚证忌用。素体阴虚或失血者及孕妇当慎用。

Fuzi *Radix Aconiti Lateralis Praeparata*

附　子

The source is from the root of *Aconitum carmichaeli* Debx., family Ranunculaceae. The medicinal material is mainly produced in the areas of Sichuan, Hubei, and Hunan, etc., collected from the last ten-day period of June to the first ten-day period of August, and they are soaked and processed into salty, black, white, bland and soaked aconiti.

为毛茛科植物乌头的子根的加工品。主产于四川、湖北、湖南等地。6 月下旬至 8 月上旬采收,加工炮制为盐附子、黑顺片、白附片、淡附片、炮附片。

Medicinal Properties Pungent and sweet in flavor, hot in nature, toxic and attributive to the heart, kidney and spleen meridians.

【药性】 味辛、甘,性热。有毒。归心、肾、脾经。

Actions Recuperate the depleted yang for resuscitation, supplement fire and strengthen yang, expel cold to relieve pain.

【功效】 回阳救逆,补火助阳,散寒止痛。

Application

【临床应用】

1. It is used for yang exhausion syndrome. It is an essential medicine for the treatment of yang-exhaustion syndrome manifested as clammy perspiration, faint breath, cold clammy limbs, indistinct and faint pulse, it is usually used in combination with Ganjiang (*Rhizoma Zingiberis*) and Gancao (*Radix Glycyrrhizae*), such as Sini Tang (Decoction); for exhaustion of qi due to yang-deficiency, it can be combined with Renshen (*Radix Ginseng*) to supplement qi to prevent prolapse of qi such as Shen Fu Tang (Decoction).

1. 用于亡阳证。本品为治亡阳证主药,症见汗出清冷、呼吸气微、四肢厥冷、脉微欲绝者,常配干姜、甘草同用,如四逆汤;若阳虚气脱,可配人参益气固脱,如参附汤。

2. It is used to treat all syndromes of yang deficiency type. For insufficiency of kidney-yang with impotence, cold and painful waist and knees, and frequent micturition,

2. 用于阳虚诸证。若治肾阳不足,阳痿宫冷,腰膝冷痛,尿频尿多,可与肉桂、山茱

it is usually combined with Rougui (*Cortex Cinnamomi*), Shanzhuyu (*Fructus Corni*), and Shudihuang (*Rhizoma Rehmanniae Praeparatae*), etc., such as Yougui Wan (Pill); for insufficiency of spleen-yang and kidney-yang and interior domination of cold and dampness with coldness and pain in epigastric abdomen, loss of appetite and diarrhea, it is combined with Dangshen (*Radix Codonopsis*), Baizhu (*Rhizoma Atractylodis Macrocephalae*), and Ganjiang (*Rhizoma Zingiberis*), etc.; for yang deficiency resulting in edema, and dysuria, usually used together with Baizhu (*Rhizoma Atractylodis Macrocephalae*), Fuling (*Poria*) and Shengjiang (*Rhizoma Zingiberis Recens*); for exogenous affection due to yang-deficiency, combined with Mahuang (*Herba Ephedrae*); for spontaneous perspiration due to yang-deficiency, combined with Huangqi (*Radix Astragali*).

萸、熟地黄等同用,如右归丸;若治脾肾阳虚,寒湿内盛的脘腹冷痛,纳少,大便泄泻,可与党参、白术、干姜等同用;治阳虚水肿,小便不利,多与白术、茯苓、生姜同用;治阳虚外感配麻黄同用;治阳虚自汗配黄芪同用。

3. It is used to treat all pain syndromes of cold type. For arthralgia of wind-cold-dampness type, pain of general joints due to domination of cold and dampness, it is combined with Guizhi (*Ramulus Cinnamomi*), Baizhu (*Rhizoma Atractylodis Macrocephalae*) and Gancao (*Radix Glycyrrhizae*); for abdominal pain due to cold accumulation and qi stagnation, combined with Dingxiang (*Flos Caryophylli*), Gaoliangjiang (*Rhizoma Alpiniae Officinarum*), etc..

3. 用于诸寒痛证。若治风寒湿痹,周身骨节疼痛,属寒湿盛者,可与桂枝、白术、甘草同用;寒凝气滞腹痛,配伍丁香、高良姜等同用。

Usage and Dosage 3 - 15 g is used in decoction for oral use and decocted at first for about a half to one hour until its narcotico-pungent taste is lost when its decoction is tasted by mouth.

【用法用量】 水煎服,3～15克,先煎0.5～1小时,至口尝无麻辣感为度。

Notes Contraindicated in a case with yin-deficiency leading to hyperactivity of yang and pregnant women because of its pungent, hot, dry and violent properties. It is incompatible with Banxia (*Rhizoma Pinelliae*), Gualou (*Fructus Trichosanthis*), Beimu (*Bulbus Fritillariae*),

【使用注意】 本品辛热燥烈,阴虚阳亢及孕妇忌用。反半夏、瓜蒌、贝母、白蔹、白及。内服须炮制后用,且须久煎,不可过量久服。

Bailian (*Radix Ampelopsis*) and Baiji (*Rhizoma Bletillae*). It must be soaked for oral use, decocted for a long time, and over dosage and long administration must be avoided.

Rougui *Cortex Cinnamomi*

The source is from the bark of *Cinnamomum cassia* Presl, family Lauraceae. The medicinal material is mainly produced in the areas of Guangdong, Guangxi, and Yunnan, etc., barked in autumn and then the bark is dried in the shade, cut into pieces or powdered and the crude form is used.

Medicinal Properties Pungent and sweet in flavor, hot in nature and attributive to the spleen, kidney and heart meridians.

Actions Supplement fire and strengthen yang, expel cold and alleviate pain, warm channels to promote the circulation of the blood.

Application

1. It is used for insufficiency syndromes of kidney-yang. For insufficiency of kidney-yang with impotence, chilliness, soreness and coldness of loins and knees, frequent micturition, seminal emission, and enuresis, etc., it is usually used in combination with Fuzi (*Radix Aconiti Lateralis Praeparata*), Shudihuang (*Rhizoma Rehmanniae Praeparatae*), and Shanzhuyu (*Fructus Corni*), etc., such as Shenqi Wan (Pill); for syndrome with deficiency and weakness of kidney-yang and up-floating of deficiency-yang, manifested as flushed face, dyspnea due to deficiency, the herbal medicine can be used in combination with Fuzi (*Radix Aconiti Praeparata*) so as to direct fire to its source.

2. It can be used to treat all pains due to accumulation of cold and stagnation of qi or stasis of the blood. For deficiency and coldness of the spleen and stomach marked

肉　桂

为樟科植物肉桂的树皮。主产于广东、广西、云南等地。秋季剥取，刮去栓皮，阴干，切片或研末。生用。

【药性】 味辛、甘，性热。归脾、肾、心经。

【功效】 补火助阳，散寒止痛，温经通脉。

【临床应用】

1. 用于肾阳不足证。治肾阳不足之阳痿宫冷、畏寒、腰膝冷痛、尿频、滑精、遗尿等，多与附子、熟地黄、山茱萸等同用，如肾气丸；若治下元虚衰，虚阳上浮之面赤、虚喘，可用本品与附子同用以引火归原。

2. 用于寒凝气滞或寒凝血瘀所致的诸痛。治脾胃虚寒，脘腹冷痛，可单用，或与干

by cold pain in epigastric abdomen, it can be used alone or together with Ganjiang (*Rhizoma Zingiberis*) and Gaoliangjiang (*Rhizoma Alpiniae Officinarum*); for colic of cold type with abdominal pain, usually used in combination with Wuzhuyu (*Fructus Evodiae*), Xiaohuixiang (*Fructus Foeniculi*); for dysmenorrhea and amenorrhea, usually combined with Danggui (*Radix Angelicae Sinensis*) and Chuanxiong (*Rhizoma Chuanxiong*), etc..

姜、高良姜等同用;治寒疝腹痛,常配吴茱萸、小茴香同用;治痛经、经闭,常与当归、川芎配伍。

3. For pudendal carbuncle and pyocutaneous disease of deficienct-cold type that has not been healed for a long time, it is combined with Lujiaojiao (*Colla Cornus Cervi*), Paojiang (*Rhizoma Zingiberis Praeparata*), and Mahuang (*Herba Ephedrae*), etc., such as Yanghe Tang (Decoction); or combined with Huangqi (*Radix Astragali*), Danggui (*Radix Angelicae Sinensis*), etc., such as Tuoli Huangqi San (Powder).

3. 用于阴疽及虚寒性疮疡,久不愈合者。可与鹿角胶、炮姜、麻黄等同用,如阳和汤;也可与黄芪、当归等同用,如托里黄芪散。

Usage and Dosage 2 - 5 g is used in decoction for oral use and decocted later or soaked in water for taking; 1 - 2 g of the powder is taken after it is mixed with water.

【用法用量】 水煎服,2～5克,宜后下或开水泡服;研末冲服,1～2克。

Notes Contraindicated for bleeding due to blood-heat, and used with caution for hypermenorrhea and in pregnant women.

【使用注意】 血热出血忌用。月经过多及孕妇慎用。

Explanation Rougui (*Cortex Cinnamomi*) and Guizhi (*Ramulus Cinnamomi*) are from same plants, the barks of which are used as medicine that is called Rougui (*Cortex Cinnamomi*); the tender branches of which are used as medicine that is called Guizhi (*Ramulus Cinnamomi*). The both medicines can expel cold and strengthen yang, Guizhi (*Ramulus Cinnamomi*) dominates going up to be a bit on the side of expelling cold to relieve exterior syndrome while Rougui (*Cortex Cinnamomi*) dominates warming the interior to enter the lower energizer, being a bit on the side of warming kidney-yang.

【说明】 肉桂与桂枝来源于同一植物。肉桂用树皮,桂枝用嫩枝。两者均能散寒助阳,桂枝主上行而偏散寒解表,肉桂主温里且入下焦,偏于温肾阳。

Ganjiang *Rhizoma Zingiberis*

The source is from the rhizome of the perennial herb, *Zingibor officinale* Rosc, family Zingiberaceae. The medicinal material is mainly produced in the areas of Sichuan, Guangdong, and Guangxi, etc., collected in winter, cut into pieces, dried in the sun or in low temperature, and the crude form is used.

Medicinal Properties Pungent in flavor, hot in nature and attributive to the spleen, stomach, heart and lung meridians.

Actions Warm the middle-energizer to expel cold, restore yang and dredge channels, warm the lung to resolve phlegm.

Application

1. It is used to treat spleen-cold and stomach-cold syndromes whether they are asthenia or sthenia. For stomach-cold with vomiting and cold and painful epigastric abdomen, it is usually used in combination with Gaoliangjiang (*Rhizoma Alpiniae Officinarum*), such as Er Jiang Wan (Pill); for deficiency and coldness of the spleen and stomach, usually combined with Dangshen (*Radix Codonopsis*), Baizhu (*Rhizoma Atractylodis Macrocephalae*), etc., such as Lizhong Wan (Pill).

2. For syndrome of yang exhaustion, it is usually combined with Fuzi (*Radix Aconiti Lateralis Praeparata*) for maximal effect to decrease the toxicity of Fuzi (*Radix Aconiti Lateralis Praeparata*) as well as to strengthen the action of Fuzi (*Radix Aconiti Lateralis Praeparata*) in recuperating the depleted yang and rescuing the patient from collapse, such as Sini Tang (Decoction).

3. For cold accumulation in the lung manifested as cough and dyspnea, body's coldness and profuse thin sputum, it is usually combined with Xixin (*Herba Asai*), Wuweizi (*Fructus Schisandrae*) and Mahuang (*Herba*

干 姜

为姜科植物姜的干燥根茎。主产于四川、广东、广西等地。冬季采收，切片，晒干或低温烘干。生用。

【药性】 味辛，性热。归脾、胃、心、肺经。

【功效】 温中散寒，回阳通脉，温肺化饮。

【临床应用】

1. 用于脾胃寒证。无论虚实均可应用。治胃寒呕吐，脘腹冷痛，多与高良姜同用，如二姜丸；治脾胃虚寒，多与党参、白术等同用，如理中丸。

2. 用于亡阳证。与附子相须为用，既能增强附子回阳救逆之力，又能减低附子的毒性，如四逆汤。

3. 用于寒饮伏肺，症见咳嗽气喘，形寒肢冷，痰多清稀。常与细辛、五味子、麻黄同用，如小青龙汤。

Ephedrae), such as Xiao Qinglong Tang (Decoction).

Usage and Dosage 3 - 10 is used in decoction for oral use.

【用法用量】 水煎服，3～10克。

Wuzhuyu *Fructus Evodiae*

吴茱萸

The source is from nearly matured fruit of *Evodia rutaecarpa* (Juss) Benth, family Rutaceae. The medicinal material is mainly produced in the areas of Guizhou, Guangxi, Hunan, Zhejiang, and Sichuan, etc., collected from August to November when the fruits are not split open, dried in the sun or in low temperature. The crude or prepared one can be used.

为芸香科植物吴茱萸、石虎或疏毛吴茱萸的将近成熟的果实。主产于贵州、广西、湖南、浙江、四川等地。8～11月果实尚未开裂时采收，晒干或低温烘干。生用或制用。

Medicinal Properties Pungent and bitter in flavor, hot in nature, mild toxic and attributive to the liver, spleen, stomach and kidney meridians.

【药性】 味辛、苦，性热。有小毒。归肝、脾、胃、肾经。

Actions Expel cold and relieve pain, warm the spleen and stomach to stop vomiting, strengthen yang and arrest diarrhea.

【功效】 散寒止痛，温中止呕，助阳止泻。

Application

1. It is used to treat all syndromes due to cold accumulation in the liver meridian. For colic of cold type with abdominal pain, it is usually combined with Xiaohuixiang (*Fructus Foeniculi*), Chuanlianzi (*Fructus Meliae Toosendan*); for jueyin headache, usually combined with Renshen (*Radix Ginseng*), Shengjiang (*Rhizoma Zingiberis Recens*), etc., such as Wuzhuyu Tang (Decoction); for dysmenorrhea due to cold accumulation, used together with Guizhi (*Ramulus Cinnamomi*), Danggui (*Radix Angelicae Sinensis*), and Chuanxiong (*Rhizoma Chuanxiong*), etc., such as Wenjing Tang (Decoction); for beriberi of cold-dampness type, used together with Mugua (*Fructus Chaenomelis*), Zisuye (*Folium Perillae*), Binglang (*Semen Arecae*), such as Jiming San (Powder).

【临床应用】

1. 用于寒凝肝脉诸证。治寒疝腹痛，常与小茴香、川楝子同用；治厥阴头痛，常与人参、生姜等同用，如吴茱萸汤；治寒凝痛经，可与桂枝、当归、川芎等同用，如温经汤；治寒湿脚气，可与木瓜、紫苏叶、槟榔同用，如鸡鸣散。

2. It is used for incoordination between the liver and

2. 用于肝胃不和，吞酸呕

stomach with acid regurgitation and vomiting. For the syndrome being a bit on the cold side, it is usually combined with Shengjiang (*Rhizoma Zingiberis Recens*), Banxia (*Rhizoma Pinelliae*), etc.; for live-fire due to depression of liver-qi with hypochondriac distention and pain, bitterness and dryness in the mouth, used together with Huanglian (*Rhizoma Coptidis*), such as Zuojin Wan (Pill).

吐。偏寒者,多与生姜、半夏等同用;若肝郁化火,伴胁肋胀痛且口苦、口干者,则与黄连同用,如左金丸。

3. For diarrhea due to deficiency and cold, it is usually combined with Buguzhi (*Fructus Psoraleae*), Roudoukou (*Semen Myristicae*) and Wuweizi (*Fructus Schisandrae*), such as Sishen Wan (Pill).

3. 用于虚寒泄泻。多与补骨脂、肉豆蔻、五味子同用,如四神丸。

In addition, powder prepared with vinegar for aphthae by local application on sole. Now it can be used to treat hypertension.

此外,本品醋调敷足心,可治口疮。现代用治高血压病。

Usage and Dosage 1.5 - 4.5 g is used in decoction for oral use and just right amount for external use.

【用法用量】 水煎服,1.5~4.5克。外用,适量。

Notes It is not suitable to be taken in large dosage and for a long time.

【使用注意】 本品辛热燥烈,易耗气动火,不宜多用、久服。

Xiaohuixiang *Fructus Foeniculi*

小茴香

The source is from the fruit of *Foeniculum Vulgare* Mill., family Umbelliferae. The medicinal material is produced in all parts of China, collected in autumn when the fruits begin to be ripe, dried in the sun. The crude herbal medicine can be used or is parched with salt water for use.

为伞形科植物茴香的成熟果实。产于中国各地。秋季果实初成熟时采收,晒干。生用或盐水炙用。

Medicinal Properties Pungent in flavor, warm in nature and attributive to the liver, kidney, spleen and stomach meridians.

【药性】 味辛,性温。归肝、肾、脾、胃经。

Actions Expel cold to alleviate pain, and regulate the stomach-qi.

【功效】 散寒止痛,理气和胃。

Application

【临床应用】

1. It is used for colic of cold type and orchidoptosis.

1. 用于寒疝腹痛,睾丸偏

It is an essential medicine to treat colic of cold type. It is usually combined with Wuyao (*Radix Linderae*), Qingpi (*Pericarpium Citri Reticulatae Viride*) and Gaoliangjiang (*Rhizoma Alpiniae Officinarum*), such as Tiantai Wuyao San (Powder).

坠。为治寒疝疼痛要药。常与乌药、青皮、高良姜同用,如天台乌药散。

2. For qi stagnation due to stomach-cold with epigastric distention and pain, vomiting and loss of appetite, combined with Ganjiang (*Rhizoma Zingiberis*) and Muxiang (*Radix Aucklandiae*).

2. 用于胃寒气滞,脘腹胀痛,呕吐食少。可配干姜、木香同用。

Usage and Dosage 3 - 6 g is used in decoction for oral use and just right amount for external use.

【用法用量】 水煎服,3～6克。外用,适量。

Huajiao *Pericarpium Zanthoxyli*

花 椒

The source is from the peel of *Zanthoxylum bungeanum* Maxim. or *Z. schinifolium* Sieb. et Zucc., family Rutaceae. The medicinal material is mainly produced in all parts of China and the quality of Huajiao (*Pericarpium Zanthoxyli*) produced in Sichuan is the best. It is collected and dried in the sun. The crude or the stir-baked one can be used.

为芸香科植物花椒或青椒的成熟果皮。产于中国各地,以四川产者为佳。秋季采收,晒干。生用或炒用。

Medicinal Properties Pungent in flavor, warm in nature and attributive to the spleen, stomach and kidney meridians.

【药性】 味辛,性温。归脾、胃、肾经。

Actions Warm the middle energizer to alleviate pain, kill worms to relieve itching.

【功效】 温中止痛,杀虫止痒。

Application

【临床应用】

1. It is used to treat syndrome of epigastric and abdominal pain, vomiting and diarrhea; for exterior cold invading the interior resulting in stomach-cold with abdominal pain and vomiting, it can be combined with Shengjiang (*Rhizoma Zingiberis Recens*), Baidoukou (*Fructus Amomi Rotundus*), etc.; for deficiency-cold of the spleen and stomach with cold epigastric pain, vomiting and loss of appetite, combined with Ganjiang (*Rhizoma Zingiberis*) and Renshen (*Radix Ginseng*), such as Da

1. 用于脘腹疼痛,呕吐泄泻。治外寒内侵,胃寒腹痛呕吐,可与生姜、白豆蔻等同用。治脾胃虚寒,脘腹冷痛,呕吐食少,可与干姜、人参同用,如大建中汤。

Jianzhong Tang (Decoction).

2. It is used to treat abdominal pain due to worms. It can relieve pain as well as kill worms. It can be used alone or combined with Wumei (*Fructus Mume*), Huanglian (*Rhizoma Coptidis*) and Ganjiang (*Rhizoma Zingiberis*), such as Wumei Wan (Pill).

3. For eczema and pruritus vulvae, it can be decocted alone for washing or used together with Kushen (*Radix Sophorae Flavescentis*), Difuzi (*Fructus Kochiae*), etc..

Usage and Dosage 3 - 6 g is used in decoction for oral use and just right amount for external use.

2. 用于蛔虫腹痛。既能杀虫又可止痛。可单用,或与乌梅、黄连、干姜同用,如乌梅丸。

3. 用于湿疹瘙痒,阴痒。单用煎水外洗,或与苦参、地肤子等同用。

【用法用量】 水煎服,3～6克。外用,适量。

6 Qi Regulating Chinese Medicinal Herbs

第六章 理气药

Any medicinal herb that acts to regulate qi-activity, disperse qi stagnation and facilitate qi flow or that takes treatment of syndrome due to abnormal rising of qi as its essential action falls under this category.

凡能疏理气机，以治疗气滞或气逆证为主的药物，称为理气药。

Most of these medicinal herbs are fragrant and warm in nature, pungent and bitter in flavor. They all have, to different degrees, the ability to regulate qi, strengthen the spleen, promote qi circulation, stop pain, facilitate qi flow, reverse rebellious qi activities, soothe the liver, disperse the depressed qi or crack qi stagnation and disperse mass, etc.. They are indicated for obstruction of pulmonary qi, failure of dispersion of the liver and the imbalance of function between the spleen and stomach. Qi stagnant syndrome is mainly manifested as oppression, fullness and pain; syndrome of abnormal rising of qi is usually manifested as nausea, hiccup or dyspnea.

理气药大多气香性温，其味辛、苦，具有调气健脾、行气止痛、顺气降逆、疏肝解郁或破气散结等功效。适用于肺失宣降，肝失疏泄，脾胃升降失司。气滞者主要表现为闷、胀、痛；气逆者常表现为恶心、呃逆或喘息。

So using these kinds of medicinal herbs, one must use other herbs flexibly and choose adaptive combination of herbs according to conditions, such as combination of the herbs for clearing away heat and resolving phlegm, clearing away heat to promote diuresis, warming the middle energizer to dry dampness, promoting digestion and relieving dyspepsia, benefiting qi and invigorating the spleen.

使用本类药物时，必须针对症候，选择相应的药物，并随证配伍其他有关药物。如配清热化痰、清热利湿、温中燥湿、消食导滞、益气健脾药。

Most of them are pungent, warm and fragrant, and may easily damage qi and yin, so one must use them with caution in cases of qi and yin deficiency.

本类药物辛温香燥者居多，易耗气伤阴，故气虚及阴虚者慎用。

Jupi *Pericarpium Citri Tangerinae*

The source is from the pericarp of *Citrus reticulate* Blanco, family Rutaceae. The medicinal material is mainly produced in the areas of Guangdong, Fujian, Sichuan, and Jiangsu, etc., collected in autumn when the fruit is ripe. The dried and stir-baked one is for medication.

Medicinal Properties Pungent and bitter in flavor, warm in nature and attributive to the spleen and lung meridians.

Actions Regulate qi and harmonize the spleen and stomach, eliminate dampness and resolve phlegm.

Application

1. It is used for stagnation of spleen-qi and stomach-qi, especially suitable for stagnation of spleen-qi and stomach-qi due to accumulation of cold and dampness in the middle energizer manifested as distention and fullness of epigastric abdomen, belching, nausea, and vomiting, etc.. It is usually used in combination with Cangzhu (*Rhizoma Atractylodis*) and Houpo (*Cortex Magnoliae Officinalis*), such as Pingwei San (Powder); for vomiting due to phlegm-heat, combined with Zhuru (*Caulis Bambusae in Taeniam*), Huanglian (*Rhizoma Coptidis*), etc.; for deficiency of spleen-qi and stomach-qi with abdominal pain that is reduced by pressure, fullness after meal, loss of appetite, usually combined with Dangshen (*Radix Codonopsis*), Baizhu (*Rhizoma Atractylodis Macrocephalae*), and Zhigancao (*Radix Glycyrrhizae, honeyfried*), etc., such as Yigong San (Powder).

2. It is used to treat cough with profuse sputum caused by dampness-phlegm and cold-phlegm. In the treatment of cough and dyspnea due to dampness-phlegm, it is usually combined with Banxia (*Rhizoma Pinelliae*) and Fuling (*Poria*) to deprive dampness and resolve phlegm, such as Erchen Tang (Decoction); for cough due

橘　皮

为芸香科橘及其栽培品种的成熟果皮。主产于广东、福建、四川、江苏等省。秋季果实成熟时收集，干燥。炒用。

【药性】 味辛、苦，性温。归脾、肺经。

【功效】 理气，调中，燥湿，化痰。

【临床应用】

1. 用于脾胃气滞证。寒湿阻中的脾胃气滞、脘腹胀满、嗳气、恶心呕吐等证尤宜。常与苍术、厚朴配伍，如平胃散；如呕吐因痰热所致者，可配竹茹、黄连等；脾胃气虚、腹痛喜按、食后饱胀、不思饮食者，常与党参、白术、炙甘草等配伍，如异功散。

2. 用于湿痰、寒痰之咳嗽痰多。治湿痰咳喘，常配半夏、茯苓以燥湿化痰，如二陈汤；若治寒痰咳嗽，多与干姜、细辛、五味子同用。

to cold-phlegm, usually combined with Ganjiang (*Rhizoma Zingiberis*), Xixin (*Flos Magnoliae*) and Wuweizi (*Fructus Schisandrae*).

Usage and Dosage 3 - 10 g is used in decoction for oral use.

【用法用量】 水煎服，3～10克。

Notes It is used with caution in cases with brushed tongue with little fluid due to exhaustion of yin and with sthenic heat in the interior.

【使用注意】 阴伤舌红少津及内有实热者慎用。

Qingpi *Pericarpium Citri Reticulatae Viride*

青　皮

The source is from the immature fruit or its pericarp of *Citrus reticuta* Blanco, family Rutaceae. The fruit or its pericarp is collected during the period of May and June, dried in the sun. The crude or the one stir-baked with vinegar can be used.

为芸香科橘及其同属植物的幼果或未成熟果实的果皮。5～6月间采集,晒干。生用或醋炒用。

Medicinal Properties Bitter and pungent in flavor, warm in nature and attributive to the liver, gallbladder and stomach meridians.

【药性】 味苦、辛,性温。归肝、胆、胃经。

Actions Soothe the liver to break qi stagnation, eliminate mass and relieve dyspepsia.

【功效】 疏肝破气,散结消滞。

Application

【临床应用】

1. It is indicated for liver-qi stagnation manifested as hypochondriac distending pain, breast distending pain, and pain due to hernia. For treatment of hypochondriac pain, it is usually used in combination with Chaihu (*Radix Bupleuri*), Yujin (*Radix Curcumae*), etc.; for swelling and pain due to breast abscess, usually combined with Gualou (*Fructus Trichosanthis*), Jinyinhua (*Flos Lonicerae*), Pugongying (*Herba Taraxaci*), and Gancao (*Radix Glycyrrhizae*), etc.; for hernia of cold type with abdominal pain, combined with Wuyao (*Radix Linderae*), Xiaohuixiang (*Fructus Foeniculi*), and Muxiang (*Radix Aucklandiae*), etc., to expel cold, regulate qi and relieve pain, such as Tiantai Wuyao San (Powder).

1. 用于肝气郁滞所致的胁肋胀痛、乳房胀痛及疝气疼痛。治胁痛,常配柴胡、郁金等品;治乳痈肿痛,常配瓜蒌、金银花、蒲公英、甘草等同用;寒疝腹痛,则配乌药、小茴香、木香等以散寒理气止痛,如天台乌药散。

2. For distention and pain of the epigastrium due to

2. 用于食积胃脘痞闷胀

indigestion, it is usually combined with Shanzha (*Fructus Crataegi*), Maiya (*Fructus Hordei Germinatus*), and Shenqu (*Massa Medicata Fermentata*), etc., such as Qingpi Wan (Pill).

痛,常与山楂、麦芽、神曲等配伍,如青皮丸。

In addition, for abdominal mass due to qi stagnation and blood stasis, and malarial nodule, it is combined with Sanleng (*Rhizoma Sparganii*), Ezhu (*Rhizoma Zedoariae*), and Yujin (*Radix Curcumae*), etc..

此外,对气滞血瘀所致的癥瘕积聚,以及疟母等证,可与三棱、莪术、郁金等同用。

Usage and Dosage 3 - 10 g is used in decoction for oral use.

【用法用量】 水煎服,3~10克。

Notes Used with caution in the patient with qi deficiency since it has violent action to damage qi.

【使用注意】 性较峻烈,易耗气、破气,气虚者慎用。

Xiangfu *Rhizoma Cyperi*

香 附

The source is from the rhizome of *Cyperus rotundus* L., family Cyperaceae. The medicinal material is mainly produced in the areas of Guangdong, Henan, and Sichuan, etc., collected during the period of December and October, dried in the sun, the hair being removed by burning. The crude or the one stir-baked with vinegar can be used.

为莎草科植物莎草的根茎。主产于广东、河南、四川等地。9~10月采收,挖取根茎,晒干,烧去须根。生用或醋炒用。

Medicinal Properties Pungent, slightly bitter and sweet in flavor, mild in nature and attributive to the liver and triple energizer meridians.

【药性】 味辛、微苦、微甘,性平。归肝、三焦经。

Actions Soothe the liver to regulate qi and regulate menstruation to relieve pain.

【功效】 疏肝理气,调经止痛。

Application

【临床应用】

1. It is used for the syndromes of stagnation of liver-qi with pain in the hypochondrium, distention and pain in epigastric abdomen and pain due to hernia, etc.. For pain in the hypochondrium, it can be combined with Chaihu (*Radix Bupleuri*), Baishaoyao (*Radix Paeoniae Alba*), Zhike (*Fructus Aurantii*), etc., such as Chaihu Shugan San (Powder); for liver-qi invading the stomach and accumulation of cold and qi stagnation with cold and pain in ep-

1. 用于肝气郁滞所致的胁肋作痛、脘腹胀痛及疝痛等证。治胁痛,可与柴胡、白芍药、枳壳等配伍,如柴胡疏肝散;肝气犯胃、寒凝气滞之胃脘冷痛,可配高良姜,即良附丸;治寒疝腹痛,则与小茴香、乌药等同用。

igastrium, combined with Gaoliangjiang (*Rhizoma Alpiniae Officinarum*) like Liang Fu Wan (Pill); for hernia of cold type with abdominal pain, combined with Xiaohuixiang (*Fructus Foeniculi*), Wuyao (*Radix Linderae*), etc..

2. For irregular menstruation, dysmenorrhea and distension and pain of the breast, especially those caused by stagnation of liver-qi, it is usually combined with Danggui (*Radix Angelicae Sinensis*), Chuanxiong (*Rhizoma Chuanxiong*), Baishaoyao (*Radix Paeoniae Alba*), and Chaihu (*Radix Bupleuri*), etc., to soothe the liver to remove stagnation and regulate qi and blood.

2. 用于月经不调,痛经及乳房胀痛。尤宜用于因肝气郁结所致者,常配当归、川芎、白芍药、柴胡等以疏肝行滞,调和气血。

Usage and Dosage 5 – 10 g is used in decoction for oral use.

【用法用量】 水煎服,5～10克。

Muxiang *Radix Aucklandiae*

木 香

The source is from the root of *Aucklandia lappa* Decne., family Compositae. The medicinal material is mainly produced in the areas of Yunnan and Sichuan, dug and collected in autumn and winter, washed cleanly, dried in the sun. The crude or roasted is used.

为菊科植物木香的根。主产于云南、四川。秋、冬季采挖,洗净,晒干。生用或煨用。

Medicinal Properties Pungent and bitter in flavor, warm in nature and attributive to the spleen, stomach, large intestine and gallbladder meridians.

【药性】 味辛、苦,性温。归脾、胃、大肠、胆经。

Actions Promote circulation of qi and alleviate pain.

【功效】 行气止痛。

Application

【临床应用】

1. It is used for stomach and spleen qi-stagnation syndrome and meanwhile is an essential medicine to activate qi circulation and alleviate pain. For epigastric fullness and pain due to stagnation of qi, it is used in combination with Jupi (*Pericarpium Citri Tangerinae*), Sharen (*Fructus Amomi*), and Tanxiang (*Lignum Santali Albi*), etc.; for the stagnation of spleen-qi due to spleen-deficiency with mass and oppression in the chest

1. 用于脾胃气滞证。为行气止痛之要药。治气滞脘腹胀痛,与橘皮、砂仁、檀香等同用。治脾虚气滞,脘腹痞闷,食少便溏,可与党参、白术、橘皮等同用,如香砂六君子汤。

and epigastric abdomen, loss of appetite, diarrhea, it is used together with Dangshen (*Radix Codonopsis*), Baizhu (*Rhizoma Atractylodis Macrocephalae*), and Jupi (*Pericarpium Citri Tangerinae*), etc., such as Xiang Sha Liujunzi Tang (Decoction).

2. For dysentery due to dampness and heat with tenesmus, usually combined with Huanglian (*Rhizoma Coptidis*), such as Xiang Lian Wan (Pill); for fullness and pain in the epigastrium due to indigestion with constipation or difficulty in diarrhea, used together with Binglang (*Semen Arecae*), Qingpi (*Pericarpium Citri Reticulatae Viride*), and Dahuang (*Radix et Rhizoma Rhei*), etc., such as Muxiang Binglang Wan (Pill).

2. 用于湿热泻痢，里急后重。常与黄连配伍，如香连丸。若治饮食积滞的脘腹胀痛、大便秘结或泻而不爽，可与槟榔、青皮、大黄等同用，如木香槟榔丸。

3. For steaming fever due to dampness and heat, and failure of the liver and gallbladder to disperse with hypochondriac distension and pain, jaundice, bitter taste in the mouth, and yellowish tongue coating, etc., it is used together with Chaihu (*Radix Bupleuri*), Yujin (*Radix Curcumae*), and Zhike (*Fructus Aurantii*), etc.. Now it has certain therapeutical effects in treatment of cholelithiasis and gallstone colic.

3. 用于湿热郁蒸，肝胆疏泄不利之胁肋胀痛、黄疸、口苦、苔黄等，可与柴胡、郁金、枳壳等配伍。现代用治胆石症、胆绞痛，有一定疗效。

In addition, it is also added to tonics with small amount for decreasing the greasy property of tonics and preventing such side effects from appearing as chest distress, abdominal distension, and loss of appetite.

此外，应用滋补药物时配用少量木香，可降低其壅滞黏腻之性，防止出现胸闷、腹胀、食欲减退等副作用。

Usage and Dosage 3 - 10 g is used in decoction for oral use. The crude herb is large in an action of circulating qi while the roasted is mild in the action and usually used for diarrhea.

【用法用量】 水煎服，3～10 g。生用行气力强，煨用行气力缓而多用于止泻。

Zhishi *Fructus Aurantii Immaturus*

枳 实

The source is from the immature fruit of *Citrus aurantium* L., or *Citrus wilsonii* Tana ka, family Rutaceae. The medicinal material is mainly produced in the provinces of Sichuan, Jiangxi, Fujian, and Zhejiang, etc.,

为芸香科植物酸橙及其栽培变种或甜橙的未成熟果实。主产于四川、江西、福建、浙江等省。5～6 月采收，晒

collected during the period of May and June, dried in the sun, the crude or the one stir-baked with bran can be used.

干。生用或麸炒用。

Medicinal Properties Bitter and pungent in flavor, slightly cold in nature and attributive to the spleen, stomach and large intestine meridians.

【药性】 味苦、辛,性微寒。归脾、胃、大肠经。

Actions Break stagnation of qi and remove food retention, resolve phlegm and eliminate mass.

【功效】 破气消积,化痰除痞。

Application

【临床应用】

1. It is indicated for the treatment of indigestion, constipation due to accumulation of heat and dysentery. For indigestion and fullness and pain in the chest and upper abdomen, it is used together with Shanzha (*Fructus Crataegi*), Maiya (*Fructus Hordei Geminatus*), and Shenqu (*Massa Medicata Fermentata*), etc.; for constipation due to accumulation of heat, abdominal mass, and fullness and pain in the epigastrium, it can be combined with Houpo (*Cortex Magnoliae Officinalis*), Dahuang (*Radix et Rhizoma Rhei*), Mangxiao (*Natrii Sulfas*), such as Da Chengqi Tang (Decoction); for stagnation of dampness and heat with dysentery and tenesmus, combined with Dahuang (*Radix et Rhizoma Rhei*), Huanglian (*Rhizoma Coptidis*), and Huangqin (*Radix Scutellariae*), etc., such as Zhishi Daozhi Wan (Pill).

1. 用于食积,热结便秘,泻痢。治饮食积滞不化,脘腹痞满胀痛,可配山楂、麦芽、神曲等;治热结便秘,腹痞胀痛,可配厚朴、大黄、芒硝,即大承气汤;湿热积滞,泻痢后重者,可配大黄、黄连、黄芩等,如枳实导滞丸。

2. It is used for turbid phlegm obstructing qi activity with fullness in the chest and epigastrium. For the syndrome due to deficiency of stomach-yang and accumulation of cold-phlegm, it can be combined with Xiebai (*Bulbus Allii Macrostemi*), Guizhi (*Ramulus Cinnamomi*), and Gualou (*Fructus Trichosanthis*), etc., such as Zhishi Xiebai Guizhi Tang (Decoction); for stagnation of dampness-phlegm in the middle energizer, fullness in the epigastric abdomen, poor appetite, combined with Houpo

2. 用于痰浊阻塞气机之胸脘痞满。属胸阳不振,寒痰内阻,可配薤白、桂枝、瓜蒌等同用,如枳实薤白桂枝汤;湿痰中阻,心下痞满,食欲不振,可配厚朴、半夏、白术等品,如枳实消痞丸。

(*Cortex Magnoliae Officinalis*), Banxia (*Rhizoma Pinelliae*), and Baizhu (*Rhizoma Atractylodis Macrocephalae*), etc., such as Zhishi Xiaopi Wan (Pill).

In addition, it can be used to treat gastroptosis, prolapse of rectum and uterus, etc., but it must be combined with Chaihu (*Radix Bupleuri*), Shengma (*Rhizoma Cimicifugae*), and Huangqi (*Radix Astragali*), etc. in order to get good therapeutic effect, and it has the action of raising blood pressure as well.

此外,还可用于胃下垂、脱肛、子宫脱垂等,但须配柴胡、升麻、黄芪等,效果才明显。本品尚有升高血压作用。

Usage and Dosage 3 - 10 g is used in decoction for oral use and a large dosage is 15 g.

【用法用量】 水煎服,3~10克;大剂量可用15克。

Notes It is used with caution in the cases with deficiency of the spleen and stomach and pregnant women.

【使用注意】 脾胃虚弱者及孕妇慎用。

Explanation Zhike (*Fructus Aurantii*) is nearly mature fruit of *Citrus aurantium* L., which is collected in autumn and removed of the pulp, the stir-baked with bran for medication or the crude being used. Its nature and flavor, meridian tropism, actions and administration are the same as Zhishi (*Fructus Aurantii Immaturus*), yet it has less powerful effect. It is mainly used to regulate qi, comfort the middle energizer and relieve distention.

【说明】 枳壳:为枳实原植物的接近成熟的果实(去瓤),生用或麸炒用。性味、归经、功用与枳实同,但作用较和缓,以行气宽中除胀为主。用法用量同枳实。

Xiebai *Bulbus Allii Macrostemi*

薤 白

The source is from the bulb of *Allium maerostemon* Bunge, family Liliaceae. The medicinal material is produced in all parts of China, collected in both summer and autumn, dried in the sun and the crude form can be used.

为百合科植物小根蒜的地下鳞茎。中国各地均产。夏、秋两季采挖,晒干。生用。

Medicinal Properties Pungent and bitter in flavor, warm in nature and attributive to the lung, stomach and large intestine meridians.

【药性】 味辛、苦,性温。归肺、胃、大肠经。

Actions Activate yang and disperse lumps, promote qi circulation and relieve the stagnation.

【功效】 通阳散结,行气导滞。

Application

【临床应用】

1. It is used to treat turbid phlegm and thoracic fullness due to deficiency of thoracic yang. It is characterized

1. 用于痰浊凝滞,胸阳不振的胸痹证。可散阴寒之结

by its dispersing, descending and warming actions and can be used to disperse accumulation of cold and activate dispersing function of yang in the chest. Therefore, it is used every time together with Gualou (*Fructus Trichosanthis*) that resolves phlegm and disperses accumulation and regulate flow of qi, such as Gualou Xiebai Baijiu Tang (Decoction) and Gualou Xiebai Banxia Tang (Decoction); for the above syndrome with blood stasis marked by stabbing pain in the epigastrium, Danshen (*Radix Salviae Miltiorrhizae*), Honghua (*Flos Carthami*), and Chishaoyao (*Radix Paeoniae Rubra*), etc., are added to the combinations.

而温通胸阳,每与化痰散结、宽胸理气的瓜蒌配伍,如瓜蒌薤白白酒汤、瓜蒌薤白半夏汤;兼有瘀血阻滞,胸脘刺痛者,可再加丹参、红花、赤芍药等。

2. For qi stagnation in the stomach and intestine manifested as dysentery with tenesmus, it is used in combination with Muxiang (*Radix Aucklandiae*), Baishaoyao (*Radix Paeoniae Alba*), and Zhishi (*Fructus Aurantii Immaturus*), etc.; for dysentery due to dampness and heat, with Huangbai (*Cortex Phellodendri*) and Qinpi (*Cortex Fraxini*).

2. 用于胃肠气滞,泻痢后重。可配木香、白芍药、枳实等;湿热泻痢,也可与黄柏、秦皮配用。

Usage and Dosage 5 - 10 g is used in decoction for oral use.

【用法用量】 水煎服,5～10克。

Notes The herb is not suitable for the cases with deficiency of qi but no stagnation, weakness of the stomach with loss of appetite and being unable to bear the smell of garlics.

【使用注意】 气虚无滞、胃弱纳呆及不耐蒜味者不宜用。

Wuyao *Radix Linderae*

乌　药

The source is from the root tuber of *Lindera strychnifolia* (Sieb. et Zucc.) Will., family Lauraceae. The medicinal material is mainly produced in the areas of Zhejiang, Anhui, and Jiangxi, etc., collected all year round, dried in the sun. The crude or the one stir-baked with bran is used for medication.

为樟科植物乌药(天台乌药)的根。主产于浙江、安徽、江西等地。全年可采挖,晒干。生用或麸炒用。

Medicinal Properties Pungent in flavor, warm in nature and attributive to the lung, spleen, kidney and

【药性】 味辛,性温。归肺、脾、肾、膀胱经。

bladder meridians.

Actions Promote the circulation of qi to relieve pain, and warm the kidney to disperse cold.

Application

1. It is indicated for stagnation of cold and qi manifested as oppression and pain in the chest, fullness and pain in the epigastrium, hernia of cold type and dysmenorrhea. For oppression in the chest and hypochondriac pain, it is combined with Xiebai (*Bulbus Allii Macrostemi*), Gualoupi (*Pericarpium Trichosanthis*), Yujin (*Radix Curcumae*), and Yanhusuo (*Rhizoma Corydalis*), etc.; for distension and pain in the epigastrium, combined with Muxiang (*Radix Aucklandiae*), Wuzhuyu (*Fructus Evodiae*), and Zhike (*Fructus Aurantii*), etc.; for hernia of cold type and low abdominal pain involving testis, combined with Xiaohuixiang (*Fructus Foeniculi*), Muxiang (*Radix Aucklandiae*), Gaoliangjiang (*Rhizoma Alpiniae Officinarum*) and others that disperse cold, circulate qi and relieve pain, such as Tiantai Wuyao San (Powder); for abdominal pain during menstruation, it can also be used together with Xiangfu (*Rhizoma Cyperi*), Danggui (*Radix Angelicae Sinensis*), and Muxiang (*Radix Aucklandiae*), etc. to regulate flow of qi and blood, such as Wuyao Tang (Decoction).

2. For insufficiency of kidney-yang, frequent urination and enuresis due to deficiency and coldness of the bladder, it is usually used in combination with Yizhiren (*Fructus Alpiniae Oxyphyllae*) and Shanyao (*Rhizoma Dioscoreae*), such as Suoquan Wan (Pill).

Usage and Dosage 3 - 10 g is used in decoction for oral use.

Binglang *Semen Arecae*

The source is from the mature seed of *Areca catechu* L., family Palmae. The medicinal material is mainly pro-

【功效】 行气止痛,温肾散寒。

【临床应用】

1. 用于寒气郁滞所致的胸闷、胁痛、脘腹胀痛、寒疝腹痛及痛经。治胸闷,胁痛,可配薤白、瓜蒌皮、郁金、延胡索等同用;脘腹胀痛,可配木香、吴茱萸、枳壳等;治寒疝、小腹痛引及睾丸,可配小茴香、木香、高良姜等散寒行气止痛,如天台乌药散;经行腹痛,也可配香附、当归、木香等以理气活血,如乌药汤。

2. 用于肾阳不足,膀胱虚寒引起的小便频数及遗尿。常合益智仁、山药同用,如缩泉丸。

【用法用量】 水煎服,3～10克。

槟 榔

为棕榈科植物槟榔的成熟种子。主产于海南、福建、

duced in the areas of Hainan, Fujian, and Yunnan, etc., collected from the end of spring to the early stage of autumn, dried after being boiled, the fruit being peeled and the seed being taken out, dried in the sun. The crude form is used for medication.

云南等地。春末至秋初采收，水煮后，干燥，剥去果皮，取出种子，晒干。生用。

Medicinal Properties Pungent and bitter in flavor, warm in nature and attributive to the stomach and large intestine meridians.

【药性】 味辛、苦，性温。归胃、大肠经。

Actions Activate circulation of qi and relieve dyspepsia, kill parasites and promote diuresis.

【功效】 行气消积，驱虫，利水。

Application

【临床应用】

1. For dyspepsia and stagnation of qi with epigastric fullness, constipation or dysentery with tenesmus, it is usually combined with Muxiang (*Radix Aucklandiae*), Qingpi (*Pericarpium Citri Reticulatae Viride*), and Dahuang (*Radix et Rhizoma Rhei*), etc., such as Muxiang Binglang Wan (Pill).

1. 用于食积气滞，胸腹胀满，便秘或泻痢后重。常与木香、青皮、大黄等同用，如木香槟榔丸。

2. It is used to treat diseases caused by all kinds of parasties such as taeniasis, ancylostomiasis, ascariasis, oxyuriasis, and fasciolopsiasis. Especially most effective for taeniasis, it can be used alone or combined with Nanguazi (*Semen Cucurbitae*); for ascariasis and oxyuriasis, usually combined with Shijunzi (*Fructus Quisqualis*), and Kulianpi (*Cortex Meliae*).

2. 用于绦虫、钩虫、蛔虫、蛲虫、姜片虫等多种寄生虫病。其中对绦虫疗效最佳，单用或与南瓜子同用取效。用治蛔虫、蛲虫证，多与使君子、苦楝皮配伍。

3. It is used for edema and painful beriberi. For edema of sthenia-syndrome and difficulty in urination and defecation, it is usually combined with Shanglu (*Radix Phytolaccae*), Zexie (*Rhizoma Alismatis*), and Mutong (*Caulis Akebiae*), etc., such as Shuzao Yinzi (Decoction); for swollen and painful beriberi of cold-dampness type, usually combined with Mugua (*Fructus Chaenomelis*), Wuzhuyu (*Fructus Evodiae*), and Jupi (*Pericarpium Citri Tangerinae*), etc., such as Jiming San (Powder).

3. 用于水肿、脚气肿痛。治水肿实证，二便不通，常与商陆、泽泻、木通等配伍，如疏凿饮子；治寒湿脚气肿痛，常与木瓜、吴茱萸、橘皮等配伍，如鸡鸣散。

Usage and Dosage 6 – 15 g is used in decoction

【用法用量】 水煎服，

for oral use.

Notes Contraindicated in the cases with diarrhea due to spleen deficiency or qi-collapse due to qi deficiency.

6～15 g。

【使用注意】 脾虚便溏或气虚下陷者忌用。

Chuanlianzi *Fructus Meliae Toosendan*

川楝子

The source is from the mature fruit of *Melia toosendan* Sieb. et Zucc., family Meliaceae. The medicinal material is produced in most parts of China, and that produced in Sichuan is the best. It is collected in winter and dried in the sun. When used, it is broken and the crude form or the one stir-baked with bran is used.

为楝科植物川楝的成熟果实。中国大部分地区均产，以四川产者为最佳。冬季采收，晒干。用时捣破，生用或麸炒用。

Medicinal Properties Bitter in flavor, cold in nature, mildly toxic and attributive to the liver, stomach, small intestine and bladder meridians.

【药性】 味苦，性寒。有小毒。归肝、胃、小肠、膀胱经。

Actions Circulate qi to relieve pain, kill parasites and treat tinea.

【功效】 行气止痛，杀虫，疗癣。

Application

【临床应用】

1. It is used for stagnation of liver-qi or hepatic qi attacking the stomach manifested as hypochondriac pain, stomachache, abdominal pain and hernia, and is more suitable for that with fever. It is usually combined with Yanhusuo (*Rhizoma Corydalis*), such as Jinlingzi San (Powder); for hernia of cold type with low abdominal pain, it is combined with Xiaohuixiang (*Fructus Foeniculi*), Wuzhuyu (*Fructus Evodiae*), and Muxiang (*Radix Aucklandiae*), etc..

1. 用于肝气郁滞或肝胃不和所致的胁肋胀痛、脘腹疼痛以及疝气疼痛等证。以证见热象者较为适宜。常与延胡索配伍，如金铃子散；配小茴香、吴茱萸、木香等，也可治寒疝少腹胀痛。

2. For ascariasis with abdominal pain, it is usually used together with Binglang (*Semen Arecae*), Shijunzi (*Fructus Quisqualis*), etc..

2. 用于蛔虫腹痛。可配槟榔、使君子等同用。

In addition, it can also be used externally for tinea capitis. It can be baked alone till it turns brown, ground into powder, mixed with lard or sesame oil and applied to the local area.

此外，外用可治头癣，可单用焙黄研末，调成油膏，涂于患处。

Usage and Dosage 3－10 g is used in decoction

【用法用量】 水煎服，

for oral use and just right amount for external use.

3～10 克。外用适量。

Notes Since the herb is toxic, overdosage or constant taking of it must be avoided. Besides, it is contraindicated for cold-deficiency type of the spleen and stomach.

【使用注意】 有毒,不可过量或持续服用。脾胃虚寒者不宜用。

Dingxiang *Flos Caryophylli*

丁 香

The source is from the flower bud of *Eugenia caryophyllata* Thunb., which is called Gongdingxiang (*Flos Caryophylli*), family Myrtaceae. The medicinal material is mainly produced in Tanzania, Malaysia, and Indonesia, etc. and also cultivated in Guangdong Province of China. It is collected usually in the period of September and March of the next year when the bud changes from the green to the red, dried in the sun and the crude form is used.

为桃金娘科植物丁香的花蕾,称公丁香。主产于坦桑尼亚、马来西亚、印度尼西亚等地。我国广东亦有栽培。通常在 9 月至次年 3 月间,花蕾由青转为鲜红时采收,干燥。生用。

Medicinal Properties Pungent in flavor, warm in nature and attributive to the spleen, stomach and kidney meridians.

【药性】 味辛,性温。归脾、胃、肾经。

Actions Warm the middle energizer and lower the adverse rising qi, warm the kidney to strengthen yang.

【功效】 温中降逆,温肾助阳。

Application

【临床应用】

1. It is used for stomach-cold syndrome with vomiting, hiccup, poor appetite and loose stool, and is an essential medicine to treat stomach-cold syndrome with vomiting and hiccup. For hiccup due to deficiency and cold, it is usually used in combination with Renshen (*Radix Ginseng*), Shengjiang (*Rhizoma Zingiberis Recens*), such as Dingxiang Shidi Tang (Decoction); for stomach-cold type with vomiting, used together with Banxia (*Rhizoma Pinelliae*); for deficiency and cold of the spleen and stomach with vomiting and diarrhea, used together with Sharen (*Fructus Amomi*) and Baizhu (*Rhizoma Atractylodis Macrocephalae*).

1. 用于胃寒呕吐、呃逆,以及少食、腹泻等。为治疗胃寒呕吐、呃逆之要药。治虚寒呃逆,常与人参、生姜同用,如丁香柿蒂汤;治胃寒呕吐,可与半夏同用;治脾胃虚寒,吐泻食少,可与砂仁、白术同用。

2. For insufficiency of kidney-yang resulting in impo-

2. 用于肾阳不足所致的

tence, premature ejaculation and soreness of back, it is used together with Fuzi (*Radix Aconiti Lateralis Praeparata*), Rougui (*Cortex Cinnamomi*), and Bajitian (*Radix Morindae Officinalis*), etc..

阳痿、早泄、腰酸。可与附子、肉桂、巴戟天等同用。

Usage and Dosage 2 - 5 g is used in decoction for oral use.

【用法用量】 水煎服，2～5 克。

Notes It is incompatible with Rougui (*Cortex Cinnamomi*).

【使用注意】 畏肉桂。

Explanation Mudingxiang (*Flos Caryophylli*) is the mature fruit of *Eugenia caryophyllata* Thunb., also called Jishexiang (*Flos Caryophylli*). Its nature, taste and action are same as those of Gongdingxiang (*Flos Caryophylli*), yet it has less powerful effect.

【说明】 母丁香为丁香的成熟果实，又名鸡舌香，性味、功用与公丁香相似而力较弱。

Chenxiang *Lignum Aquilariae Resinatum*

沉 香

The source is from the dark brown resinous wood of *Aquilaria sinensis* (Lour) Gilg, family Thymelaeaceae. The medicinal material is mainly produced in the areas of Guangdong, Guangxi and Taiwan of China. The resinous wood or the root part is cut, collected and dried in shade, ground into powder for medication.

为瑞香科植物白木香含有黑色树脂的木材。主产于广东、广西、台湾。割取含有树脂的木部和根部，阴干。锉末或磨粉服。

Medicinal Properties Pungent and bitter in flavor, warm in nature and attributive to the spleen, stomach and kidney meridians.

【药性】 味辛、苦，性温。归脾、胃、肾经。

Actions Send down adverse flow of qi to regulate the function of the middle energizer, promote the circulation of qi to relieve pain, warm the kidney to improve inspiration.

【功效】 降逆调中，行气止痛，温肾纳气。

Application

【临床应用】

1. For stomach-cold with vomiting and hiccup, it can be combined with Dingxiang (*Flos Caryophylli*) and Baidoukou (*Fructus Amomi Rotundus*).

1. 用于胃寒呕吐，呃逆。可配丁香、白豆蔻同用。

2. For syndrome of stagnation of cold and qi with fullness and oppression in the chest and epigastric abdomen, it is usually combined with Wuyao (*Radix Lin-*

2. 用于寒凝气滞，胸腹胀闷作痛之证。常与乌药、木香、槟榔配伍，即沉香四磨汤。

derae), Muxiang (*Radix Aucklandiae*) and Binglang (*Semen Arecae*), such as Chenxiang Simo Tang (Decoction).

3. For syndrome with extreme asthenia of kidney-yang and failure of the kidney to promote inspiration with dyspnea and cough due to retention of phlegm, and syndrome of hypersthenia and hypoasthenia; for the former, it can be combined with Fuzi (*Radix Aconiti Lateralis Praeparata*), Rougui (*Cortex Cinnamomi*), and Buguzhi (*Fructus Psoraleae*), etc.; for the latter, usually combined with Zisuzi (*Fructus Perillae*), Qianhu (*Radix Peucedani*), Houpo (*Cortex Magnoliae Officinalis*), Jupi (*Pericarpium Citri Tangerinae*), Banxia (*Rhizoma Pinelliae*) and others that resolve phlegm to relieve cough and lower the adverse-rising qi and relieve dyspnea.

3. 用于下元虚冷，肾不纳气之虚喘，以及痰饮咳喘，上盛下虚之证。对于前者，可与附子、肉桂、补骨脂等配伍；对于后者，常与紫苏子、前胡、厚朴、橘皮、半夏等化痰止咳、降气平喘之品同用。

Usage and Dosage 1-1.5 g of the powder is swallowed with water or the herb is pounded into juice for oral use.

【用量用法】 研末冲服，1～1.5克；亦可用原药磨汁服。

Notes The herb is pungent and warm to support heat, therefore it is used with caution in cases with hyperactivity of fire due to yin deficiency.

【使用注意】 本品辛温助热，阴虚火旺者慎用。

Shidi *Calyx Kaki*

柿　蒂

The source is from the persistent calyx of *Diospyro Kaki* L.f., family Ebenaceae. The medicinal material is mainly produced in the areas of Sichuan, Guangdong, Fujian, Shandong, and Henan, etc., collected during the period of August and September, dried in the sun and the crude form is used.

为柿科植物柿树的宿存花萼。主产于四川、广东、福建、山东、河南等地。8～9月收集花萼，晒干。生用。

Medicinal Properties Bitter in flavor, bland in nature and attributive to the stomach meridians.

【药性】 味苦，性平。归胃经。

Actions Lower the adverse rising qi and relieve hiccup.

【功效】 降气止呃。

Application

It is used to treat syndrome of hiccup, and can be combined with relevant medicinal herbs according to symptoms and signs. For hiccup due to stomach-cold, it is combined with Dingxiang (*Flos Caryophylli*) and Shengjiang (*Rhizoma Zingiberis Recens*), that is, Shidi Tang (Decoction) to warm the stomach and lower the adverse-rising qi and relieve hiccup; for that due to stomach-heat, combined with Lugen (*Rhizoma Phragmitis*), Zhuru (*Caulis Bambusae in Taeniam*) and others that clear away heat from the stomach.

Usage and Dosage 5 - 10 g is used in decoction for oral use.

【临床应用】

用于呃逆之证。可视证情不同而选配相应的药物。如胃寒气逆者,可配丁香、生姜以温中降逆止呃,即柿蒂汤;若属胃热呃逆,亦可与芦根、竹茹等清胃药配伍同用。

【用法用量】 水煎服,5～10克。

7 Food Retention Relieving Chinese Medicinal Herbs

第七章 消食药

Any Chinese medicinal herb that takes promoting digestion and relieving dyspepsia, restoring transportation and transformation of the spleen and stomach as the dominant actions, and meanwhile can treat the syndrome of indigestion is considered as food retention relieving Chinese medicinal herbs.

凡以消食化积，恢复脾胃运化为主要功效，治疗食积证的药物，称为消食药。

In addition to digesting and relieving food accumulation and stagnation, most of them have the actions of increasing appetite and harmonizing the stomach and spleen. They are indicated for indigested syndrome with epigastric and abdominal fullness, belching, acid regurgitation, nausea, vomiting, lack of appetite, and irregular bowel movement such as constipation or diarrhea, etc., which are all due to food accumulation.

消食药除能消化饮食积滞外，多数具有开胃和中的作用。可以治疗饮食积滞、脘腹胀满、嗳腐吞酸、恶心呕吐、不思饮食、大便失常等消化不良证。

When they are used, they are usually combined wtih qi regulating medicinal herbs to promote digestion and relieve dyspepsia, and meanwhile other appropriate medicinal herbs must be combined with separately according to different conditions, such as those for warming the spleen and stomach, clearing away heat or eliminating dampness. For indigestion due to deficiency of the spleen and stomach, those for nourishing the spleen and stomach must be taken as dominants and the digestive herbs as assistants.

使用时，常配理气药，可助消食化滞，并根据病情分别配伍温中、清热、化湿药。食积因脾胃虚弱者，应以补养脾胃为主，辅以消导。

Shanzha *Fructus Crataegi*

山 楂

The source is from the fruit of *Crataegus cuneata* Sieb. et Zucc., or *C. pinnatifida* Bunge, family Rosaceae. The medicinal material is mainly produced in the

为蔷薇科植物山里红或山楂的果实。主产于河南、江苏、浙江、安徽等省。秋末冬

provinces of Henan, Jiangsu, Zhejiang, and Anhui, etc., collected in the end of autumn and the early stage of winter, dried in the sun. The raw or the stir-baked one can be used.

初采收,晒干。生用或炒用。

Medicinal Properties Sour and sweet in flavor, slightly warm in nature, and attributive to the spleen, stomach and liver meridians.

【药性】 味酸、甘,性微温。归脾、胃、肝经。

Actions Digest food and dissipate the food accumulation, circulate the blood and disperse blood stasis.

【功效】 消食化积,活血散瘀。

Application

【临床应用】

1. It is indicated for syndrome of indigestion manifested as epigastric fullness and distention, abdominal pain with diarrhea, especially improperly eating meats and fat. For indigestion of food and meats, it can be decocted alone or combined with Shenqu (*Massa Medicata Fermentata*), and Maiya (Fructus Hordei Germanatus), etc.; for obvious fullness and pain in epigastrium, it is combined with Muxiang (*Radix Aucklandiae*), Zhike (*Fructus Aurantii*), etc.; for abdominal pain with diarrhea due to improper diet, the charred one can be ground into powder, which is mixed with water for oral use.

1. 用于食滞不化,脘腹胀满,腹痛泄泻。擅长于消化油腻肉食积滞。治食肉不消,单用煎服即可;也常与神曲、麦芽等配伍;脘腹胀痛明显者,可配木香、枳壳等;伤食腹痛泄泻,可用焦山楂研末,开水调服。

2. It is used for blood-stasis syndrome manifested as postpartum abdominal pain with lochiostasis, hernia with bearing-down distending pain; for postpartum blood-stasis, it is usually combined with Danggui (*Radix Angelicae Sinensis*), Chuanxiong (*Rhizoma Chuanxiong*), and Yimucao (*Herba Leonuri*); for pain due to hernia, combined with Xiaohuixiang (*Fructus Foeniculi*), Juhe (*Semen Citri Reticulatae*), etc..

2. 用于产后瘀阻腹痛、恶露不尽,疝气偏坠胀痛。治产后血瘀证,常与当归、川芎、益母草等配伍;治疝气,可与小茴香、橘核等同用。

Besides, it can also be used for hypertension, coronary heart disease and hyperlipemia.

此外,本品生用还可治疗高血压病、冠心病及高脂血症。

Usage and Dosage 10 - 12 g is used in decoction for oral use, the raw is a bit on the side of promoting

【用法用量】 水煎服,10～12 克。生山楂偏于消食

digestion and relieving dyspepsia, and the charred one is a bit on the side of relieving diarrhea and dysentary.

散结,焦山楂偏于止泻止痢。

Shenqu　*Massa Medicata Fermentata*

神　曲

This medicinal herb consists of the mixture of fermented powders of wheat flour, *Semen Armeniacae Amarum*, sprout of *Semen Phaseoli*, *Herba Artmisiae Annuae*, *Fructus Xanthii*, and *Herba Polygoni Hydropiperis*, etc.. The medicinal material is produced in all parts of China. The crude or the stir-baked is used for medication.

为面粉和杏仁泥、赤小豆粉、鲜青蒿、鲜苍耳、鲜辣蓼自然汁等混合后经发酵而成的加工品。中国各地均产。长出菌丝(生黄衣)后,取出晒干。生用或炒用。

Medicinal Properties　Sweet and pungent in flavor and warm in nature and attributive to the spleen and stomach meridians.

【药性】 味甘、辛,性温。归脾、胃经。

Actions　Promote digestion and harmonize the stomach.

【功效】 消食和胃。

Application

【临床应用】

For dyspepsia with epigastric distention, poor appetite and diarrhea, it is usually combined with Shanzha (*Fructus Crataegi*), Maiya (*Fructus Hordei Germinatus*), etc.. Furthermore, it has a little the action of relieving exterior syndrome, so it's more suitable for dyspepsia due to exogenous pathogenic factors.

用于食积不化,脘腹胀满,不思饮食及肠鸣泄泻。常与山楂、麦芽等同用。又本品略有解表之功,故外感食滞者有之尤宜。

In addition, if a pill includes mineral and shell medicine that is difficult to be absorbed, Shenqu (*Massa Medicata Fermentata*) can be added so as to promote digestion and is a excipient as well, such as Ci Zhu Wan (Pill).

此外,丸剂中有矿物、贝壳药物,难于消化吸收者,可用神曲糊丸,以助消化并赋形,如磁朱丸。

Usage and Dosage　5 – 15 g is used in decoction for oral use.

【用法用量】 水煎服,5～15克。

Maiya　*Fructus Hordei Germinatus*

麦　芽

The source is from the germinant fruit of *Hordeum vulgare* L., family Gramineae. The medicinal material is produced in all parts of China, the crude or the one stir-baked into yellow is used for medication.

为禾本科植物大麦的成熟果实经发芽干燥而成,中国各地均产。随时制备。生用或炒黄用。

Medicinal Properties　Sweet in flavor, bland in

【药性】 味甘,平。归

nature and attributive to the spleen, stomach and liver meridians.

脾、胃、肝经。

Actions Digest the accumulated food and harmonize the middle energizer, and help stop lactation.

【功效】 消食和中，回乳。

Application

【临床应用】

1. It is used for food accumulation and indigestion, epigastric distress and abdominal distention, especially for helping digest starch food, it is usually combined with Shanzha (*Fructus Crataegi*), Shenqu (*Massa Medicata Fermentata*), and Jineijin (*Endothelium Corneum Gigeriae Galli*), etc.; for poor transportation and transformation due to deficiency of the spleen and stomach, the tonics can be combined with the herb.

1. 用于食积不化、脘闷腹胀等。擅于助淀粉类食物消化。常与山楂、神曲、鸡内金等同用。脾胃虚弱而运化不良者，可以在补气药中配用本品。

2. It can be used for delactation for breast-feeding women or for distention and pain of the breast due to galactostasis, 30 -60 g of the crude one and same amount of the fried one can be decocted and taken separately every day.

2. 用于妇女断乳，或乳汁郁积所致的乳房胀痛等证。麦芽有回乳之功。可每天用生、炒麦芽各 30～60 克煎汁分服。

Usage and Dosage 10 - 15 g is used in decoction for oral use, large dose can be increased to 30 - 120 g.

【用法用量】 水煎服，10～15 克，大剂量 30～120 克。

Notes It is not suitable to be used in breast-feeding period.

【使用注意】 授乳期不宜用。

Jineijin *Endothelium Corneum Gigeriae Galli*

鸡内金

The source is from the membrane of the gizzard of *Gallus domesticus* Brisson, family Phasianidae. The medicinal material, after being cleaned, is dried in the sun and then ground into powder that can be used or the stir-baked for being used.

为雉科动物鸡的沙囊的角质内壁。剥离后洗净晒干。研末生用或炒用。

Medicinal Properties Sweet in flavor, bland in nature and attributive to the spleen, stomach, small intestine and bladder meridians.

【药性】 味甘，性平。归脾、胃、小肠、膀胱经。

Actions Strengthen the spleen to improve digestion, arrest seminal emission and relieve enuresis.

【功效】 运脾消食，固精止遗。

Application

1. It is used for indigestion, food accumulation, and infantile malnutrition. For milder cases, it is stir-baked singly and ground into powder for oral use; for the syndrome with food accumulation and fullness of epigastrium, it is combined with Shanzha (*Fructus Crataegi*), Maiya (*Fructus Hordei Germinatus*), etc.; for infantile malnutrition due to spleen-deficiency, combined with Baizhu (*Rhizoma Atractylodis Macrocephalae*), Shanyao (*Rhizoma Dioscoreae*), and Fuling (*Poria*), etc..

2. It is used for syndromes of enuresis and emission. For enuresis, it is used in combination with Sangpiaoxiao (*Ootheca Mantidis*), Fupenzi (*Fructus Rubi*), etc.; for emission, used in combination with Lianzi (*Semen Nelumbinis*), Tusizi (*Semen Cuscutae*), etc..

In addition, it also has the action of eliminating stones, so it can be used for urinary and gall stones and usually combined with Jinqiancao (*Herba Lysimachiae*).

Usage and Dosage 3 - 10 g is used in decoction for oral use; 1.5 - 3 g of the powder being taken with better effect.

【临床应用】

1. 用于消化不良,食积不化,及小儿疳积。病情较轻者,单用炒研末服有效;用治食积不化,脘腹胀满,可与山楂、麦芽等配伍;治小儿脾虚疳积,可与白术、山药、茯苓等同用。

2. 用于遗尿、遗精等证。治遗尿,与桑螵蛸、覆盆子等配伍;治遗精,可配莲子、菟丝子等同用。

此外,尚有消结石作用,可用于尿路结石及胆结石,常与金钱草配用。

【用法用量】 水煎服,3～10克。研末服,1.5～3克。研末服效果较好。

8 Hemostatic Chinese Medicinal Herbs

第八章 止血药

Any medicines that mainly stop various bleeding internally or externally are called hemostatic Chinese medicinal herbs. They separately have the different actions of cooling the blood and stopping bleeding, stopping bleeding by their astringent property, by removing obstructions and by warming channels, etc.. They are mainly indicated for bleeding from all parts of the body, such as hemoptysis, haematemesis, epistaxis, hematuria, bloody stools, metrorrhagia and metrostaxis, purpura and traumatic bleeding.

凡以制止体内外出血为主要作用的药物，称为止血药。

止血药分别具有凉血止血、收敛止血、化瘀止血、温经止血等不同作用。主要适用于全身各部分出血，如咯血、吐血、衄血、尿血、便血、崩漏、紫癜及外伤出血。

So, clinically, one must choose proper hemostatic Chinese medicinal herbs that are combined with each other, according to the bleeding causes and specific symptoms and signs, so as to enhance the effects. For example, for bleeding due to blood heat, blood cooling hemostatic herbs should be selected, and combined with those for clearing away heat and cooling the blood; for hyperactivity of yang due to deficiency of yin, those for nourishing yin and suppressing the sthenic yang should be used together; for bleeding due to blood stasis, those for removing blood stasis to stop bleeding should be mainly selected, and used together with those for circulating qi and the blood; for bleeding due to deficiency and cold, those for warming yang, replenishing qi and strengthening the function of the spleen should be used together; for excessive bleeding followed by exhaustion of qi, those for supplementing primordial qi should be used so as to supplement qi.

临床使用时，须根据出血的原因和具体的证候，辨证选用，并进行适当的配伍，以增强疗效。如血热妄行者，应选用凉血止血药，并配伍清热凉血药；阴虚阳亢者，应与滋阴潜阳药同用；瘀血阻滞而出血不止者，应选用化瘀止血药为主，并酌配行气活血药；虚寒性出血，应与温阳、益气、健脾等药同用；出血过多而导致气虚欲脱者，应急予大补元气之药，以益气固脱。

When one applies the blood cooling hemostatic and astringent hemostatic herbs, he/she must pay attention to whether there is blood stasis or not. If bleeding is caused by remaining of blood stasis, one must add herbs for circulating blood to remove blood stasis according to the conditions, and cannot simply use herbs for relieving bleeding and further cannot choose astringent hemostatic and blood cooling hemostatic herbs so as to prevent blood stasis.

使用凉血止血和收敛止血药时,必须注意有无瘀血。瘀血未尽之出血,应酌加活血去瘀药,不能单纯止血,更不宜选用收敛止血及凉血止血药,以免有留瘀之弊。

Daji *Radix Cirsii Japonici*

大 蓟

The source is from the root and herb of *Cirsium japonicum* DC., family Compositae. The medicinal material is mainly produced in all parts of China, collected in summer and autumn when the flower opens, and the root is dug in the end of autumn, dried in the sun, cut into segments. The crude or the stir-baked can be used.

为菊科植物蓟的根及全草。中国各地均产。夏、秋花期时采集全草,秋末采挖根部,晒干,切段。生用或炒用。

Medicinal Properties Sweet and bitter in flavor, cool in nature and attributive to the heart and liver meridians.

【药性】 味甘、苦,性凉。归心、肝经。

Actions Cool the blood and stop bleeding, remove blood stasis to treat carbuncle.

【功效】 凉血止血,散瘀消痈。

Application

【临床应用】

1. For hemoptysis, epistaxis, metrorrhagia and metrostaxis, and hematuria, etc. of blood-heat type, it can be used alone or combined with Xiaoji (*Herba Cephalanoploris*), Cebaiye (*Cacumen Biotae*), etc..

1. 用于血热咯血、衄血、崩漏、尿血等。可单味应用,也可与小蓟、侧柏叶等同用。

2. For sore and carbuncle, it is effective whether it is used internally or externally, the fresh being best in action. Also it can be combined with Jinyinhua (*Flos Lonicerae*), Daqingye (*Folium Isatidis*), and Chishaoyao (*Radix Paeoniae Rubra*), etc..

2. 用于疮痈肿毒。无论内服、外敷,皆有效,以鲜品为佳。也可配金银花、大青叶、赤芍药等同用。

In addition, it can also be used to treat hypertension and hepatitis, and has the actions of lowering blood pressure and draining the gallbladder to relieve jaundice.

此外,亦用于治高血压病及肝炎,有降血压及利胆退黄作用。

Usage and Dosage 10 – 15 g is used in decoction

【用法用量】 水煎服,

for oral use; 30 - 60 g of the fresh; just right amount for external application on the wounded area.

Xiaoji *Herba Cephalanoploris*

The source is from the whole plant of the perennial herbage, *Cephalanoplos segetum* (Bunge) kitam., family Compositae. The medicinal material is produced in all parts of China, collected during flowering period in summer, dried in the sun. The crude one, especially the fresh can be used.

Medicinal Properties Sweet in flavor, cool in nature and attributive to the heart and liver meridians.

Actions Cool the blood and stop bleeding, eliminate toxic materials to treat carbuncle.

Application

1. For bleeding due to blood heat manifested as hemoptysis, epistaxis, haematemesis, hematuria, and metrorrhagia and metrostaxis. Because of its action of promoting diuresis as well, it is usually used together with Puhuang (*Pollen Typhae*), Huashi (*Talcum*), etc., such as Xiaoji Yinzi (Decoction).

2. For sore and carbuncle due to toxic heat, it can be used alone orally, or the fresh can be pounded for external application. The action of eliminating toxic materials and treating carbuncle is the same as that of Daji (*Radix Cirsii Japonici*) while the efficacy is weaker, so they are usually combined with each other.

Usage and Dosage 5 - 15 g is used in decoction for oral use; 30 - 60 g of the fresh, just right amount for external use.

Diyu *Radix Sanguisorbae*

The source is from the root of the perennial herbage, *Sanguisorba officinalis* L., family Rosaceae. The medicinal material is mainly produced in the areas of Zhejiang, Anhui, Hubei, Hunan, and Shandong, etc., dug in

10～15克;鲜品可用至30～60克。外用适量,捣敷患处。

小　蓟

为菊科植物刺儿菜的全草及地下茎。中国各地均产。夏季花期采集,晒干。生用,尤以鲜品为佳。

【药性】 味甘,性凉。归心、肝经。

【功效】 凉血止血,解毒消痈。

【临床应用】

1. 用于血热妄行之咯血、衄血、吐血、尿血及崩漏。因兼能利尿,故擅治尿血。常与蒲黄、滑石等同用,如小蓟饮子。

2. 用于热毒疮痈。可单用内服,亦可取鲜品捣烂外敷。其解毒消痈之功,与大蓟相似而力量较弱,常相须为用。

【用法用量】 水煎服,5～15克;鲜品可用30～60克。外用适量。

地　榆

为蔷薇科植物地榆或长叶地榆的根。主产于浙江、安徽、湖北、湖南、山东等地区。春、秋季采挖,晒干,切片。生

spring and autumn, dried in the sun, cut into slices, the crude or stir-baked one can be used.

用或炒用。

Medicinal Properties　Bitter and sour in flavor, slightly cold in nature, and attributive to the liver, stomach and large intestine meridians.

【药性】 味苦、酸,性微寒。归肝、胃、大肠经。

Actions　Cool the blood and stop bleeding, eliminate toxic materials and treat pyogenic infection.

【功效】 凉血止血,解毒敛疮。

Application

【临床应用】

1. It is used for all kinds of bleeding due to various blood-heat, especially for hematochezia, hemorrhoids, dysentery with bloody stools and metrorrhagia and metrostaxis due to blood-heat in the lower energizer, etc.. For hematochezia and hemorrhoids, it is usually combined with Huaihua (*Flos Sophorae*); for metrorrhagia and metrostaxis due to blood-heat, used in combination with Shengdihuang (*Radix Rehmanniae*), Huangqin (*Radix Scutellariae*), Chaopuhuang (*Pollen Typhae*, fried), etc.; for chronic dysentery with bloody stools, usually combined with Huanglian (*Rhizoma Coptidis*), Muxiang (*Radix Aucklandiae*), and Wumei (*Fructus Mume*), etc., such as Diyu Wan (Pill).

1. 用于各种血热出血,尤其适用于下焦血热所致的便血、痔血、血痢及崩漏等。治便血、痔血,常与槐花合用;治血热崩漏,可与生地黄、黄芩、炒蒲黄等配伍;治血痢经久不愈,常与黄连、木香、乌梅等同用,如地榆丸。

2. For scald, eczema, and skin ulcer, etc., especially for scald, it can be ground into powder that is mixed with sesame oil for application or used together with powder of Dahuang (*Radix et Rhizoma Rhei*); for eczema and skin ulcer, etc., the crude form being decocted into thick decoction for external application; also being combined with Duanshigao (*Gypsum Fibrosum Usta*) and Mingfan (*Alumen*), which are ground together into powder for application.

2. 用于烫伤、湿疹、皮肤溃烂等。为治疗烫伤的要药,可单味研末,麻油调敷,或配大黄粉同用。治湿疹、皮肤溃烂等,可用生地榆煎浓液,浸湿外敷;也可加煅石膏、明矾,研末撒或调敷。

Usage and Dosage　10 – 15 g is used in decoction for oral use, just right amount for external use.

【用法用量】 水煎服,10～15克。外用,适量。

Notes　It is not suitable for large burn with external application so as to prevent the herb from being taken

【使用注意】 大面积烧伤,不宜使用地榆制剂外涂,

largely causing toxic hepatitis.

以防所含水解型鞣质被大量吸收而引起中毒性肝炎。

Huaihua *Flos Sophorae*

槐 花

The source is from the flower bud of *Sophora japonica* L., family Leguminosae. The medicinal material is cultivated in most parts of China. The flower bud is collected from June to July, dried in the sun. The crude or stir-baked one can be used.

为豆科植物槐的花蕾，中国大部分地区均有栽培。6～7月采摘花蕾，晒干。生用或炒用。

Medicinal Properties Bitter in flavor, slightly cold in nature and attributive to the liver and large intestine meridians.

【药性】 味苦，性微寒。归肝、大肠经。

Actions Cool the blood and stop bleeding, clear away liver-heat and lower the fire.

【功效】 凉血止血，清肝降火。

Application

【临床应用】

1. It is used for bleeding due to blood-heat, especially for bleeding from the lower part of the body. The carbonized form is usually used. For hematochezia and hemorrhoids, it is usually combined with Diyu (*Radix Sanguisorbae*); for hemoptysis and epistaxis, usually used together with Xianhecao (*Herba Agrimoniae*), Baimaogen (*Rhizoma Imperatae*), and Cebaiye (*Cacumen Biotae*), etc..

1. 用于血热出血证。尤善于治下部出血。多炒炭用，用于便血、痔血，常与地榆相须配伍；治咯血、衄血，则多与仙鹤草、白茅根、侧柏叶等同用。

2. For headache and conjunctivitis due to flaming-up of the dominant liver-fire, it can be decocted as tea or used together with Xiakucao (*Spica Prunellae*), Juhua (*Flos Chrysanthemi*).

2. 用于肝火上炎之头痛目赤。可单用煎汤代茶，或配夏枯草、菊花等同用。

Usage and Dosage 10－15 g is used in decoction for oral use.

【用法用量】 水煎服，10～15克。

Cebaiye *Cacumen Biotae*

侧柏叶

The source is from the tender branch and leaf of *Biota orientalis* (L.) endl., family Cupressaceae. The plants are cultivated in all parts of China. The medicinal material can be collected all year round. The crude or charred one can be used.

为柏科植物侧柏的嫩枝及叶。中国各地有栽培。全年均可采收。生用或炒炭用。

Medicinal Properties Bitter and astringent in flavor, slightly cold in nature and attributive to the lung, liver and large intestine meridians.

【药性】 味苦、涩,性微寒。归肺、肝、大肠经。

Actions Cool the blood and stop bleeding, eliminate phlegm and relieve cough.

【功效】 凉血止血,祛痰止咳。

Application

【临床应用】

1. It is used for all kinds of internal or external bleedings. For bleeding due to blood-heat manifested as hemoptysis, haematemesis, epistaxis, hematuria, and metrorrhagia and metrostaxis, it can be combined with Daji (*Radix Cirsii Japonici*), Xiaoji (*Herba Cephalanoploris*), Baimaogen (*Rhizoma Imperatae*); for bleeding due to trauma injures, the fresh is used alone externally. Otherwise, in treating bleeding due to deficiency and cold, it is often combined with Aiye (*Folium Artemisiae Argyi*), Paojiang (*Rhizoma Zingiberis Praeparata*) and others that warm channels to stop bleeding.

1. 用于各种内外出血证。治血热妄行之咯血、吐血、鼻衄、尿血、崩漏,可与大蓟、小蓟、白茅根等同用;治外伤出血,单味鲜品外用。与艾叶、炮姜等温经止血药同用,还可治虚寒性出血。

2. For cough with plenty of sputum, especially for cough with yellowish and thick sputum, and dyspnea due to lung-heat, it can be used alone or combined with Huangqin (*Radix Scutellariae*), Shashen (*Radix Adenophorae Strictae*), etc..

2. 用于咳喘痰多。对肺热咳喘,痰黄质稠者尤宜,可单用,或配黄芩、沙参等同用。

In addition, it is also prepared into tincture for external application to treat loss of hair.

此外,还可制成酊剂外搽治脱发。

Usage and Dosage 10 - 15 g is used in decoction for oral use, and just right amount for external use.

【用法用量】 水煎服,10～15克。外用,适量。

Baimaogen *Rhizoma Imperatae*

白茅根

The source is from Rhizome of *Imperata cylindrica* (L.) beauv. var. major (Nees) C. E. Hubb., family Gramineae. The medicinal material is produced in most parts of China, dug and collected in spring when the seedling is not out of soil and after autumn when the plant is withered, and dried in the sun. The crude form is used.

为禾本科植物白茅的根茎。中国多数地区均有分布。春季苗未出土或秋后苗枯时采挖,晒干。生用。

Medicinal Properties Sweet in flavor, cold in

【药性】 味甘,性寒。归

nature and attributive to the lung, stomach and bladder meridians.

肺、胃、膀胱经。

Actions Cool the blood to stop bleeding, clear away heat and promote diuresis.

【功效】 凉血止血,清热利尿。

Application

【临床应用】

1. It is used for bleeding due to blood-heat. For haematemesis and epistaxis, it is usually combined with Xianhecao (*Herba Agrimoniae*); especially for hematuria because of its action of promoting diuresis, usually combined with Cebaiye (*Cacumen Biotae*), Xiaoji (*Herba Cephalanoploris*), and Puhuang (*Pollen Typhae*), etc..

1. 用于血热妄行的出血证。治吐血、衄血,常与仙鹤草配伍;因又能利尿,故治尿血,效果更好,常与侧柏叶、小蓟、蒲黄等合用。

2. For stranguria of heat type, dysuria, edema, and jaundice of dampness-heat type, it is usually combined with Cheqianzi (*Semen Plantaginis*), Jinqiancao (*Herba Lysimachiae*) and others that promote diuresis and eliminate dampness.

2. 用于热淋,小便不利,水肿及湿热黄疸。多配车前子、金钱草等利水渗湿药同用。

In addition, it is usually combined with Lugen (*Rhizoma Phragmitis*) to treat febrile diseases with excessive thirst, vomiting due to stomach-heat and cough due to lung-heat since it can clear away heat from the lung and stomach.

此外,尚能清泄肺胃之热,用治热病烦渴、胃热呕吐及肺热咳嗽等证,常与芦根合用。

Usage and Dosage 15 – 30 g is used in decoction for oral use and 30 g of the fresh is used.

【用法用量】 水煎服,15～30克,鲜品30克。

Baiji *Rhizoma Bletillae*

白 及

The source is from the tuber of *Bletilla striata* (Thunb.) Reichb. f., family Orchidaceae. The medicinal material is mainly produced in the reaches of Yangtze River to the provinces of its south and southwest. It is dug and collected in summer and autumn before the plant is dried, boiled in boiling water, dried in the sun, cut into pieces or pounded into powder for medication.

为兰科植物白及的地下块茎。主产于长江流域至南部及西南各省。夏、秋季苗枯前采挖,沸水煮,晒干,切片或打粉用。

Medicinal Properties Bitter, sweet and astringent in flavor, slightly cold in nature and attributive to the lung, liver and stomach meridians.

【药性】 味苦、甘、涩,性微寒。归肺、肝、胃经。

Actions Stop bleeding by astringing, remove swelling and promote granulation.

【功效】 收敛止血,消肿生肌。

Application

【临床应用】

1. It can be used for hemoptysis, haematemesis and bleeding due to trauma injures. It can be powdered alone and then mixed with water for oral use. It can be used in combination with Pipaye (*Folium Eriobotryae*), Ejiao (*Colla Corii Asini*), and Shengdihuang (*Radix Rehmanniae*), etc. to treat insufficiency of lung-yin with dry cough and hemoptysis; in treating bleeding of stomach, combined with Wuzeigu (*Os Sepiellae seu Sepiae*), etc.; in treating bleeding due to trauma, it can be used alone or combined with Duanshigao (*Gypsum Fibrosum Usta*), which is ground into powder and applied to the local area.

1. 用于咯血、吐血及外伤出血。可单味研末调服。肺阴不足,干咳咯血,也可配枇杷叶、阿胶及生地黄等;治胃出血,多配乌贼骨;外伤出血,单用或配煅石膏研末外敷。

2. It can be used for sores and carbuncle, and rhagadia of hands and feet. For the early stage of carbuncle, it is usually combined with Jinyinhua (*Flos Lonicerae*), Beimu (*Bulbus Fritillariae Thunbergii*), Tianhuafen (*Radix Trichosanthis*), Zaojiaoci (*Spina Gleditsiae*), etc., such as Neixiao San (Powder); for ulcerated and unhealed carbuncle, its powder is usually used externally; for rhagadia of hands and feet, the powder can be mixed with sesame oil and then applied to the local area.

2. 用于疮痈肿毒,手足皲裂。治疮痈初起,常配金银花、贝母、天花粉、皂角刺等,如内消散;如疮痈已溃,久不收口,常研末外用。用于手足皲裂,可研末用麻油调涂。

Besides, it is also used for pulmonary abscess with cough out of fishy sputum, pus and blood that reduce day by day, it is usually combined with Jinyinhua (*Flos Lonicerae*), Jiegeng (*Radix Platycodi*), Shashen (*Radix Adenophorae Strictae*) and Gancao (*Radix Glycyrrhizae*), etc..

此外,本品还可用于肺痈,以咳吐腥痰,脓血日渐减少时为宜,常配金银花、桔梗、沙参、甘草等同用。

Usage and Dosage 3 - 10 g is used in decoction for oral use; 1.5 - 3 g of the powder is used and just right amount for external use.

【用法用量】 水煎服,3～10克;研末服,1.5～3克。外用适量。

Notes It is incompatible with Wutou (*Rhizoma Aconiti*).

【使用注意】 反乌头。

Xianhecao *Herba Agrimoniae*

仙鹤草

The source is from the herb of *Agrimonia pilosa* ledeb., family Rosaceae. The medicinal material is produced in all parts of China, collected in summer and autumn, cut into segments and the crude form is used.

为蔷薇科植物龙芽草的全草。中国各地均产。夏、秋季采收，切段。生用。

Medicinal Properties Bitter and astringent in flavor, bland in nature and attributive to the lung, liver and spleen meridians.

【药性】 味苦、涩，性平。归肺、肝、脾经。

Actions Stop bleeding by astringing, relieve dysentery, restore qi and kill trichomonad.

【功效】 收敛止血，止痢，补虚，杀虫。

Application

【临床应用】

1. For various kinds of bleedings, it can be used alone or in combination according to syndrome. For the bleeding due to blood-heat, it can be used in combination with Shengdihuang (*Radix Rehmanniae*), Mudanpi (*Cortex Moutan Radicis*) and Shanzhizi (*Fructus Gardeniae*); endless metrorrhagia due to deficiency and cold, usually with Dangshen (*Radix Codonopsis*), Huangqi (*Radix Astragali*), Shudihuang (*Rhizoma Rehmanniae Praeparatae*), and Paojiang (*Rhizoma Zingiberis Praeparate*), etc..

1. 用于出血证。可单味应用，亦可随证配伍。属于血热妄行者，可与鲜生地黄、牡丹皮、栀子同用；崩漏不止，证属虚寒，则常与党参、黄芪、熟地黄、炮姜等药同用。

2. It is used for diarrhea and dysentery, especially chronic dysentery and that with bloody stool, since it has action to stop bleeding by astringing. It can be used alone or in combination according to syndrome.

2. 用于腹泻、痢疾。因有收敛止血之性，故多治慢性泻痢及血痢，可单用，也可随证配伍。

3. For patients with internal injury caused by over strain manifested as fatigue and sallow complexion, it can be decocted with same amount of Chinese date into thick decoction, which is taken orally, helping restore health.

3. 用于劳力过度所致的脱力劳伤，见神疲乏力，面色萎黄，可用本品与等量红枣水煎浓汁服用，有助于体力恢复。

Besides, it can also be used to treat itching pudendus, it is usually decocted alone into thick decoction for washing.

此外，还可治阴部瘙痒，常单味煎浓汁冲洗。

Usage and Dosage 10 - 15 g is used in decoction

【用法用量】 水煎服，

for oral use, large dose is 30 - 60 g and just right amount for external use.

10～15克,大剂量可用30～60克。外用,适量。

Sanqi *Radix Notoginseng*

三 七

The source is from the root of *Panax notoginseng* (Burk.) T. H. Chen, family Araliaceae. The medicinal material is mainly produced in the areas of Yunnan, Guangxi, etc.. The root that has grown for over three years is collected. The one that is dug during the first ten days of August, after or before 10 days of the beginning of Autumn is called "Chunsanqi", which is better in quality; The one that is dug in November of winter when the seed is ripe is called "Dongsanqi", which is poorer in quality. The root collected is exposed to the sun until it becomes half dryness, and then it is rubbed with the hands as it is in the sun so as to make its surface smooth and the body somewhat conical and solid, and then dried in the sun. The crude is used.

为五加科植物三七的根。主产于云南、广西等地。采收栽培3年以上的植株。在8月上旬立秋前后10天结籽前采挖的为"春三七",根饱满、质较好;在冬季11月种籽成熟后采挖的为"冬三七",质较差。先曝晒至半干,边晒边搓,使其表皮光滑,体形圆整坚实,晒干。生用。

Medicinal Properties Sweet and slightly bitter in flavor, warm in nature and attributive to the liver and stomach meridians.

【药性】 味甘、微苦,性温。归肝、胃经。

Actions Remove blood stasis to stop bleeding, promote blood circulation and alleviate pain.

【功效】 化瘀止血,活血定痛。

Application

【临床应用】

1. It is used for various kinds of internal and external bleedings, especially for the bleeding with blood stasis, since it has very good action of stopping bleeding, can promote blood circulation to remove blood stasis, and has the advantage of arresting bleeding without stasis and removing blood stasis while healthy qi can be kept. It can be ground singly into powder that is swallowed or combined with Huaruishi (*Ophicalcitum*), Xueyutan (*Crinis Carbonisatus*), such as Huaxue Dan (Pill). For bleeding due to trauma, its powder is used externally on local area to arrest bleeding and alleviate pain.

1. 用于体内外各种出血证。三七止血作用甚佳,并能活血化瘀,具有止血不留瘀,化瘀不伤正气的优点,故对出血兼有瘀滞者尤为适宜。可单味研末吞服;也可配合花蕊石、血余炭同用,即化血丹。创伤出血,可研末外敷,能止血定痛。

2. It is used for trauma with blood-stasis syndrome and painful swelling. It has the actions of promoting blood circulation to remove blood stasis, relieving swelling and especially alleviating pain. It can be used alone or combined with herbs that promote circulation of blood and qi.

2. 用于跌打损伤，瘀滞肿痛。有活血祛瘀、消肿止痛之功，尤长于止痛。可单独应用，亦可配合活血、行气药同用。

In addition, it can circulate the blood and alleviate pain and is used in the treatment of coronary heart disease with angina pectoris and ischemic cerebrovascular disease, etc., also used for chronic hepatitis due to blood stasis.

此外，本品活血定痛用治冠心病心绞痛、缺血性脑血管病等。还可用治血瘀型慢性肝炎等。

Usage and Dosage 3 - 10 g is used in decoction for oral use. 1 - 3 g of the powder is swallowed; just right amount for external use.

【用法用量】 水煎服，3～10克。研粉吞服，1～3 克。外用，适量。

Qiancaogen *Radix Rubiae*

茜草根

The source is from the root of *Rubia Cordifolia* L., family Rubiaceae. The medicinal material is produced in all parts of China, dug and collected in spring and autumn, dried in the sun and the crude or fried one is used.

为茜草科植物茜草的根及根茎。中国各地均产。春、秋两季均可采挖，晒干。生用或炒用。

Medicinal Properties Bitter in flavor, cold in nature and attributive to the liver meridian.

【药性】 味苦，性寒。归肝经。

Actions Cool the blood to stop bleeding, promote blood circulation to remove blood stasis.

【功效】 凉血止血，活血祛瘀。

Application

【临床应用】

1. It is used for various kinds of bleedings due to blood-heat and blood stasis. The crude one is used for cooling blood to stop bleeding; the fried one can stop bleeding as well as promote blood circulation and remove blood stasis, but the carbonized one is used for bleeding without blood stasis. It is usually used in combination with Daji (*Radix Cirsii Japonici*), Xiaoji (*Herba Cephalanoploris*), and Cebaiye (*Cacumen Biotae*), etc., such as Shihui San (Powder)

1. 用于血热夹瘀所致的各种出血证。生用凉血止血；炒用既能活血化瘀，又能止血。凡无瘀滞者宜炒炭用。常与大蓟、小蓟、侧柏叶等同用，如十灰散。

2. It is used for amenorrhea due to blood stasis, traumatic pain, Bi-syndrome with arthralgia. Amenorrhea

2. 用于血滞经闭、跌打损伤及瘀滞作痛及痹证关节疼

can be treated with it in combination with Danggui (*Radix Angelicae Sinensis*), Xiangfu (*Rhizoma Cyperi*), and Chishaoyao (*Radix Paeoniae Rubra*), etc.; traumatic pain can be treated with the single soaked in wine or that in combination with Honghua (*Flos Carthami*), Danggui (*Radix Angelicae Sinensis*) and Chuanxiong (*Rhizoma Chuanxiong*), etc.; Arthralgia can be treated with it in combination with Jixueteng (*Caulis Spatholobi*), Haifengteng (*Caulis Piperis Futokadsurae*) and Yanhushuo (*Rhzoma Corydalis*).

痛。经闭,常配当归、香附、赤芍药等同用;跌打伤痛,可单味泡酒服,亦可与红花、当归、川芎等配伍;关节疼痛,可配鸡血藤、海风藤、延胡索等合用。

Usage and Dosage 10 - 15 g is used in decoction for oral use; the carbonized one is used for stopping bleeding; the crude one or the one stir-baked with wine is used for promoting circulation of the blood; just right amount for external use.

【用法用量】 水煎服,10~15克。止血炒炭用;活血生用或酒炒用。外用,适量。

Puhuang *Pollen Typhae*

蒲　黄

The source is from the pollen of *Typha angustifolia* L., or other species of the same genus, family Typhaceae. The medicinal material is produced in all parts of China. The male one on the flower is collected during May and June when the flower just opens, dried in the sun, ground and the fine power being sieved. The crude or fried one can be used.

为香蒲科植物水烛香蒲或东方香蒲的花粉。中国各地均产。5~6月花刚开放时,采收花序上的雄花,晒干碾压,筛取粉末。生用或炒用。

Medicinal Properties Sweet in flavor, mild in nature and attributive to the liver and pericardium meridians.

【药性】 味甘,性平。归肝、心包经。

Actions Stop bleeding and remove blood stasis, and promote diuresis.

【功效】 化瘀止血,利尿。

Application

【临床应用】

1. It is used for all interior and exterior bleeding syndromes, whether the syndromes are due to cold or heat, with or without blood stasis. The crude can stop bleeding and meanwhile can promote circulation of the blood and remove blood stasis. The carbonized one can

1. 用于内外出血证,无论属寒、属热,有无瘀血均可使用。生用止血而兼能行血化瘀,有止血而不留瘀的优点;炒炭则收涩止血。可单味应

stop bleeding with the astringent action. It can be used alone or together with Xianhecao (*Herba Agrimoniae*), Hanliancao (*Herba Ecliptae*), and Cebaiye (*Cacumen Biotae*), etc.. External application is used for bleeding due to trauma.

用,也可配合仙鹤草、旱莲草、侧柏叶等同用。外敷可用于创伤出血。

2. For angina pectoris, postpartum abdominal pain, and dysmenorrhea, etc., it is usually combined with Wulingzhi (*Faeces Trogopterori*), that is, Shixiao San (Powder).

2. 用于心腹瘀痛、产后瘀痛、痛经等证。常配合五灵脂同用,即失笑散。

3. For stranguria complicated by hematuria, it can be combined with Dongkuizi (*Semen Malvae Verticillatae*) and Shengdihuang (*Radix Rehmanniae*), such as Puhuang San (Powder).

3. 用于血淋涩痛。可配冬葵子、生地黄同用,如蒲黄散。

Besides, it can be used for hyperlipemia in clinic.

此外,临床还用本品治高脂血证。

Usage and Dosage 3 - 10 g is wrapped and used in decoction for oral use and just right amount for external use.

【用法用量】 水煎服,3～10克。包煎。外用适量。

Notes Contraindicated in pregnant women but can be used for postpartum bleeding caused by abnormal uterine contraction.

【使用注意】 孕妇忌服,但可用于产后子宫收缩不良的出血。

Aiye *Folium Artemisiae Argyi*

艾 叶

The source is from the leaf of *Artemisia argyi* levl. et Vant., family Compositae. The medicinal material is produced in all parts of China, collected in the period between spring and summer when the flower is not open, dried in the sun or in shade. The crude or the carbonized one can be used. The plant is cut, dried in the sun and pounded into wool, which is called dry moxa which moxa stick is made of.

为菊科植物艾的叶片。产于我国中部各省。春夏间花未开时采摘;晒干或阴干。生用或炒炭用。若连枝割下,晒干捣绒,名艾绒,供作艾条。

Medicinal Properties Bitter and pungent in flavor, warm in nature and attributive to the liver, spleen and kidney meridians.

【药性】 味苦、辛,性温。归肝、脾、肾经。

Actions Stop bleeding by warming meridians,

【功效】 温经止血,散寒

expel cold and alleviate pain, and prevention of miscarriage.

止痛,安胎。

Application

【临床应用】

1. For bleeding syndrome due to deficiency and cold, especially for metrorrhagia and metrostaxis. It can be carbonized for use or in combination with Ejiao (*Colla Corii Asini*), Dihuang (*Radix Rehmanniae*), etc., such as Jiao'ai Tang (Decoction); for bleeding due to blood heat, such as hemoptysis and epistaxis, the fresh should be used together with fresh Shengdihuang (*Radix Rehmanniae*), Xiancebaiye (*Cacumen Biotae*, fresh) and Heye (*Folium Nelumbinis*).

1. 用于虚寒性出血证,对妇女崩漏下血尤宜。炒炭用,并可与阿胶、地黄等药配伍,如胶艾汤;血热妄行所致的衄血、咯血,也可用鲜艾叶配合大量凉血止血的鲜生地黄、鲜侧柏叶、鲜荷叶等同用。

2. For asthenia-cold of the lower energizer or cold attacking uterus manifested as abdominal pain and cold, irregular menstruation, abdominal pain during menstruation and abnormal leukorrhea, it is usually combined with Danggui (*Radix Angelicae Sinensis*), Xiangfu (*Rhizoma Cyperi*), etc..

2. 用于下焦虚寒或寒客胞宫所致的腹中冷痛,月经不调,经行腹痛,带下。常与当归、香附等同用。

3. For vaginal bleeding during pregnancy and threatened abortion, it is usually combined with Chuanxuduan (*Radix Dipsaci*), Sangjisheng (*Ramulus Taxilli*), etc..

3. 用于胎漏下血,胎动不安。常配伍川续断、桑寄生等同用。

In addition, it is decocted for washing to treat eczema and itching of the skin; the moxa stick made of dry moxa is put over the acupoints and ignited, which can send heat into the interior and has the action of promoting circulation of qi and the blood in the channels by warming. Volatile oil has the actions of relieving cough, removing phlegm and relieving asthma.

此外,本品煎汤外洗,可治皮肤湿疹瘙痒;将艾绒制成艾条、艾柱等,用以烧灸,能使热气内注,具有温煦气血、透达经络的作用。艾叶油有止咳、祛痰、平喘作用。

Usage and Dosage 3 - 10 g is used in decoction for oral use; the stir-baked one is used for warming channels to stop bleeding and other syndromes are treated with the crude; just right amount is used externally.

【用法用量】 水煎服,3～10克。温经止血宜炒用,余则生用;外用,适量。

Paojiang *Rhizoma Zingiberis Praeparata*

The source is from the dried rhizome of *Zingiber officinale* (Willed.) Rosc., family Zingiberaceae. The medicinal herb is prepared by cutting dry ginger into pieces which is stir-baked with strong-fire into burnt-yellow or blackish of the surface and dark brown of the interior.

Medicinal Properties Bitter and astringent in flavor, warm in nature and attributive to the spleen and liver meridians.

Actions Warm channels to stop bleeding and warm the middle energizer to alleviate pain.

Application

1. It is used for haematemesis, hematochezia and metrorrhagia and metrostasis of asthenia-cold type. For asthenia-cold of the thoroughfare and conception vessels and metrorrhagia and metrostaxis, it is combined with Zonglütan (*Petiolus Trachycarpi*, charred), Wumei (*Fructus Mume*) and others that stop bleeding by astringents; besides, it is usually combined with Renshen (*Radix Ginseng*), Huangqi (*Radix Astragali*), and Fuzi (*Radix Aconiti Lateralis Praeparata*), etc. to replenish qi and yang and stop bleeding by warming channels.

2. For abdominal pain and diarrhea of asthenia-cold type, it is used alone or together with Fuzi (*Radix Aconiti Praeparata*); for postpartum deficiency of blood and stagnation of cold with lower abdominal pain, also with Danggui (*Radix Angelicae Sinensis*), Chuanxiong (*Rhizoma Chuanxiong*), etc., such as Shenghua Tang (Decoction).

Usage and Dosage 3 - 6 g is used in decoction for oral use.

炮 姜

为姜科植物姜的干燥根茎的炮制品。将姜块置于锅中,用武火急炒至起泡鼓起,表皮呈焦黄色,或炒炭至外表色黑,内呈棕褐色入药。

【药性】 味苦、涩,性温。归脾、肝经。

【功效】 温经止血,温中止痛。

【临床应用】

1. 用于虚寒性吐血、便血、崩漏等。治冲任虚寒、崩漏下血,配棕榈炭、乌梅等收敛止血药同用;另常配人参、黄芪、附子等同用,以益气助阳,温经止血。

2. 用于虚寒腹痛、腹泻等。可单用或配附子同用;产后血虚寒凝,小腹疼痛,还可配当归、川芎等同用,如生化汤。

【用法用量】 水煎服,3~6克。

9 Chinese Medicinal Herbs for Invigorating the Blood and Removing Blood Stasis

第九章 活血化瘀药

Chinese medicinal herbs with the main action of facilitating blood flow and removing blood stasis are called medicinal herbs for invigorating the blood and removing blood stasis, in which those with strong power of promoting blood circulation and removing blood stasis are also called drastic medicinal herbs for removing blood stasis.

凡以通畅血行，消除瘀血为主要作用的药物，称活血化瘀药，或称活血祛瘀药。其中活血逐瘀作用较强者，又称破血药。

They are mostly pungent and bitter in flavor and mainly attributive to the liver and heart meridians and xuefen.

They can facilitate blood flow and remove blood stasis so as to achieve the therapeutic effects of stimulating the menstrual flow, treating arthralgia and trauma and relieving swelling and pain. They are indicated for unsmooth blood flow and blood stasis manifested as fixed pain or numbness; for internal or external lumps, bleeding with darkish blood and purple-dark masses and ecchymosis on the skin and tongue.

活血化瘀药，味多辛、苦，主归肝、心经，入血分。善于走散，通过活跃血行，消散瘀血，而能达到通经、利痹、消肿、定痛、疗伤等功效，适用于血行失畅，瘀血阻滞之证。症见疼痛(痛处固定不移)或麻木；身体内外部肿块，出血色暗，夹有紫黯色血块；皮肤、粘膜或舌质瘀斑等。

There are various causes of forming blood stasis, therefore the causes should be found out by differentiation of syndromes and proper combination of medicinal herbs worked out when they are used. For example, if blood stasis is caused by cold obstruction and qi stagnation, the medicinal herbs warming the interior and dissipating cold should be combined; if by heat invading yingfen and xuefen and blood stasis in the interior, those clearing away

形成瘀血证的原因颇多，在运用活血祛瘀药时，应辨证审因，选择适当的药物，并作适宜的配伍。如属寒凝气滞者，须配温里祛寒药同用；属热伤营血，瘀血内阻者，配清热凉血药同用；风湿痹痛，须与祛风湿药合用；如跌打损

heat and cooling the blood should be combined; if by obstructive pain due to wind-dampness, wind-dampness eliminating ones should be combined; if by trauma, those that can promote qi circulation and dredge collaterals should be combined; if by abdominal mass, those that resolve phlegm, soften hardness and disperse stagnation should be used together; if the blood stasis syndrome is accompanied by insufficiency of healthy qi, those that supplement qi should be used together.

伤,宜与行气和络之品配伍;对癥瘕痞块,应与化痰软坚散结药配用;兼有正气不足之证者,又当配伍相应的补虚药同用。

Since qi and blood are closely related to each other, i.e. free flow of qi leads to free flow of the blood and stagnation of qi results in blood stasis and vice versa, they are usually used in combination with qi regulating medicinal herbs so as to enhance the action of invigorating the blood and removing stagnation.

人体气血之间有着密切的关系,气行则血行,气滞则血凝,故在使用活血祛瘀药时,常配合行气药,以增强行血散瘀的作用。

They are not suitable for excessive menstruation and used with great caution or contraindicated in pregnant women.

本类药物不宜用于妇女月经过多,对于孕妇,尤当慎用或忌用。

Danshen *Radix Salviae Miltiorrhizae*

丹 参

The source is from the root and rhizome of *Salvia miltiorrhiza* Bunge, family Labiatae. The medicinal herb is produced in most parts of China, mainly in areas of Hebei, Anhui, Jiangsu, and Sichuan, etc., dug and collected in spring and winter, dried in the sun and the crude or the stir-baked with wine is used.

为唇形科植物丹参的根及根茎。中国大部分地区均产。主产于河北、安徽、江苏、四川等地。春、秋季采挖,晒干。生用或酒炒用。

Medicinal Properties Bitter in flavor, slightly cold in nature and attributive to the heart, pericardium and liver meridians.

【药性】 味苦,性微寒。归心、心包、肝经。

Actions Promote blood circulation to remove blood stasis, regulate menstruation to relieve pain, cool the blood to relieve carbuncle, and clear away heat from the heart and tranquilize the mind.

【功效】 活血祛瘀,调经止痛,凉血消痈,清心安神。

Application

【临床应用】

1. It is indicated for irregular menstruation,

1. 用于血滞月经不调,经

amenorrhea, postpartum abdominal pain resulting from blood stasis, abdominal masses and pain of limbs. Since it is cold in nature, it is especially suitable for syndrome of blood stasis with heat. It is also good at regulating menstruation, therefore it is an essential medicine in maternity department. For women's syndromes due to blood stasis, it is usually combined with Honghua (*Flos Carthami*), Taoren (*Semen Persicae*), and Yimucao (*Herba Leonuri*), etc.; for the pains in the chest and epigastric abdomen resulting from blood stasis and stagnation of qi, combined with Tanxiang (*Lignum Santali Albi*) and Sharen (*Fructus Amomi*), such as Danshen Yin (Decoction); for abdominal masses, combined with Sanleng (*Rhizoma Sparganii*), Ezhu (*Rhizoma Zedoariae*), Zelan (*Herba Lycopi*), and Biejia (*Carapax Trionycis*), etc.; for trauma with pain due to blood stasis, usually combined with Danggui (*Radix Angelicae Sinensis*), Honghua (*Flos Carthami*) and Chuanxiong (*Rhizom Chuanxiong*); for Bi-syndrome of wind-damp-heat type with red, swollen and painful joints, combined with Rendongteng (*Caulis Lonicerae*), Chishaoyao (*Radix Paeoniae Rubra*) and Qinjiao (*Radix Gentianae Macrophyllae*).

闭，产后瘀滞腹痛，心腹疼痛，癥瘕积聚以及肢体疼痛等证。因其性属寒，故对瘀血兼热的病证尤为适宜。又善调妇女经水，为妇产科要药。对妇女经产诸证因瘀血者，常与红花、桃仁、益母草等配伍；用于血瘀气滞所致的心腹、胃脘疼痛，可与檀香、砂仁配伍，如丹参饮；治癥瘕积聚，可与三棱、莪术、泽兰、鳖甲等配伍；跌打损伤、瘀滞作痛，常与当归、红花、川芎同用；风湿热痹，关节红肿疼痛，与忍冬藤、赤芍药、秦艽同用。

2. For carbuncle with swelling and pain, it is combined with medicinal herbs that clear away heat and eliminate toxic materials, which can help relieve carbuncle. For example, for breast abscess with swelling and pain, combined with Ruxiang (*Olibanum*), Jinyinhua (*Flos Lonicerae*) and Lianqiao (*Flos Forsythiae*), that is, Xiaoru Tang (Decoction).

2. 用于疮痈肿痛。与清热解毒药相配，有助于消除痈肿。如乳痈肿痛与乳香、金银花、连翘等同用，即消乳汤。

3. It is used for febrile disease with restlessness, coma, palpitation and insomnia; for pathogenic factors invading yingfen and xuefen in the seasonal febrile disease, it is usually combined with Shengdihuang (*Radix Reh-*

3. 用于热病烦躁昏迷及杂病心悸失眠。治温热病，邪入营血，常与生地黄、玄参、竹叶心等同用，如清营汤；对于

manniae), Xuanshen (*Radix Scrophulariae*), Zhuyexin (the centre of *Folium Phyllostachydis Nigrae*), such as Qingying Tang (Decoction); for palpitation and insomnia due to preponderant heart-fire or blood failing to nourish the heart, usually combined with Suanzaoren (*Semen Ziziphi Spinosae*) and Baiziren (*Semen Biotae*).

心火偏旺或血不养心的心悸失眠，常配酸枣仁、柏子仁同用。

But now, clinically, it is usually prepared into tablet or injection to treat hepatosplenomegaly and anginal attack in coronary heart disease.

临床现常以之制成片剂、注射液，用治肝脾肿大及冠心病心绞痛发作。

Usage and Dosage 9 - 15 g is used in decoction for oral use. The stir-baked one with wine can strengthen the action of promoting blood circulation.

【用法用量】 水煎服，9～15克。酒炒可增强活血作用。

Notes It is incompatible with Lilu (*Rhizoma et Radix Veratra*).

【使用注意】 反藜芦。

Chuanxiong *Rhizoma Chuanxiong*

川　芎

The source is from the rhizome of *Ligusticum chuanxiong* Hort., family Umbelliferae. The medicinal material is a special one of Sichun, being cultivated artificially. It is dug and collected in May, dried by fire and cut into pieces. The crude one or the one stir-baked with wine can be used.

为伞形科植物川芎的根茎。为四川特产药材，系人工栽培。5月下旬采挖，烘干，切片。生用或酒炒用。

Medicinal Properties Pungent in flavor, warm in nature and attributive to the liver, gallbladder and pericardium meridians.

【药性】 味辛，性温。归肝、胆、心包经。

Actions Promote the circulation of the blood and qi, expel wind and alleviate pain.

【功效】 活血行气，祛风止痛。

Application

【临床应用】

1. It is indicated for stagnation of the blood and qi resulting in irregular menstruation, dysmenorrhea, amenorrhea and postpartum abdominal pain due to blood stasis, hypochondriac pain, numbness of limbs, trauma and carbuncle with swelling and pain. It is used together with Danggui (*Radix Angelicae Sinensis*) every time. On the basis of the combination, other medicinal herbs are

1. 用于血瘀气滞的月经不调，痛经，闭经，产后瘀阻腹痛，胁肋疼痛，肢体麻木，以及跌打损伤、疮痈肿痛等病证。每与当归配伍同用。以之为基础，根据不同病证再配伍其他药物。如用以调经，可配合

combined with according to different syndromes. If the combination is used to regulate menstruation, it is used together with Chishaoyao (*Radix Paeoniae Rubra*), Xiangfu (*Rhizoma Cyperi*) and others; for postpartum abdominal pain due to blood stasis, Yimucao (*Herba Leonuri*), Taoren (*Semen Persicae*), etc. are combined; for hypochondriac pain due to stagnation of liver-qi resulting in unsmooth circultion of blood, Chaihu (*Radix Bupleuri*), Xiangfu (*Rhizoma Cyperi*), etc. are combined; for numbness of limbs or wound pain, every time Chishaoyao (*Radix Paeoniae Rubra*), Honghua (*Flos Carthami*), etc. are combined; for carbuncle and ulcer disease of skin with pus that is ulcerated due to weakness of the healthy qi, Huangqi (*Radix Astragali*), Jinyinhua (*Flos Lonicerae*), and Zaojiaoci (*Spina Gleditsiae*), etc. can also be combined.

赤芍药、香附等药；治产后瘀阻腹痛，与益母草、桃仁等同用；对肝郁气滞血行失畅的胁痛，与柴胡、香附等合用；肢体麻木或伤痛，每与赤芍药、红花等配用；疮痈化脓，体虚不溃者，又可与黄芪、金银花、皂角刺等同用，

2. It is an essential medicinal herb to be used in the treatment of headache. For headache due to exogenous wind and dampness, it is combined with Baizhi (*Radix Angelicae Dahuricae*), Fangfeng (*Radix Saposhnikoviae*), and Xixin (*Herba Asari*), such as Chuanxiong Chatiao San (Powder); for headache due to wind and heat, combined with Juhua (*Flos Chrysanthemi*), Shigao (*Gypsum Fibrosum*) and Baijiangcan (*Bombyx Batryticatus*), such as Chuanxiong San (Powder); for headache due to wind and dampness, combined with Qianghuo (*Rhizoma et Radix Notopterygii*), Gaoben (*Rhizoma Ligustici*) and Fangfeng (*Radix Saposhnikoviae*), such as Qianghuo Shengshi Tang (Decoction); for headache due to blood stasis, combined with Chishaoyao (*Radix Paeoniae Rubra*), Honghua (*Flos Carthami*), Danshen (*Radix Salviae Miltiorrhizae*) and Baizhi (*Radix Angelicae Dahuricae*); for headache due to blood deficiency, combined with Danggui (*Radix Angelicae Sinensis*),

2. 用于头痛。为治头痛之要药。外感风寒头痛，配白芷、防风、细辛，如川芎茶调散；风热头痛，配菊花、石膏、白僵蚕同用，即川芎散；风湿头痛，配羌活、藁本、防风等，如羌活胜湿汤；血瘀头痛，与赤芍药、红花、丹参、白芷同用；血虚头痛，与当归、熟地黄、白芍药、菊花等同用。

Shudihuang (*Rhizoma Rehmanniae Praeparatae*), Baishaoyao (*Radix Paeoniae Alba*), Juhua (*Flos Chrysanthemi*), etc..

3. For Bi-syndrome of wind and damp type with painful joints, it is combined with wind-dampness eliminating herbs such as Qianghuo (*Rhizoma et Radix Notopterygii*), Duhuo (*Radix Angelicae Pubescentis*), Sangzhi (*Ramulus Mori*) and Haifengteng (*Caulis Piperis Futokadsurae*) to strengthen the therapeutic effects.

3. 用于风湿痹痛，肢节疼痛。与祛风湿药羌活、独活、桑枝、海风藤等同用，可增强疗效。

Besides, it can also be used for coronary heart disease with angina pectoris and ischemic brain disease.

此外，也可用治冠心病心绞痛及缺血性脑病。

Usage and Dosage 3 - 10 g is used in decoction for oral use, 1 - 1.5 g of the powder being swallowed with water.

【用法用量】 水煎服，3～10 克。研末吞服，1～1.5 克。

Notes It is pungent, warm, lifting and dispersing in properties, therefore it is contraindicated in the cases with yin deficiency leading to hyperactivity of fire marked by red tongue and dryness in the mouth; used with caution in women with excessive menstruation and cases with bleeding.

【使用注意】 本品辛温升散，凡阴虚火旺、舌红口干者忌用；妇女月经过多及出血性疾病患者，慎用。

Yanhusuo *Rhizoma Corydalis*

延胡索

The source is from the tuber of the perennial herbage *Corydalis Yanhusuo* W. T. Wang, family Papaveraceae. The medicinal material is mainly produced in the areas of Zhejiang, Jiangsu, Hunan and Hubei, collected in the beginning of summer, cleaned and then boiled in boiling water, dried in the sun and pounded into pieces when it is used. The crude one or the one prepared with vinegar is used.

为罂粟科植物延胡索的块茎。主产于浙江、江苏、湖南、湖北。夏初采挖，洗净，入沸水中烫煮(无白心时)捞起，晒干。用时捣碎。生用或醋制用。

Medicinal Properties Pungent and bitter in flavor, warm in nature and attributive to the heart, liver and spleen meridians.

【药性】 味辛、苦，性温。归心、肝、脾经。

Actions Promote the circulation of blood and qi to relieve pain.

【功效】 活血，行气，止痛。

Application

It is an essential medicine to relieve pain and used for painful syndrome due to stagnation of qi and stasis of the blood, and widely used for pain in all parts of the body. The powder is effective to be taken alone and in order to increase the therapeutic effect, it can also be used in combination according to the painful location and properties. For example, it is combined with Chuanlianzi (*Fructus Meliae Toosendan*) to treat pains in the epigastric abdomen; combined with Xiaohuixiang (*Fructus Foeniculi*) to treat pain due to hernia; combined with Danggui (*Radix Angelicae Sinensis*), Chuanxiong (*Rhizoma Chuanxiong*), Baishaoyao (*Radix Paeoniae Alba*), and Xiangfu (*Rhizoma Cyperi*), etc., to treat abdominal pain during menstruation; combined with Gualou (*Fructus Trichosanthis*), Xiebai (*Bulbus Allii Macrostemi*), Yujin (*Radix Curcumae*), and Wuyao (*Radix Linderae*), etc., to treat hypochondriac pain; combined with Danggui (*Radix Angelicae Sinensis*), Guizhi (*Ramulus Cinnamomi*), Chishaoyao (*Radix Paeoniae Rubra*), etc., in the treatment of pain of limbs or general pain due to blood stasis, and trauma.

【临床应用】

用于气滞血瘀所致的痛证。本品为止痛要药,可广泛应用于身体各部位的多种疼痛。单味研末服有效,为增强疗效,也可根据疼痛部位、性质适当配伍。如配川楝子,治脘腹疼痛;配小茴香,治疝气痛;配当归、川芎、白芍药、香附等,用于经行腹痛;配瓜蒌、薤白、郁金、乌药等,用于胸胁作痛;配当归、桂枝、赤芍药等,用于四肢或周身血滞疼痛及跌打伤痛。

Usage and Dosage 3 - 10 g is used in decoction for oral use and 1.5 - 3 g of the powder is taken.

【用法用量】 水煎服,3~10 克。研末服,1.5~3 克。

Explanation After being prepared with vinegar, it can raise solubility of its effective components in decoction so as to strengthen the effect of arresting pain.

【说明】 醋制后可使其有效成分的溶解度大大提高,而加强止痛效果。

Yujin *Radix Curcumae*

郁　金

The source is from the tuberous root of the perennial herbage *Curcuma aromatica* Salisb., and *C. zedoaria* (Berg) Rosc. or *C. longa* L. or *C. kwangsiensis* S. lee et C. F. Liang, family Zingiberaceae. The medicinal material is dug and collected in autumn and winter, cleaned, dried in the sun and cut into pieces after being boiled thor-

为姜科植物郁金、姜黄或广西莪术的块根。秋、冬季采挖,洗净,入沸水中煮透,晒干,切片。生用。

oughly in boiling water. The raw can be used.

Medicinal Properties Pungent and bitter in flavor, cold in nature and attributive to the heart, liver and gallbladder meridians.

【药性】 味辛、苦，性寒。归心、肝、胆经。

Actions Circulate the blood, arrest pain, promote flow of qi and disperse the stagnated qi, cool the blood and clear away heat from the heart, normalize the gallbladder to cure jaundice.

【功效】 活血止痛，行气解郁，凉血清心，利疸退黄。

Application

1. It is indicated for distention and pain in the chest and hypochondrium, irregular menstruation, dysmenorrhea and abdominal masses, etc., due to qi stagnation and blood stasis. For pain in the chest and hypochondrium, it is combined with Danshen (*Radix Salviae Miltiorrhizae*), Chaihu (*Radix Bupleuri*), Xiangfu (*Rhizoma Cyperi*), and Zhike (*Fructus Aurantii*), etc.; for depression of liver-qi with fever, abdominal pain before menstruation, combined with Chaihu (*Radix Bupleuri*), Xiangfu (*Rhizoma Cyperi*), Danggui (*Radix Angelicae Sinensis*) and Baishaoyao (*Radix Paeoniae Alba*); for mass in the hypochondrium, combined with Danshen (*Radix Salviae Miltiorrhizae*), Biejia (*Carapax Trionycis*) and Qingpi (*Pericarpium Citri Reticulatae Viride*).

【临床应用】

1. 用于气滞血瘀的胸腹胁肋胀痛、月经不调、痛经及癥瘕痞块等证。治胸腹胁肋胀痛，可与丹参、柴胡、香附、枳壳等配用；治肝郁有热，经前腹痛，可与柴胡、香附、当归、白芍药等配伍；胁下癥块不消，可配丹参、鳖甲、青皮等同用。

2. It is used for damp febrile disease, mental confusion due to turbid phlegm, fullness and oppression in the epigastrium, unconsciousness; and epilepsy and mania due to phlegmatic mental confusion. For the former, it is usually combined with Shichangpu (*Rhizoma Acori Graminei*), Zhizi (*Fructus Gardeniae*), and Lianqiao (*Fructus Forsythiat*), etc., such as Changpu Yujin Tang (Decoction); for the latter, usually combined with Mingfan (*Alumen*), such as Baijin Wan (Pill).

2. 用于湿温病痰浊蒙蔽清窍，胸脘痞闷，神志不清，以及痰阻心窍所致的癫痫或癫狂。对于前者，常与石菖蒲、栀子、连翘等配伍，如菖蒲郁金汤；对于后者，常与明矾配用，如白金丸。

3. For bleeding due to blood-heat manifested as

3. 用于血热妄行的吐血、

haematemesis, epistaxis, hematuria and unsmooth menstruation, etc., which is accompanied by blood stasis, it is combined with Shengdihuang (*Radix Rehmanniae*), Mudanpi (*Cortex Moutan Radicis*), Zhizi (*Fructus Gardeniae*), and Niuxi (*Radix Achyranthis Bidentatae*), etc..

衄血、尿血及妇女经血逆行等证兼有瘀滞者，可配生地黄、牡丹皮、栀子、牛膝等同用。

4. For jaundice of dampness-heat type, it is usually combined with Yinchen (*Herba Artemisiae Scopariae*), Zhizi (*Fructus Gardeniae*), etc..

4. 用于湿热黄疸。常与茵陈、栀子等配伍。

Usage and Dosage 3 - 10 g is used in decoction for oral use, and 2 - 5 g of the powder is taken.

【用法用量】 水煎服，3～10 克；研末服，2～5 克。

Notes It's incompatible with Dingxing (*Flos Caryophylli*).

【使用注意】 畏丁香。

Jianghuang *Rhizoma Curcumae Longae*

姜　黄

The source is from the rhizome of the perennial herbage *Curcuma longa* L., family Zingiberaceae. The medicinal material is mainly produced in the areas of Sichuan and Fujian, dug and collected in winter. The impurity is removed, boiled in water, dried in the sun, cut into pieces and the crude is used.

为姜科植物姜黄的根茎。主产于四川、福建。冬季采挖，除去杂质，水煮或蒸至透心，晒干，切片。生用。

Medicinal Properties Pungent and bitter in flavor, warm in nature and attributive to the liver and spleen meridians.

【药性】 味辛、苦，性温。归肝、脾经。

Actions Promote circulation of the blood and qi, dredge the meridian passage to arrest pain.

【功效】 活血行气，通经止痛。

Application

【临床应用】

1. For epigastric and hypochondriac pain due to qi stagnation and blood stasis and abdominal pain resulting from amenorrhea, it is combined each time with Danggui (*Radix Angelicae Sinensis*), Baishaoyao (*Radix Paeoniae Alba*), Honghua (*Flos Carthami*), and Yanhusuo (*Rhizoma Corydalis*), etc..

1. 用于气滞血瘀所致的胸胁疼痛、经闭腹痛等证。每与当归、白芍药、红花、延胡索等配伍。

2. For pain in the Bi-syndrome of wind-dampness type, especially for that of arms and shoulders, it is combined

2. 用于风湿痹痛。尤宜治上肢臂肩痹痛。每与羌活、

each time with Qianghuo (*Rhizoma et Notopterygii*), Haitongpi (*Cortex Erythrinae*) and Danggui (*Radix Angelicae Sinensis*), such as Shujin Tang (Decoction).

海桐皮、当归同用,如舒筋汤。

In addition, Jianghuang (*Rhizoma Curcume Longae*) is used in combination with Dahuang (*Radix et Rhizoma Rhei*), Baizhi (*Radix Angelicae Dahuricae*), Tiannanxing (*Rhizoma Arisaematis*), and Tianhuafen (*Radix Trichosanthis*), etc., which are ground into powder for external application on the local area to treat early stage of abscess, ulcer, sore, and furuncle with redness, swelling, feverish sensation and pain, such as Ruyi Jinhuang San (Powder), and now it is used for hyperlipemia.

此外,姜黄与大黄、白芷、天南星、天花粉等合用,研末外敷,可治痈疡疮疖初起,红肿热痛,方如如意金黄散。近代还用治高血脂症。

Usage and Dosage 3 - 10 g is used in decociton for oral use, and just right amount for external use.

【用法用量】 水煎服,3～10克。外用,适量。

Ruxiang *Olibanum*

乳　香

The source is from the resin from the dark of *Boswellia carterii* Birdw and other species in the same genus, family Burseraceae. The medicinal material is mainly produced in Somalia, Ethiopia of Africa. In spring and autumn, the bark is cut with knife from the bottom to the upper along the tree so that the resin can made to ooze out of the cut and coagulate into solid after several days, the solid being collected. It is often stir-baked for medication.

为橄榄科植物卡氏乳香树及其同属植物皮部渗出的树脂。产于非洲的索马里、埃塞俄比亚等地。春、夏季将树干的皮部由下而上用刀顺序切伤,使树脂由伤口渗出,数天后凝成硬块,收集即得。入药多炒用。

Medicinal Properties Pungent and bitter in flavor, warm in nature and attributive to the heart, liver and spleen meridians.

【药性】 味辛、苦,性温。归心、肝、脾经。

Actions Circulate the blood and qi to alleviate pain, subside swelling and promote tissue regeneration.

【功效】 活血行气止痛,消肿生肌。

Application

【临床应用】

1. It is indicated for various pains due to stasis of blood. For dysmenorrhea and amenorrhea, it is usually combined with Danggui (*Radix Angelicae Sinensis*), Chuanxiong (*Rhizoma Chuanxiong*), and Xiangfu (Rhi-

1. 用于内、妇、外、伤各科瘀滞疼痛证。治痛经、经闭,常配当归、川芎、香附等品;胃脘疼痛,配川楝子、延胡索等;

zoma Cyperi), etc.; for epigastric pain, combined with Chuanlianzi (*Fructus Meliae Toosendan*), Yanhusuo (*Rhizoma Corydalis*), etc.; for Bi-syndrome of wind-cold-dampness type, combined with Qianghuo (*Rhizoma et Radix Notopterygii*), Qinjiao (*Radix Gentianae Macrophyllae*), and Danggui (*Radix Angelicae Sinensis*), etc., such as Juanbi Tang (Decoction); for trauma with pain due to blood stasis, combined with Moyao (*Myrrha*), Xuejie (*Resina Draconis*), Honghua (*Flos Carthami*), and Shexiang (*Moschus artifactus*), etc., such as Qili San (Powder); for large carbuncle with hardness and pain, combined with Moyao (*Myrrha*), Xionghuang (*Realgar*), and Shexiang (*Moschus artifactus*), that is, Xingxiao Wan (Pill); for periappendicular abscess, combined with Hongteng (*Caulis Sargentodoxae*), Zihuadiding (*Herba Violae*), Lianqiao (*Fructus Forsythiae*), and Jinyinhua (*Flos Lonicerae*), etc., such as Hongteng Jian (Decoction).

风寒湿痹,配羌活、秦艽、当归等,如蠲痹汤;治跌打损伤瘀痛,配没药、血竭、红花、麝香等,如七厘散;治痈疽肿毒、坚硬疼痛者,配没药、雄黄、麝香,即醒消丸;治肠痈,可配红藤、紫花地丁、连翘、金银花等,如红藤煎。

2. It is used for pyocutaneous disease after rupture, which is not yet healed for a long time. Its combination with Moyao (*Myrrha*) is ground into powder for application on a sore and the powder has the actions of subsiding swelling and alleviating pain, removing the necrotic tissue and promoting tissue regeneration.

2. 用于疮疡溃破久不收口。以本品配合没药,共研细末,外敷患处,有消肿止痛,去腐生肌之效。

Usage and Dosage 3 - 10 g is used in decoction for oral use. It can be usually prepared into plaster to be used for application, or put in decoction for washing.

【用法用量】 水煎服,3～10克。外用,多制成膏药用作敷贴剂,或入洗剂。

Notes Its decoction looks turbid that it easily makes a case with weakness of stomach vomit, therefore the large dosage should be avoided. It is contraindicated in a case without blood satsis, and pregnant women.

【使用注意】 本品入煎剂汤液混浊,胃弱者多服易致呕吐,故用量不宜过多。无瘀滞者及孕妇忌用。

Moyao *Myrrha*

没　药

The source is from the resin from the bark of *Commiphora myrrha* Engl. or other species in the same ge-

为橄榄科植物没药树或其他同属植物茎干皮部渗出

nus, family Burseraceae. The medicinal material is mainly produced in Somalia and Ethiopia of Africa and in India, etc.. The resin oozes out of crevices in the tree and changes into redbrown but hard one in the air that is collected. So it is broken and stir-baked until it changes into burned black for being used.

的油胶树脂。主产于非洲索马里、埃塞俄比亚以及印度等地。采集树皮裂缝处渗出，于空气中变成红棕色而坚硬的油胶树脂。打碎，炒至焦黑色应用。

Medicinal Properties Bitter in flavor, mild in nature, and attributive to the liver, heart and spleen meridians.

【药性】 味苦，性平。归心、肝、脾经。

Actions Promote circulation of the blood to alleviate pain, subside swelling and promote tissue regeneration.

【功效】 活血止痛，消肿生肌。

Application

It is used for amenorrhea due to blood stasis, dysmenorrhea, epigastric pain, trauma, carbuncle and periappendicular abscess. Its actions are similar to those of Ruxiang (*Olibanum*), so far for the above syndromes, they are usually combined with each other so that they can strengthen the action of promoting circulation of the blood and alleviating pain.

In addition, it can also be used for hyperlipemia.

【临床应用】

用于血瘀经闭，痛经，胃脘疼痛，跌打伤痛，痈疽肿痛及肠痈。功用与乳香相似，故对上述之证，常与乳香相须为用，可增强活血止痛之功。

此外，本品亦可用于高脂血证的治疗。

Usage and Dosage 5 - 10 g is used in decoction for oral use, the usage being same as Ruxiang (*Olibanum*).

【用法用量】 水煎服，5～10 克。用法与乳香相同。

Notes The notes are same as those of Ruxiang (*Olibanum*). If the both herbs are used together, their dosage must be decreased accordingly.

【使用注意】 与乳香同。若与乳香同用，两药的用量须相应减少。

Taoren *Semen Persicae*

桃 仁

The source is from the seed of *Prunus persica* (L.) Batsch or *P. davidiana* Franch., family Rosaceae. The medicinal material is mainly produced in the areas of Sichuan, Shaanxi, Hebei, Shandong and Guizhou. The ripe fruits are picked from July to September, the flesh of fruit

为蔷薇科植物桃或山桃的种仁。主产于四川、陕西、河北、山东、贵州。7～9 月摘下成熟果实，除去果肉，击破果核，取出种子，晒干。除去

is removed, the centre of fruit is broken and the seed is fetched out and dried in the sun. The seed peeled, the crude or pounded one being used.

种皮,生用或捣碎用。

Medicinal Properties Bitter in flavor, mild in nature, mildly toxic and attributive to the heart, liver, lung and large intestine meridians.

【药性】 味苦,性平。有小毒。归心、肝、肺、大肠经。

Actions Promote blood circulation, remove blood stasis, moisten the intestine and relax the bowels.

【功效】 活血祛瘀,润肠通便。

Application

【临床应用】

1. It is usually used for a lot of blood-stasis syndromes. For irregular menstruation, amenorrhea, dysmenorrhea, postpartum abdominal pain due to blood stasis and abdominal mass, it is combined with Honghua (*Flos Carthami*), Danggui (*Radix Angelicae Sinensis*), Chuanxiong (*Rhizoma Chuanxiong*), and Chishaoyao (*Radix Paeoniae Rubra*), etc., such as Tao Hong Siwu Tang (Decoction); for trauma, swelling and pain due to blood stasis, usually combined with Danggui (*Radix Angelicae Sinensis*), Dahuang (*Radix et Rhizoma Rhei*), and Honghua (*Flos Carthami*), etc.; for the early stage of pulmonary abscess, periappendicular abscess, while heat clearing herbs are used, Taoren (*Semen Persicae*) is usually used to assist them to remove blood stasis, purge heat and subside carbuncle, such as Weijing Tang (Decoction) and Dahuang Mudanpi Tang (Decoction).

1. 用于多种瘀血证。治妇女经行不畅,经闭,产后瘀滞腹痛及癥瘕痞块,可与红花、当归、川芎、赤芍药等同用,如桃红四物汤;跌打损伤,瘀肿疼痛,常与当归、大黄、红花等配伍。肺痈、肠痈初起,在使用清热药同时,常佐桃仁以祛瘀泄热消痈。如苇茎汤、大黄牡丹皮汤。

2. For constipation due to dry intestine, it is usually combined with Huomaren (*Fructus Cannabis*) and Gualouren (*Fructus Trichosanthis*).

2. 用于肠燥便秘。常配火麻仁、瓜蒌仁同用。

In addition, it can relieve cough and dyspnea, so it can be used as an assistant to treat cough and dyspnea.

此外,本品尚能止咳平喘,用治咳嗽气喘,可作为辅助之品。

Usage and Dosage 6 – 10 g is used in decoction for oral use, being broken to be put in decoction.

【用法用量】 水煎服,6~10克,捣碎,入煎剂。

Notes Contraindicated in pregnant women.

【使用注意】 孕妇忌服。

Honghua *Flos Carthami*

红 花

The source is from the flower of *Carthamus tinctorius* L., family Compositae. The medicinal material is mainly produced in the areas of Henan, Hubei, Sichuan, and Zhejiang, etc.. The medicinal material is picked in summer when the flower changes from the yellow into the bright red, dried in shade and the crude is used.

为菊科植物红花的花冠。主产于河南、湖北、四川、浙江等地。夏季花色由黄转为鲜红时采摘，阴干。生用。

Medicinal Properties Pungent in flavor, warm in nature and attributive to the heart and liver meridians.

【药性】 味辛，性温。归心、肝经。

Actions Promote blood circulation to remove blood stasis, promote menstruation and alleviate pain.

【功效】 活血祛瘀，通经止痛。

Application

【临床应用】

1. For blood-stasis syndrome with dysmenorrhea, amenorrhea, postpartum abdominal pain and mass, trauma and pain of joints, etc., it is usually combined with Taoren (*Semen Persicae*), Danggui (*Radix Angelicae Sinensis*), Chuanxiong (*Rhizoma Chuanxiong*), and Chishaoyao (*Radix Paeoniae Rubra*), etc..

1. 用于血瘀痛经、血滞经闭、产后瘀阻腹痛、癥瘕积聚、跌打损伤瘀痛以及关节疼痛等证。常与桃仁、当归、川芎、赤芍药等配用。

2. For darkish skin eruptions due to stagnation of heat and blood stasis, it is combined with Danggui (*Radix Angelicae Sinensis*), Zicao (*Radix Amebiae seu Lithospermi*), and Daqingye (*Folium Isatidis*), etc., such as Danggui Honghua Yin (Decoction).

2. 用于斑疹色暗，因热郁血滞所致者。可与当归、紫草、大青叶等配伍，如当归红花饮。

In addition, it can be used for angina pectoris of coronary heart disease, thromboangiitis obliterans and erythema multiforme, etc..

此外，本品亦可用治冠心病心绞痛、血栓闭塞性脉管炎及多形性红斑等。

Usage and Dosage 3 - 10 g is used in decoction for oral use and just right amount for external use.

【用法用量】 水煎服，3～10克。外用，适量。

Notes Contraindicated in pregnant women and over dose is not suitable for cases with tendancy of bleeding.

【使用注意】 孕妇忌用，有出血倾向者不宜多用。

Explanation Fanhonghua (*Stigma Croci*) is from the dried flower of the perennial herbage *Crocus sativus*

【说明】 番红花为鸢尾科植物番红花（藏红花）的花

L. family Iridaceae. It is mainly produced in Europe and Middle Asia, sweet in flavor, cold in nature and attributive to the heart and liver meridians. Its effect is similar to but stronger than that of Honghua (*Flos Carthami*) in circulating the blood and removing blood stasis, and promoting menstruation. Besides, it also has the effect of cooling the blood and removing toxins and is especially suitable for heat invading yingfen and xuefen, general eruption whose color is not redish, etc.. 1.5 - 3 g is decocted for oral use.

柱。主产于欧洲及中亚。味甘,性寒。归心、肝经。有与红花相似的活血祛瘀、通经作用,且作用更强。又兼有凉血解毒之功,尤宜于热入营血、身发斑疹、疹色不红等证。水煎服,用量1.5～3克。

Yimucao *Herba Leonuri*

益母草

The source is from the aerial parts of *Leonurus heterophyclus* Sweet, family Labiatae. The medicinal material is produced in all areas of China, cut in summer, dried in the sun. The crude is used or decocted into extract for being used.

为唇形科植物益母草的地上部分。中国各地均产。夏季割取,晒干。生用或熬膏用。

Medicinal Properties Pungent and bitter in flavor, slightly cold in nature and attributive to the heart, liver and bladder meridians.

【药性】 味辛、苦,性微寒。归心、肝、膀胱经。

Actions Promote blood circulation and regulate menstruation, promote diuresis and relieve edema.

【功效】 活血调经,利尿消肿。

Application

【临床应用】

1. For blood stasis syndrome with unsmooth menstruation, dysmenorrhea, amenorrhea, postpartum abdominal pain and lochiostasis, it is usually combined with Chuanxiong (*Rhizoma Chuanxiong*), Danggui (*Radix Angelicae Sinensis*), and Chishaoyao (*Radix Paeoniae Rubra*).

1. 用于妇女血脉阻滞之经行不畅,痛经,经闭,产后瘀阻腹痛,恶露不尽。常配川芎、当归、赤芍药同用。

2. For dysuria and edema, especially for edema and dysuria due to stagnation of water, it can be used alone or together with Baimaogen (*Rhizoma Imperatae*) and Zelan (*Herba Lycopy*) so as to strengthen the effects of promoting diuresis and relieving edema.

2. 用于小便不利,水肿。尤宜于水瘀互阻之水肿,小便不利。可单味煎服,也可与白茅根、泽兰合用,以增强利尿消肿之效。

Besides, it is also used to treat ulcer and carbuncle,

此外,又可用于疮痈肿毒,

and skin itching rash. It may be used orally or externally.

皮肤痒疹。内服、外用均可。

Usage and Dosage 10 – 15 g is used in decoction for oral use, large dosage may be 30 g and just right amount is for external use.

【用法用量】 水煎服，10～15克，大剂量可用 30 克。外用适量。

Notes Contraindicated for pregnant women and used with caution for deficiency of the blood without stasis.

【使用注意】 孕妇忌用，血虚无瘀者慎用。

Niuxi *Radix Achyranthis Bidentatae*

牛　膝

The source is from the root of the perennial herbage *Achyrantes bidentata* Blume (Huainiuxi) and *C. officinalis* Kuan (Chuanniuxi), family Amaranthaceae. The former is cultivated in large amount in Henan Province and the latter is mainly produced in the areas of Sichuan, Yunnan, and Guizhou, etc.. Their roots are dug in winter, stored after being dried or smoked with sulphur. The crude is cut into small sections or stir-baked with wine for medication.

为苋科植物牛膝（怀牛膝）和川牛膝的根。怀牛膝大量栽培于河南省，川牛膝主产于四川、云南、贵州等地；冬季采挖，干燥或经硫黄熏后保存。切片生用或酒炒用。

Medicinal Properties Bitter and sour in flavor, mild in nature and attributive to the liver and kidney meridians.

【药性】 味苦、酸，性平。归肝、肾经。

Actions Promote blood circulation to remove blood stasis, nourish the liver and kidney, strengthen bones and muscles, induce diuresis to treat stranguria and ensure proper downward flow of blood.

【功效】 活血祛瘀，补肝肾，强筋骨，利尿通淋，引火（血）下行。

Application

【临床应用】

1. It is used for blood stasis syndrome with irregular menstruation, dysmenorrhea, amenorrhea, postpartum abdominal pain, and trauma with pain. For irregular menstruation, dysmenrrhea, amenorrhea and postpartum abdominal pain, it is usually combined with Honghua (*Flos Carthami*), Taoren (*Semen Persicae*) and Danggui (*Radix Angelicae Sinensis*); for trauma with pain, combined with Danggui (*Radix Angelicae Sinensis*), Ruxiang (*Olibanum*), Moyao (*Myrrha*), and Xuduan

1. 用于瘀血阻滞的月经不调，痛经，闭经，产后瘀阻腹痛，以及跌打伤痛等证。治月经不调，痛经，闭经，产后腹痛，多配红花、桃仁、当归同用；治跌打伤痛，可与当归、乳香、没药、续断等同用。

(*Radix Dipsaci*), etc..

2. It is used for pains of the loins and knees and weakness of lower limbs, especially for pains of the low back and knee joints. For those due to insufficiency of the liver and kidney, it is used every time in combination with Duzhong (*Cortex Eucommiae*), Xuduan (*Radix Dipsaci*), and Sangjisheng (*Ramulus Taxilli*), etc.; for those due to wind and dampness, combined with Mugua (*Fructus Chaenomelis*), Fangji (*Radix Stephaniae Tetrandrae*), and Duhuo (*Radix Angelicae Pubescentis*), etc.; for those due to dampness and heat blended attacking the lower energizer, usually combined with Cangzhu (*Rhizoma Atractylodis*), Huangbai (*Cortex Phellodendri*) and Yiyiren (*Semen Coicis*), that is, Simiao Wan (Pill).

2. 用于腰膝酸痛,下肢无力。尤宜治下半身腰膝关节酸痛,属肝肾不足者。每与杜仲、续断、桑寄生等配伍。风湿所致者,可与木瓜、防己、独活等同用;湿热下注所致者,常与苍术、黄柏、薏苡仁配用,即四妙丸。

3. For hematuria, dysuria and urethralgia, it is used in combination with Danggui (*Radix Angelicae Sinensis*), Mutong (*Caulis Akebiae*), and Huashi (*Talcum*), etc..

3. 用于尿血,小便不利,尿道涩痛。与当归、木通、滑石等配用。

4. It is used for haematemesis, epistaxis, toothache, aphthae, headache and dizziness. Of those, for haematemesis and epistaxis caused by flaming-up of fire and bleeding due to blood-heat, it is combined with Baimaogen (*Rhizoma Imperatae*), Xiaoji (*Herba Cephalanoploris*) and Zhizi (*Fructus Gardeniae*) to lead fire downward flow, to cool the blood and stop bleeding; for toothache and aphthae caused by hyperactivity of fire due to deficiency of yin, usually combined with Dihuang (*Radix Rehmanniae*), Shengshigao (*Gypsum Fibrosum*), and Zhimu (*Rhizoma Anemarrhenae*), etc. to moisten yin and lower fire; for headache and dizziness caused by hyperactivity of yang due to deficiency of yin, and liver-wind stirring inside, often combined with Daizheshi (*Haematitum*), Shengmuli (*Concha Ostreae*), Shenglonggu (*Os Draconis*),

4. 用于吐血,衄血,齿痛,口舌生疮,以及头痛眩晕等证。对火热炎上,迫血妄行之吐血、衄血,可配白茅根、小蓟、栀子等引火下行,凉血止血;对阴虚火旺引起的齿痛、口疮,常配地黄、生石膏、知母等以滋阴降火;对阴虚阳亢、肝风内动所致的头痛眩晕,昏仆,常配代赭石、生牡蛎、生龙骨、白芍药等以潜阳摄阴,镇肝熄风,

and Baishaoyao (*Radix Paeoniae Alba*), etc. to suppress the sthenia-yang and astringe yin, and eliminate liver-wind.

Usage and Dosage 5 - 15 g is used in decoction for oral use. The crude one is used for promoting blood circulation and diuresis, and leading fire downward, but the one parched with wine is used for nourishing the liver and kidney, and strengthening bones and muscles.

【用法用量】 水煎服，5～15克。活血、利水、引火下行宜生用，补肝肾强筋骨宜酒炙用。

Notes Contraindicated in pregnant women and women with profuse menstruation.

【使用注意】 孕妇及月经过多者忌用。

Explanation The actions of Huainiuxi and Chuanniuxi are similar. But Huainiuxi is a bit on the side of nourishing the liver and kidney, and strengthening the back. It is often used to treat pains of the loins and knees, and weakness of lower limbs. Chuanniuxi is a bit on the side of promoting blood circulation to remove blood stasis, and mostly used for syndrome of blood stasis.

【说明】 怀牛膝和川牛膝，两者功效相似。但怀牛膝偏于补肝肾强腰脊，多用治腰膝酸痛，下肢无力。川牛膝偏于活血祛瘀，多用于瘀血阻滞证。

Jixueteng *Caulis Spatholobi*

鸡血藤

The source is from the vine of *Spatholobus suberectus* Dunn, family Leguminosaae. The medicinal material is mainly produced in Guangxi, cut in autumn, dried in the sun, moistened thoroughly and then cut into pieces. The crude form or paste steamed is used.

为豆科植物密花豆的藤茎。主产于广西。秋季割取藤茎，晒干，润透切片。生用，或熬成膏用。

Medicinal Properties Bitter and slightly sweet in flavor, warm in nature and attributive to the liver meridian.

【药性】 味苦、微甘，性温。归肝经。

Actions Promote blood circulation and enrich the blood, regulate menstruation, relax tendons and activate the meridians.

【功效】 行血补血，调经，舒筋活络。

Application

【临床应用】

1. It is used for irregular menstruation, unsmooth menstruation, dysmenorrhea and amenorrhea due to blood deficiency no matter whether the symptoms are caused by stasis or deficiency of blood or blood deficiency concur-

1. 用于月经不调，经行不畅，痛经，血虚经闭。无论血瘀、血虚或血虚而兼有瘀滞之证皆可适用。

rently having stasis.

2. For soreness, numbness and palsy of extremities and pain in the Bi-syndrome due to wind-damp, etc., it can be combined with according to syndromes.

Recently paste of Jixueteng (*Caulis Spatholobi*) is used for leukocytopenia.

Usage and Dosage 10 - 15 g is used in decoction for oral use and large amount of 30 g may be used. Or it can be soaked in wine or decocted into paste.

2. 用于关节酸痛、手足麻木、肢体瘫痪、风湿痹痛等证。可随证配伍。

近代以鸡血藤膏治疗白细胞减少症,有一定疗效。

【用法用量】 水煎服,10～15克,大剂量可用至30克。或浸酒服,或熬成膏服。

Sanleng *Rhizoma Sparganii*

三 棱

The source is from the tuber of *Sparganium stoloniferum* Buch. Ham., family Sparganiaceae. The medicinal material is mainly produced in the areas of Jiangsu, Henan, Shandong, Jiangxi and Anhui, dug and collected in winter and spring, peeled, dried in the sun, moistened thoroughly and then cut into pieces. The crude form or the one stir-baked with vinegar is used.

为黑三棱科植物黑三棱的块茎。产于江苏、河南、山东、江西、安徽等地。冬、春两季采挖,去皮,晒干,润透切片。生用或醋炒用。

Medicinal Properties Bitter in flavor, mild in nature and attributive to the liver and spleen meridians.

【药性】 味苦,性平。归肝、脾经。

Actions Remove blood stasis, activate circulation of qi and alleviate pain.

【功效】 破血行气,消积止痛。

Application

【临床应用】

1. It is used for stagnation of qi and stasis of blood manifested as amenorrhea, abdominal pain and mass. Since it can promote circulation of qi to alleviate pain as well as remove blood stasis, it can be used in combination with Ezhu (*Rhizoma Zedoariae*) every time to treat the above syndrome. For example, Sanleng Wan (Pill) is used for amenorrhea and abdominal pain due to blood stasis.

1. 用于气滞血瘀所致的经闭腹痛及癥瘕积聚等证。既能破血祛瘀,又能行气止痛。每与莪术配伍,以治上述证候。如用于血瘀经闭腹痛之三棱丸。

2. For stagnation of food with fullness and pain of epigastric abdomen, it is usually combined with Ezhu (*Rhizoma Zedoariae*), Qingpi (*Pericarpium Citri Reticulatae Viride*) and Maiya (*Fructus Hordi Germinatus*),

2. 用于食积气滞,脘腹胀痛。常与莪术、青皮、麦芽等配伍;若兼见脾胃虚弱之证,当配合党参、白术等益气补脾

etc. ;if the syndrome is accompanied by weakness of the spleen and stomach, Dangshen (*Radix Codonopsis*), Baizhu (*Rhizoma Atractylodis Macrocephalae*) and others that enrich qi and nourish the spleen should be combined with.

药同用。

Usage and Dosage 3 - 10 g is used in decoction for oral use. That prepared with vinegar can strengthen the action of alleviating pain.

Notes Contraindicated in excessive menstruation and pregnant women.

【用法用量】 水煎服，3～10克。醋制能加强止痛作用。

【使用注意】 月经过多者及孕妇忌用。

Ezhu *Rhizoma Zedoariae*

The source is from axial rhizome of *Curcuma Kwangsinensis* S. G. Lee et C. F. Liang, *C. aromatica* Salisb. and *C. zedoaria* Rosc., family Zingiberaceae. The medicinal material is mainly produced in areas of Guangxi, Sichuan, Guangdong and Yunan, dug and collected in autumn and winter, steamed or boiled until to its center, and then dried and cut into pieces. The crude or the prepared with vinegar is used.

Medicinal Properties Pungent and bitter in flavor, warm in nature and attributive to the liver and spleen meridians.

Actions Remove blood stasis, activate qi and alleviate pain.

Application

1. It is used for amenorrhea and abdominal pain and mass caused by stagnation of qi and blood stasis. Its action is similar to that of Sanleng (*Rhizoma Sparganii*), but the action of removing blood stasis is weaker and the action of circulating qi to arrest pain is stronger than that of Sanleng (*Rhizoma Sparganii*). For the former, combined with Sanleng (*Rhizoma Sparganii*), Chuanxiong (*Rhizoma Chuanxiong*), and Niuxi (*Radix Achyranthis Bidenatatae*), etc.; for the latter, it is combined

莪 术

为姜科植物莪术、郁金或广西莪术的根茎。主产于广西、四川、广东、云南等地。秋、冬两季均可采挖。蒸或煮至透心，干燥，切片。生用或醋制用。

【药性】 味辛、苦，性温。归肝、脾经。

【功效】 破血祛瘀，行气止痛。

【临床应用】

1. 用于气滞血瘀所致的经闭腹痛及癥瘕积聚。本品功效与三棱相似，破血作用比三棱弱，但行气止痛之力则较强。用于前者，可与三棱、川芎、牛膝等配伍；用于后者，可配三棱、丹参、鳖甲等同用。

with Sanleng (*Rhizoma Sparganii*), Danshen (*Radix Salviae Miltiorrhizae*), and Biejia (*Carapax Trionycis*), etc..

2. For stagnation of food and fullness and distention of epigastric abdomen due to irregular diet and failure of spleen's transportation and transformation, it is usually combined with Sanleng (*Rhizoma Sparganii*), Muxiang (*Radix Aucklandiae*), Zhishi (*Fructus Aurantii Immaturus*), and Shanzha (*Fructus Crataegi*), etc.; for the above syndrome accompanied by weakness of spleen-qi, yet combined with Dangshen (*Radix Codonopsis*), Baizhu (*Rhizoma Atractylodis Macrocephalae*) and others that can enrich spleen-qi.

2. 用于饮食不节，脾运失常所致的食滞不化，脘腹胀满疼痛。常与三棱、木香、枳实、山楂等配伍；兼见脾虚气弱者，还应配合补气健脾药党参、白术等同用。

Usage and Dosage 3 - 10 g is used in decoction, and the herb prepared with vinegar can strengthen the action of alleviating pain.

【用法用量】 水煎服，3～10克。醋制能加强止痛作用。

Notes Contraindicated in women with excessive menstruation and pregnant women.

【使用注意】 月经过多者及孕妇忌用。

Shuizhi *Hirudo*

水　蛭

The source is from the whole body of *Annelid whitmania* pigra (whitman), *Whitmania acranulae* (whitman), *Hirudo nipponica* whitman, etc., family Hirudinidae. The medicinal material is produced in all parts of China, caught in summer from May to June or in autumn, dried in the sun to avoid moth-eating. The powder or the one roasted with weak fire is used.

为水蛭科动物蚂蟥、水蛭及柳叶蚂蟥等的全体。中国各地均产。夏季5～6月或秋季捕捉，晒干，防蛀。用时研末或微火炙黄。

Medicinal Properties Salty and bitter in flavor, mild in nature, mildly toxic and attributive to the liver meridian.

【药性】 味咸、苦，性平。有小毒。归肝经。

Action Remove blood stasis.

【功效】 破血逐瘀。

Application

【临床应用】

It is used for blood-stasis syndromes such as amenorrhea, abdominal mass and trauma. For amenorrhea and abdominal mass, it is usually combined with Taoren (*Se-*

用于血滞经闭，癥瘕积聚，以及跌打损伤等瘀血阻滞证。治经闭，癥瘕，常与桃仁、

men Persicae), Sanleng (*Rhizoma Sparganii*) and Sumu (*Lignum Sappan*), etc.; for those with general weakness, medicinal herbs tonifying qi and nourishing blood should be combined as assistants, such as Huazheng Huisheng Dan (Bolus); for blood stasis in the interior due to trauma with chest pain and constipation, combined with Dahuang (*Radix et Rhizoma Rhei*) and Qianniuzi (*Semen Pharbitidis*), that is, Duoming San (Powder).

三棱、苏木等配伍;体虚者尚须佐以益气养血药,如化癥回生丹;治伤损瘀血内阻,心腹疼痛,大便不通,可与大黄、牵牛子同用,即夺命散。

Besides, it can also be used to treat thrombocythemia, intracranial hematoma, angina pectoris and onset of pulmonary heart disease.

此外,本品可用于治疗血小板增多症、颅内血肿、冠心病心绞痛以及肺心病急性发作。

Usage and Dosage 1.5 – 3 g is used in decoction for oral use; 0.3 – 0.5 g of the powder is swallowed.

【用法用量】 水煎服,1.5～3 克;焙干研末吞服,0.3～0.5 克。

Notes Contraindicated in pregnant women.

【使用注意】 孕妇忌服。

Mengchong *Tabanus*

虻 虫

The source is from the female insect *Tabanus bivittatus* Mats., family Tabanidane. The medicinal materials are in all parts of China and most in animal areas. They are caught during May and June, boiled or slightly steamed, dried and their wing and foot must be removed. The crude form or the one stir-baked is used.

为虻科动物复带虻的雌虫体。中国各地均有,以畜牧区最多。5～6 月捕捉,沸水烫或稍蒸,晒干,去翅足。生用或炒用。

Medicinal Properties Bitter in flavor, slightly cold in nature, mildly toxic and attributive to the liver meridian.

【药性】 味苦,性微寒。有小毒。归肝经。

Action Remove blood stasis.

【功效】 破血逐瘀。

Application

【临床应用】

It is used for amenorrhea due to blood stasis, abdominal mass and trauma. It is similar in actions to Shuizhi (*Hirudo*) but its nature is violent. For amenorrhea and mass due to blood stasis, it is usually combined with Shuizhi (*Hirudo*) and Taoren (*Semen Persicae*); for trauma and pain due to blood stasis, usually combined with

用于血滞经闭,癥瘕积聚及跌打损伤,与水蛭功效相似,而性尤峻猛。治经闭,瘀结成块,常配水蛭、桃仁同用;对跌打损伤,瘀滞疼痛之证,常与大黄、水蛭、乳香、没药等

Dahuang (*Radix et Rhizoma Rhei*), Shuizhi (*Hirudo*), Ruxiang (*Olibanum*) and Moyao (*Myrrha*), etc., such as Huazheng Huisheng Dan (Pill).

配伍，如化癥回生丹。

Usage and Dosage 1 - 1.5 g is used in decoction for oral use. 0.3 g of the powder is swallowed with water.

【用法用量】 水煎服，1～1.5 克。研末吞服，0.3 克。

Notes Contraindicated in pregnant women.

【使用注意】 孕妇忌服。

10 Phlegm Resolving, Antitussive and Antiasthmatic Chinese Medicinal Herbs

第十章 化痰止咳平喘药

Any Chinese medicinal herb that helps to dissolve and excrete phlegm out of the lung and takes treatment of phlegm-syndnome as its main action is considered as phlegm resolving Chinese medicinal herbs while any Chinese medicinal herb with the main actions of relieving cough and asthma is called antitussive and antiasthmatic Chinese medicinal herbs. Phlegm resolving herbs concurrently have the action of arresting cough and stopping asthma, and antitussive and antiasthmatic herbs can also concurrently have the effect of dissolving phlegm, so these two kinds of medicinal herbs fall into one chapter, known as phlegm resolving, antitussive and antiasthmatic Chinese medicinal herbs. Phlegm resolving Chinese medicinal herbs are mainly used for cough due to excessive phlegm or asthma due to phlegm-retention, unsmooth coughing sputum, etc.. Antitussive and antiasthmatic Chinese medicinal herbs are mainly indicated for cough and asthma caused by internal injury and external affection. Syndromes such as epilepsy, infantile convulsion, goiter, scrofula, yin furuncle and suppurative tissue disease are closely related to phlegm in pathogenesis, therefore, they are also treated by phlegm resolving Chinese medicinal herbs.

凡具祛痰或消痰作用,以治疗“痰证”为主要作用的药称化痰药;以减轻或制止咳嗽和喘息为主要作用的药物,叫止咳平喘药。化痰药多兼止咳、平喘之功,止咳平喘药亦多兼化痰之效。所以,两类药合于一章,总称为化痰止咳平喘药。化痰药,主要用于痰多咳嗽或痰饮气喘,咯痰不爽之证。止咳平喘药,主要用于内伤、外感所引起的咳嗽和喘息。癫痫惊厥、瘿瘤瘰疬、阴疽流注等证,在病机上均与痰有密切的关系,故亦可用化痰药治之。

External affection and internal damage can all cause cough and excessive sputum, so clinically, besides choosing these kinds of medicinal herbs according to each

外感、内伤均可引起咳喘或多痰,因而在应用时除根据各药的特点加以选择外,还须

property of them, one must combine them appropriately with each other according to the pathogenic factors, signs and symptoms. For example, for cough or asthma accompained by exterior syndrome, diaphoretic Chinese medicinal herbs must be combined; for that with internal heat, heat clearing herbs must be combined; for that with internal cold, the interior warming Chinese herbs must be combined; and for that due to asthenia of viscera, tonics must be combined. Besides, for epilepsy and infantile convulsion, Chinese medicinal herbs for calming the mind and liver should be combined; for goiter and scrofula, Chinese medicinal herbs for softening hardness and dispersing lumps should be combined; for yin furuncle and suppurative tissue disease, Chinese medicinal herbs for eliminating cold to remove stagnation should be combined.

根据致病的原因和证型作适当的配伍。例如,兼有表证者配解表药,兼有里热者配清热药,兼有里寒者配温里药,虚劳咳喘者配补益药。此外,如癫痫惊厥者,配安神药和平肝熄风药;瘿瘤瘰疬者,配软坚散结药;阴疽流注者,配散寒通滞药。

Expectorants with violent and stimulative property are not suitable for cough accompanied by hemoptysis, otherwise bleeding can be induced. Cough at the early stage of measles is usually treated with the medicinal herbs with the main actions of clearing away lung-heat and opening inhibited lung-qi but is not suitably arrested with the medicinal herbs with warm and astringent property so as to avoid assisting heat or affecting smooth eruptions of measles.

咳嗽兼咯血者,不宜用强烈而有刺激性的化痰药,否则有促进出血之虞;对于麻疹初期的咳嗽,一般以清宣肺气为主,不宜止咳,不宜用温性或带有收敛性质的化痰止咳药,以免助热或影响麻疹的透发。

Banxia *Rhizoma Pinelliae*

半　夏

The source is from rhizome of *Pinellia ternata* (Thunb.) Breit, family Araceae. The medicinal material is produced in all parts of China and mostly in the reaches of the Yangtze River, dug and collected in summer and autumn, prepared by being dried in the sun after the cortex is removed and the fibrous root is got rid of. The crude or the one prepared by being soaked in ginger juice and alum water is used.

为天南星科植物半夏的块茎。中国各地均产,长江流域产量最多。夏、秋间采挖,去皮及须根,晒干。生用或用生姜、明矾等炮制后用。

Medicinal Properties Pungent in flavor, warm in

【药性】 味辛,性温。有

nature, toxic and attributive to the spleen, stomach and lung meridians.

毒。归脾、胃、肺经。

Actions Dry dampness and eliminate phlegm, lower the adverse rising qi to stop vomiting, disperse stagnation and lumps and externally disperse swelling and relieve pains.

【功效】 燥湿化痰,降逆止呕,消痞散结;外用消肿止痛。

Application

【临床应用】

1. It is used for dampness or cold phlegm syndrome and is an essential medicinal herb to treat dampness-phlegm syndrome. For cough and asthma with plenty of sputum caused by accumulation of phlegm and dampness in the lung, it is usually combined with Jupi (*Pericarpium Citri Tangerinae*) and Fuling (*Poria*), such as Erchen Tang (Decoction); for that accompanied by cold, profuse and thin sputum, Xixin (*Herba Asari*) and Ganjiang (*Rhizoma Zingiberis*) may be added to the above combination; for that with fever, thick and yellowish sputum, it must be combined with Huangqin (*Radix Scutellariae*), Zhimu (*Rhizoma Anemarrhenae*) and Gualou (*Fructus Trichosanthis*); for dizzines caused by damp turbidity up-attacking, it is usually combined with Baizhu (*Rhizoma Atractylodis Macrocephalae*), Tianma (*Rhizoma Gastrodiae*), etc., such as Banxia Baizhu Tianma Tang (Decoction).

1. 用于湿痰、寒痰证。为治痰湿证要药。治痰湿壅肺之咳嗽气喘,痰多,常与橘皮、茯苓同用,如二陈汤;兼见寒象,痰多清稀,可加配细辛、干姜;若见热象,痰稠色黄者,则需与黄芩、知母、瓜蒌同用;湿浊上犯清阳,致头昏目眩者,常配白术、天麻等,如半夏白术天麻汤。

2. For vomiting due to the adverse-rising of stomach-qi, it is usually combined with Shengjiang (*Rhizoma Zingiberis Recens*); for that due to stomach-deficiency, combined with Renshen (*Radix Ginseng*) and Baimi (White Honey), named Da Banxia Tang (Decoction); for that due to stomach-heat, combined with Huanglian (*Rhizoma Coptidis*), Zhuru (*Caulis Bambusae in Taeniam*), etc.; for that during pregnancy, used together with Zisugen (*Caulis Perillae*), Sharen (*Fructus Amomi*) and others that regulate qi and prevent fetus from miscar-

2. 用于胃气上逆呕吐。常与生姜同用。胃虚呕吐,配人参、白蜜,名大半夏汤;胃热呕吐,则可配黄连、竹茹等;妊娠呕吐,可与紫苏梗、砂仁等理气安胎、和胃止呕之品同用。

riaging and regulate the function of the stomach to stop vomiting.

3. It is used for stagnation and oppression in the chest and epigastric abdomen, and globus hystcricus. For the former syndrome and vomiting due to co-stagnation of phlegm and heat, it is usually combined with Huanglian (*Rhizoma Coptidis*) and Gualou (*Fructus Trichosanthis*), named Xiao Xianxiong Tang (Decoction); for the latter due to stagnation of qi and phlegm or stagnation of something or so in the throat, used together with Houpo (*Cortex Magnoliae Officinalis*), Zisuye (*Folium Perillae*) and Fuling (*Poria*), etc., such as Banxia Houpo Tang (Decoction).

3. 用于胸脘痞闷，梅核气。治痰热互结所致的胸脘痞闷、呕吐，常与黄连、瓜蒌同用，名小陷胸汤；治气郁痰结、咽中如有物阻的梅核气，可与厚朴、紫苏叶、茯苓等同用，如半夏厚朴汤。

4. It is used for goiter, subcutaneous nobule, large carbuncle and mammary sores. For goiter and subcutaneous nobule, it is used together with Kunbu (*Thallus laminariae seu Eckloniae*), Zhebeimu (*Bulbus Fritillariae Thunbergii*), Haizhao (*Sargassum*) and others that soften hardness and disperse lumps; for large carbuncle, its crude powder mixed with egg white is applied on the wounded area, which can also be used to treat poisonous snake bite.

4. 用于瘿瘤痰核，痈疽发背及乳疮。治瘿瘤痰核，可与昆布、海藻、浙贝母等软坚散结药同用；治痈疽，可将生半夏研末，用鸡蛋清调敷患处。此法也可用于治疗毒蛇咬伤。

Usage and Dosage 3-10 g is used in decoction for oral use. Just right amount of the raw is used externally and ground into powder that is mixed for application.

【用法用量】 水煎服，3～10克。外用，生品适量，研末调敷。

Notes Since it is warm and dry in nature, it is contraindicated or used with caution for dry cough due to yin deficiency, hemorrhagic diseases and heat-phlegm. It is incompatible with Wutou (*Rhizoma Aconiti*).

【使用注意】 其性温燥，对阴亏燥咳、血证、热痰等证，当忌用或慎用。反乌头。

Explanation The prepared Banxia is usually taken orally, that is, Jiangbanxia, *Rhizoma Pinelliae* prepared with ginger and alum, Fabanxia, that prepared with Gancao (*Radix Glycyrrhizae*) and lime, and Zhulibanxia, that prepared with Zhuli (*Succus Bambusae*) and alum.

【说明】 内服一般制用，主要有姜半夏、法半夏、竹沥半夏等，姜半夏长于降逆止呕，多用于治呕吐；法半夏长于燥湿且温性较弱，多用于湿

Jiangbanxia is effective in lowering the adverse-rising qi to stop vomiting, so it is usually used for vomiting; Fabanxia is effective in eliminating dampness but its warm nature is weaker, so it is usually used for syndrome of dampness-phlegm; Zhulibanxia is cool in nature and can eliminate phlegm-heat, so it is mainly used for phlegm of heat and wind types.

痰证；竹沥制半夏，使药性由温变凉，能清化痰热，主治热痰、风痰之证。

Tiannanxing *Rhizoma Arisaematis*

天南星

The source is from the tuber of the perennial herbage *Arisaema Consanguineum* Schott, *Arisaema amurense* Maxim., or *Arisaema heterophyllum* Bl., family Araceae. Tiannanxing (*Rhizoma Arisaematis*) is mainly produced in the areas of Henan, Hebei, and Sichuan, etc.; Arisaema amurense Maxim. is mainly produced in Northeast China and Arisaema heterophyllum Bl. is mainly produced in the areas of Jiangsu, Zhejiang, etc.. The medicinal materials are dug and collected in autumn and winter, the impurity being got rid of, and then dried in the sun, that is, Shengnanxing (*Rhizoma Arisaematis*, crude). The medicinal herb prepared by soaking it in the alum solution, decocting it together with ginger, cutting it into slices and drying it in the sun is called Zhinanxing (*Rhizoma Arisaematis Praeparata*).

为天南星科植物天南星、东北天南星或异叶天南星的块茎。天南星主产于河南、河北、四川等地；东北天南星主产于东北地区，异叶天南星主产于江苏、浙江等地。秋、冬两季采挖，去杂质，晒干，即为生南星。经白矾水浸泡，再与生姜共煮，切片晒干，即为制南星。

Medicinal Properties Bitter and pungent in flavor, warm in nature, toxic and attributive to the lung, liver and spleen meridians.

【药性】 味苦、辛，性温。有毒。归肺、肝、脾经。

Actions Eliminate dampness and resolve phlegm, expel wind and relieve spasm, and disperse swelling and arrest pain externally.

【功效】 燥湿化痰，祛风止痉，外用消肿止痛。

Application

1. It is used for chronic phlegm-syndrome with cough and chest distension and distress. Its action of eliminating dampness and resolving phlegm is dominative to that of Banxia (*Rhizoma Pinelliae*). For stagnation of

【临床应用】

1. 用于顽痰咳嗽，胸膈胀闷。燥湿化痰作用胜于半夏。治痰湿阻肺证，每与橘皮、半夏、茯苓、枳实等同用，如导痰

phlegm-dampness in the lung, it is used every time in combination with Jupi(*Pericarpium Citri Tangerinae*), Banxia (*Rhizoma Pinelliae*), Fuling (*Poria*), and Zhishi (*Fructus Aurantii Immaturus*), etc., such as Daotan Tang (Decoction); for cough of lung-heat type with yellowish and thick sputum, must be used in combination with Huangqin (*Radix Scutellariae*), Gualou (*Fructus Trichosanthis*) and others that clear away lung-heat and resolve phlegm.

汤;如属肺热咳嗽,咯痰黄稠,须配黄芩、瓜蒌等清肺化痰之品。

2. For dizziness due to wind-phlegm, apoplexy with distortion of the face, epilepsy and tetanus. It dominates to expel wind-phlegm and relieve spasm. For dizziness due to wind-phlegm, it can be used together with Banxia (*Rhizoma Pinelliae*), Tianma (*Rhizoma Gastrodiae*), etc.; for numbness of extremities, hemiplegia and distortion of face due to stagnation of phlegm in the channels, it can be combined with Baifuzi (*Rhizoma Typhonii*), Banxia (*Rhizoma Pinelliae*), and Chuanwu (*Radix Aconiti*), etc., such as Qingzhou Baiwanzi (Pill); for epilepsy, it can be used together with Yujin (*Radix Curcumae*) and Shichangpu (*Rhizoma Acori Graminei*); for that with severe convulsion, Wugong (*Scolopendra*), Quanxie (*Scorpio*) and others should be added to; for tetanus, it can be combined with Fangfeng (*Radix Saposhnikoviae*), Baizhi (*Radix Angelicae Dahuricae*), and Tianma (*Rhizoma Gastrodiae*), etc..

2. 用于风痰眩晕,中风后口眼歪斜,癫痫及破伤风。善祛风痰而止痉。治风痰眩晕,可配半夏、天麻等药;对于风痰留滞经络引起的手足顽麻、半身不遂、口眼歪斜,可配白附子、半夏、川乌等同用,如青州白丸子;治癫痫,可与郁金、石菖蒲同用,抽搐甚者,可再加蜈蚣、全蝎等止痉药;治破伤风,可配防风、白芷、天麻等使用。

3. For large carbuncle and subcutaneous nodule with swelling and pain, Shengnanxing (*Rhizoma Arisaematis*, crude) can be applied on wounded areas and recently, it can be taken orally or used externally on local area to treat cancer, having certain therapeutic effect, especially in cancer of uterine cervix.

3. 用于痈疽,痰核肿痛。可取生南星外敷。近年来以生南星内服、局部外用用治癌肿有一定效果,尤以子宫颈癌多用。

Usage and Dosage 3 – 10 g of prepared Tiannanxing is used in decoction for oral use, or 0.3 – 1 g of that is

【用法用量】 水煎服,制南星,3~10克;或入丸、散,

used in pill or powder, crude Tiannanxing is generally not taken orally. Just right amount of it is for external use.

0.3～1 克。生南星一般不作内服。外用，适量。

Notes Contraindicated in pregnant women and used with caution in cases with yin deficiency and dry-phlegm.

【使用注意】 孕妇忌用。阴虚燥痰者慎用。

Baiqian *Rhizoma Cynanchi Stauntonii*

白 前

The source is the root and rhizome of *Cynanchum stauntonii* (Decne.) Schltr. ex levl. or *C. glaucescens* (Decne.) Hand.-Mazz., family Asclepiadaceae. The medicinal material is mainly produced in areas of Zhejiang, Anhui, Hunan, and Fujian, etc., dug and collected in autumn, dried in the sun and cut into segments. The crude one or the one roasted with honey is used.

为萝摩科植物柳叶白前和芫花叶白前的根茎及根。主产于浙江、安徽、湖南、福建等地。秋季采挖，晒干，切段。生用或蜜炙用。

Medicinal Properties Pungent and sweet in flavor, slightly warm in nature and attributive to the lung meridian.

【药性】 味辛、甘，性微温。归肺经。

Actions Descend the adverse-rising qi, resolve phlegm, relieve cough and asthma.

【功效】 降气化痰，止咳平喘。

Application

【临床应用】

It is used for cough with excessive sputum, fullness in the chest and dyspnea whether the syndrome is due to cold, heat, exogenous affection or interior injury. For the syndrome that is a bit on cold side, it is combined with Ziwan (*Radix Asteris*) and Banxia (*Rhizoma Pinelliae*); for the syndrome that is a bit on heat side, combined with Sangbaipi (*Cortex Mori Radicis*) and Digupi (*Cortex Lycii Radicis*); for cough due to exogenous wind and cold, usually combined with Jingjie (*Herba Schizonepetae*), Jiegen (*Radix Platycodi*) and Jupi (*Pericarpium Citri Tangerinae*).

用于咳喘痰多，胸满气急。无论属寒、属热，外感、内伤均可用。偏寒者，配紫菀、半夏；偏热者配桑白皮、地骨皮；外感风寒咳嗽，常与荆芥、桔梗、橘皮同用。

Usage and Dosage 3 - 10 g is used in decoction for oral use.

【用法用量】 水煎服，3～10 克。

Qianhu *Radix Peucedani*

前 胡

The source is from the root of *Peucedanum*

为伞形科植物白花前胡

praeruptorum Dunn and *P. decurisivum* Maxim., family Umbelliferae. They are separately produced in the areas of Zhejiang, Hunan and Sichuan; or the areas of Jiangxi, Anhui, etc.. They are dug and collected in winter and spring and dried in the sun after the stem and leaves are got rid of. The crude one is cut into pieces for being used or the one roasted with honey is used.

和紫花前胡的根。白花前胡主产于浙江、湖南及四川；紫花前胡主产于江西、安徽等地。冬、春季间采挖，去茎叶，晒干，切片。生用或蜜炙用。

Medicinal Properties Bitter and pungent in flavor, slightly cold in nature and attributive to the lung meridian.

【药性】 味苦、辛，性微寒。归肺经。

Actions Lower the adverse-rising qi and resolve phlegm, expel wind and heat.

【功效】 降气化痰，宣散风热。

Application

【临床应用】

1. For undescending of lung-qi with cough, dyspnea and thick sputum, it is usually combined with Sangbaipi (*Cortex Mori Radicis*), Beimu (*Bulbus Fritillariae*) and Xingren (*Semen Pruni Armeniacae*), etc.; for cold-phlegm and dampness-phlegm syndrome, used in combination with Baiqian (*Rhizoma Cynanchi Stauntonii*).

1. 用于肺气不降，喘咳，痰稠。常与桑白皮、贝母、杏仁等同用；亦可用于寒痰、湿痰证，可与白前相须配用。

2. For exogenous wind and heat, especially for stagnation of wind and heat in the lung with cough and sputum, it is usually combined with Bohe (*Herba Menthae*), Niubangzi (*Fructus Arctii*) and Jiegeng (*Radix Platycodi*).

2. 用于外感风热证。尤宜于风热郁肺咳嗽有痰者。常与薄荷、牛蒡子、桔梗同用。

Usage and Dosage 3－10 g is used in decoction for oral use.

【用法用量】 水煎服，3～10克。

Gualou *Fructus Trichosanthis*

瓜 蒌

The source is from the mature fruit of *Trichosanthes kirilowii* Maxim. or several species of the same genus, family Cucurbitaceae. The medicinal material is produced in all parts of China, collected in autumn when the fruits are ripe, dried in shade or the peel and seed are dried separately. The peel or the seed can be used in raw

为葫芦科植物栝楼和双边栝楼的成熟果实。中国各地均产。秋季果实成熟时连柄剪下，晾干，或剖开去瓤，将壳与种子分别干燥。瓜蒌皮(壳)、瓜蒌仁(种子)生用或炒

or in stir-baked form. When the peel and seed are used together or the whole fruit is used, the medicinal herb is called the whole Fructus Trichosanthis (Quangualou).

用,皮、仁合用称全瓜萎。

Medicinal Properties Sweet and slightly bitter in flavor and cold in nature and attributive to the lung, stomach and large intestine meridians.

【药性】 味甘、微苦,性寒。归肺、胃、大肠经。

Actions Clear away lung-heat and resolve phlegm, ease the chest and disperse lumps, lubricate the intestine and relax the bowels.

【功效】 清肺化痰,宽胸散结,滑肠通便。

Application

【临床应用】

1. For lung-heat syndrome manifested as cough with thick sputum, it is usually combined with Zhimu (*Rhizoma Anemarrhenae*), Beimu (*Bulbus Fritillariae*), etc.; for accumulation of phlegm-heat in the interior manifested as yellow and thick sputumn, chest distress but difficulty in defecation, Gualouren (*Semen Trichosanthis*) is combined with Huangqin (*Radix Scutellariae*), Dannanxing (*Arisaema cum Bile*) and Zhishi (*Fructus Aurantii Immaturus*), such as Qingqi Huatan Wan (Pill).

1. 用于痰热咳嗽,痰稠不易咯出。常与知母、贝母等同用;痰热内结,痰黄稠,胸闷而大便不畅者,以瓜蒌仁配黄芩、胆南星、枳实同用,如清气化痰丸。

2. It is used for chest pain and accumulation of phlegm-heat in the chest manifested as feeling of oppression or pains in the chest and hypochondrium. If a case has a chest pain but can't lie, he should be treated with the herb in combination with Xiebai (*Bulbus Allii Macrostemi*), Banxia (*Rhizoma Pinelliae*); for accumulation of phlegm-heat in the chest and pain by pressure, combined with Banxia (*Rhizoma Pinelliae*) and Huanglian (*Rhizoma Coptidis*).

2. 用于胸痹,结胸,症见胸膈痞闷或作痛。治胸痹不得卧,可配薤白、半夏等宽胸化痰;痰热结胸,按之则痛者,可与半夏、黄连同用。

3. For constipation due to dry intestine, it is usually combined with Huomaren (*Fructus Cannabis*), Yuliren (*Semen Pruni*) and Zhike (*Fructus Aurantii*), etc..

3. 用于肠燥便秘。常配火麻仁、郁李仁、枳壳等同用。

Besides, Quangualou can also be used for mammary abscess with swelling and pain, it is usually combined with

此外,全瓜蒌还可用于乳痈肿痛,常与蒲公英、乳香、没

Pugongying (*Herba Taraxaci*), Ruxiang (*Olibanum*), and Moyao (*Myrrha*), etc..

药等合用。

Usage and Dosage Usually, 5 - 15 g of the whole herb, 6 - 9 g of Gualoupi (*Pericarpium Trichosanthis*), 10 - 15 g of Gualouren (*Semen Trichosanthis*) are used in decoction for oral use. Gualoupi (*Pericarpium Trichosanthis*) is a bit on side of resolving phlegm while Gualouren (*Semen Trichosanthis*) is a bit on side of moistening intestine and relaxing bowels.

【用法用量】 水煎服,全瓜蒌5～15克,瓜蒌皮6～9克,瓜蒌仁10～15克。瓜蒌皮偏于化痰,瓜蒌仁偏于润肠通便。

Notes Contraindicated for loose stool due to spleen deficiency and phlegm of dampness and cold types. It is incompatible with Wutou (*Rhizoma Aconiti*).

【使用注意】 脾虚便溏及湿痰、寒痰忌用。反乌头。

Beimu　*Bulbus Fritillariae*

贝　母

Beimu (*Bulbus Fritillariae*) is divided into two kinds: Chuanbeimu (*Bulbus Fritillarae Cirrhosae*) and Zhebeimu (*Bulbus Fritillariae Thunbergii*).

贝母分为两种:川贝母和浙贝母。

1. Chuanbeimu (*Bulbus Fritillariae Cirrhosae*) is the bulb of *Fritillaria cirrhosa* D. Don, *F. unibracteata* Hsiao et K. C. Hsia and *F. Przewalskii* Maxim., family Liliaceae. It is mainly produced in the areas of Sichuan, Yunnan, Gansu, Tibet of China, etc., dug and collected in summer and dried in the sun.

1. 川贝母为百合科植物川贝母、暗紫贝母和甘肃贝母,或棱砂贝母的地下鳞茎。主产四川、云南、甘肃及西藏等地。夏季采挖,晒干。

2. Zhebeimu (*Bulbus Fritillariae Thunbergii*) is the bulb of the same genus, *Fritillaria Thunbergii*, mainly produced in Xiangshan and Jinxian counties of Zhejiang Province, and cultivated artificially. The bulb is dug after the plant is withered and dried in the sun after it is cleaned. The crude one is used.

2. 浙贝母为同科植物浙贝母的地下鳞茎。主产浙江象山县、槿县。均为人工栽培。立夏植株枯萎后采挖,洗净,晒干。生用。

Medicinal Properties Chuanbeimu (*Bulbus Fritillariae Cirrhosae*) is bitter and sweet in flavor, slightly cold in nature; Zhebeimu (*Bulbus Fritillariae Thunbergii*) is bitter in flavor and cold in nature. They are attributive to the lung and heart meridians.

【药性】 川贝母味苦、甘,性微寒;浙贝母味苦,性寒。归肺、心经。

Actions Resolve phlegm and arrest cough, clear

【功效】 化痰止咳,清热

away heat and disperse stagnation.

散结。

Application

【临床应用】

1. It is used for chronic cough due to lung deficiency with less sputum and dry throat, and cough due to exogenous wind and heat or cough due to stagnation of phlegm-heat with yellowish and thick sputum. Chuanbeimu (*Bulbus Fritillarae Cirrhosae*) and Zhebeimu (*Bulbus Fritillariae Thunbergii*) can all clear away lung-heat, resolve phlegm to treat cough due to phlegm-heat. They are usually combined with Zhimu (*Rhizoma Anemarrhenae*), such as Ermu San (Powder). Whereas, Chuanbeimu (*Bulbus Fritillarae Cirrhosae*) is companied with the action of moistening the lung, so it is usually used for chronic cough due to lung deficiency with less sputum and dry throat and can be combined with Shashen (*Radix Glehniae*), Maimendong (*Radix Ophiopogonis*), Tianmendong (*Radix Asparagi*) and others that can nourish yin and moisten the lung; the action of Zhebeimu (*Bulbus Fritillariae Thunbergii*) to clear away fire and disperse stagnation is stronger, so it is usually used for exogenous wind and heat or cough due to stagnation of phlegm-heat and combined with Sangye (*Folium Mori*), Niubangzi (*Fructus Arctii*), Qianhu (*Radix Peucedani*), Xingren (*Semen Pruni Armeniacae*) and others that can disperse the lung to eliminate phlegm.

1. 用于肺虚久咳，痰少咽燥，以及外感风热咳嗽，或痰火郁结，咯痰黄稠等。川贝母与浙贝母都能清肺化痰止咳而治痰热咳嗽。常与知母同用，如二母散。但川贝兼有润肺之功，多用于肺虚久咳、痰少咽燥等证，可与沙参、麦门冬、天门冬等养阴润肺药配伍；浙贝清火散结作用较强，多用于外感风热或痰火郁结的咳嗽，常与桑叶、牛蒡子、前胡、杏仁等宣肺祛痰药同用。

2. It is used for scrofula, carbuncle, mammary abscess and pulmonary abscess. Chuanbeimu (*Bulbus Fritillarae Cirrhosae*) and Zhebeimu (*Bulbus Fritillariae Thunbergii*) both have the actions of clearing away heat and disperse stagnation but Zhebeimu (*Bulbus Fritillariae Thunbergii*) is more effective in treating scrofula, it is usually combined with Xuanshen (*Radix Scrophulariae*) and Muli (*Concha Ostreae*), that is Xiaoluo Wan (Pill); For carbuncle and mammary abscess, it is usually

2. 用于瘰疬疮痈肿毒及乳痈、肺痈等证。川贝母、浙贝母皆有清热散结的功效，浙贝母治瘰疬较优，常配玄参、牡蛎，即消瘰丸；治疮痈、乳痈，常与蒲公英、天花粉、连翘等配伍；治肺痈，可与鱼腥草、鲜芦根、薏苡仁等同用。

combined with Pugongying (*Herba Taraxaci*), Tianhuafen (*Radix Trichosanthis*), and Lianqiao (*Fructus Forsythiae*), etc.; for pulmonary abscess, combined with Yuxingcao (*Herba Houttuyniae*), Xianlugen (*Rhizoma Phragmitis*, fresh), and Yiyiren (*Semen Coicis*), etc..

Usage and Dosage 3 - 10 g is used in decoction for oral use and 1 - 2 g is used in the powder.

Notes It is incompatible with Wutou (*Rhizoma Aconiti*).

【用法用量】 水煎服，3～10 克。研末服，1～2 克。

【使用注意】 反乌头。

Xingren *Semen Armeniacae Amarum*

The source is from the mature seed of *Prunus armeniaca* L., or *P. armeniaca* L. var. ansu Maxim, family Rosaceae. The medicinal material is produced in the areas of Northeast, North and Northwest China, Xinjiang, and the reaches of the Yangtze River of China, collected in summer when the fruit is ripe and dried in the sun after it is shelled. The crude one is used.

Medicinal Properties Bitter in flavor, slightly warm in nature, mildly toxic and attributive to the lung and large intestine meridians.

Actions Relieve cough and dyspnea, moisten the intestine and relax the bowels.

Application

1. It is used for cough and dyspnea, is an essential medicine of treating them and can be used to treat all kinds syndromes of cough and dyspnea in combination with other herbs according to syndrome. For cough and dyspnea of wind-cold type, it can be used in combination with Mahuang (*Herba Ephedrae*) and Gancao (*Radix Glycyrrhizae*), such as San'ao Tang (Decoction); for cough of wind-heat type, used with Sangye (*Folium Mori*), Juhua (*Flos Chrysanthemi*), etc.; for that of dryness-heat type, used together with Sangye (*Folium Mori*), Beimu

杏 仁

为蔷薇科植物山杏、东北杏、西伯利亚杏或杏的成熟种子。产于东北、华北、西北、新疆及长江流域。夏季果实成熟时采收种子，除去果肉及核壳，晒干。生用。

【药性】 味苦，性微温。有小毒。归肺、大肠经。

【功效】 止咳平喘，润肠通便。

【临床应用】

1. 用于咳嗽气喘。为治咳喘要药，随证配伍可用治各种咳喘证。治风寒咳喘，可配麻黄、甘草，如三拗汤；治风热咳嗽，每与桑叶、菊花等配伍；治燥热咳嗽，与桑叶、贝母、沙参等同用；治肺热咳喘，与麻黄、生石膏等合用，如麻杏石甘汤。

(*Bulbus Fritillariae*), and Shashen (*Radix Glehniae*), etc.; for that of lung-heat type, used together with Mahuang (*Herba Ephedrae*), Shengshigao (*Gypsum Fibrosum*, unprepared), etc.; such as Ma Xing Shi Gan Tang (Decoction).

2. For constipation due to dryness of intestine, it is usually combined with Huomaren (*Semen Cannabis*), Danggui (*Radix Angelicae Sinensis*), Zhike (*Fructus Aurantii*) and others, such as Runchang Wan (Pill).

2. 用于肠燥便秘。常与火麻仁、当归、枳壳等同用,如润肠丸。

Usage and Dosage 3 - 10 g is used in decoction for oral use, which is usually broken.

【用法用量】 水煎服,3~10 克,宜打碎入煎。

Notes Since it is mildly toxic, overdosage should be avoided and it is used in infants with caution.

【使用注意】 本品有毒,用量不宜过大,婴儿慎服。

Jiegeng *Radix Platycodi*

桔 梗

The source is from the root of *Platycodon grandiflorum* (Jacq.) A. DC., family Campanulaceae. The medicinal material is produced in the areas of Anhui, Jiangsu, and Shandong, etc., dug and collected in both spring and autumn, dried in the sun after the impurity is got rid of. The raw is cut into pieces for being used.

为桔梗科植物桔梗的根。主产安徽、江苏及山东等地。春秋两季采挖。去杂质,晒干,切片。生用。

Medicinal Properties Bitter and pungent in flavor, bland in nature and attributive to the lung meridian.

【药性】 味苦、辛,性平。归肺经。

Actions Disperse the lung to resolve phlegm, ease the throat and drain the pus.

【功效】 宣肺化痰,利咽,排脓。

Application

【临床应用】

1. It is indicated for cough with excessive phlegm, sore throat and aphonia due to failure of the lung to disperse. It can be used for cough with excessive phlegm no matter whether it is due to lung-cold or lung-heat. For cough of wind-cold type, it is combined with Xingren (*Semen Pruni Armeniacae*), Zisuye (*Folium Perillae*) and Jupi (*Pericarpium Citri Tangerinae*), etc.; for that of wind-heat type, usually combined with Sangye (*Folium Mori*), Juhua (*Flos Chrysanthemi*), and Xingren

1. 用于肺气不宣之咳嗽痰多,咽痛音哑。治咳嗽痰多,不论肺寒、肺热,俱可应用。治风寒咳嗽,配杏仁、紫苏叶、橘皮等;治风热咳嗽,常配桑叶、菊花、杏仁等;咽痛音哑因热邪犯肺,则可配薄荷、牛蒡子、蝉蜕等;热毒盛者配射干、马勃、板蓝根等。

(*Semen Pruni Armeniacae*), etc.; for sore throat and aphonia due to pathogenic heat invading the lung, combined with Bohe (*Herba Menthae*), Niubangzi (*Fructus Arctii*), and Chantui (*Periostracum Cicadae*), etc.; for domination of pathogenic heat, combined with Shegan (*Rhizoma Belamcandae*), Mabo (*Lasiosphaera seu Calvatia*) and Banlangen (*Radix Isatidis*), etc..

2. For pulmonary abscess with chest pain, cough with pus, blood and yellow sputum with stinking smell, it is combined with Gancao (*Radix Glycyrrhizae*), such as Jiegeng Tang (Decoction); if the herb is combined with Yuxingcao (*Herba Houttuyniae*), Yiyiren (*Semen Coicis*), Dongguazi (*Semen Benincasae*) and Beimu (*Bulbus Fritillariae*), its action of clearing away heat and draining the pus is even stronger.

2. 用于肺痈胸痛,咳吐脓血,痰黄腥臭。可配伍甘草同用,如桔梗汤;若与鱼腥草、薏苡仁、冬瓜子、贝母同用,清热排脓之力更强。

Usage and Dosage 3-6 g is used in decoction for oral use. Large dosage untill 10 g can be used in draining pus.

【用法用量】 水煎服,3~6 克。排脓可用至10 克。

Notes It is lifting and dispersing in property, therefore, it is not suitable for functional activities of qi going upward resulting in vomiting, chocking cough and dizziness. Over dosage easily results in nausea and vomiting. It is not suitable to be used as injection because of the hemolyzation of its platycodoside.

【使用注意】 本品性升散,凡气机上逆、呕吐、呛咳、眩晕者不宜用。用量过大易致恶心呕吐;所含桔梗皂苷有溶血作用,不宜作注射给药。

Zisuzi *Fructus Perillae*

紫苏子

The source is from the mature fruit of *Perilla frutescens* (L.) Britt. var. acuta (Thunb.) Kudo, family Labiatae. The medicinal material is mainly produced in the areas of Jiangsu, Anhui, etc.. They are collected in autumn when the fruits are ripe, dried in the sun. The crude one or the one stir-baked slightly is used, broken when used.

为唇形科植物紫苏的成熟果实。主产于江苏、安徽等地。秋季果实成熟时采收,晒干。生用或微炒,用时捣碎。

Medicinal Properties Pungent in flavor, warm in nature and attributive to the lung and large intestine me-

【药性】 味辛,性温。归肺、大肠经。

ridians.

Actions Lower the adverse-rising qi, resolve phlegm, relieve cough and dyspnea, moisten the intestine and relax bowels.

【功效】 降气化痰,止咳平喘,润肠通便。

Application

【临床应用】

1. It is used for accumulation of phlegm and the adverse-rising of qi manifested as cough and dyspnea, it is usually combined with Baijiezi (*Semen Sinapis*) and Laifuzi (*Semen Raphani*), such as Sanzi Yangqin Tang (*Decoction*); for phlegm-fluid accumulation with dyspnea and cough, and chest distress, it is combined with Houpo (*Cortex Magnoliae Officinalis*), Jupi (*Pericarpium Citri Tangerinae*) and Banxia (*Rhizoma Pinelliae*), etc., such as Suzi Jiangqi Tang (Decoction).

1. 用于痰壅气逆,咳嗽气喘。常与白芥子、莱菔子同用,如三子养亲汤;治痰涎壅盛,喘咳上气,胸闷,可与厚朴、橘皮、半夏等配用,如苏子降气汤。

2. For constipation due to dryness of the intestine, it is usually combined with Huomaren (*Fructus Cannabis*), Gualouren (*Semen Trichosanthis*), and Xingren (*Semen Pruni Armeniacae*), etc..

2. 用于肠燥便秘。常与火麻仁、瓜蒌仁、杏仁等同用。

Usage and Dosage 5-10 g is used in decoction for oral use.

【用法用量】 水煎服,5～10 克。

Notes It is used with caution in the cases with cough due to yin deficiency and loose stool due to spleen deficiency.

【使用注意】 阴虚喘咳及脾虚便溏者慎用。

Tinglizi *Semen Lepidii seu Descurainiae*

葶苈子

The source is from the mature seed of *Lepidum apetalum* Willd., (Nantinglizi) or *Descurainia sophia* (L.) Webb ex Prantl (Beitinglizi), family Cruciferae. *Descurainia sophia* (L.) Webb ex Prantl is mainly produced in the areas of Jiangsu and Shandong; *Lepidium apetalum* Willd. is mainly produced in the areas of Hebei and Liaoning. Before or after the beginning of summer, when the fruits are ripe, the whole plants are cut, dried and then the seeds are collected. The crude one or the one stir-baked slightly is used.

为十字花科植物播娘蒿(南葶苈子)和独行菜(北葶苈子)的成熟种子。播娘蒿主产于江苏、山东;独行菜主产于河北、辽宁。立夏前后果实成熟时,割取全株,干燥,打下种子。生用或微炒用。

Medicinal Properties Bitter and pungent in flavor, extreme cold in nature and attributive to the lung and bladder meridians.

【药性】 味苦、辛,性大寒。归肺、膀胱经。

Actions Purge lung-fire, relieve dyspnea, promote diuresis and reduce edema.

【功效】 泻肺平喘,利水消肿。

Application

【临床应用】

1. It is indicated in a case with phlegm-fluid accumulation, cough with excessive sputum, dyspnea and being unable to lie, and general swelling. It especially purges the retention of fluid and phlegm-fire in the lung so as to relieve dyspnea and cough. It is usually combined with Dazao (*Fructus Ziziphi Jujube*) to moderate herbal property, such as Tingli Dazao Xiefei Tang (Decoction).

1. 用于痰涎壅滞,咳逆痰多,喘息不得卧,一身面目浮肿。本品专泻肺中水饮、痰火而平喘止咳。多配大枣以缓和药性,如葶苈大枣泻肺汤。

2. It is also used for edema, pleural effusion and ascites, and dysuria. For abdominal edema due to dampness and heat, it is combined with Fangji (*Radix Stephaniae Tetrandrae*), Jiaomu (*Semen Zanthoxyli*), and Dahuang (*Radix et Rhizoma Rhei*), that is, Ji Jiao Li Huang Wan (Pill); for syndrome resulting from pathogenic factors accumulating in the thorax with pleural effusion and ascites, combined with Xingren (*Semen Pruni Armeniacae*), Dahuang (*Radix et Rhizoma Rhei*), and Mangxiao (*Natrii Sulfas*), such as Da Xianxiong Tang (Decoction).

2. 用于水肿、悬饮、胸腹积水、小便不利。治腹水肿满属湿热者,配防己、椒目、大黄,即己椒苈黄丸;治结胸证之胸胁积水,配杏仁、大黄、芒硝,即大陷胸丸。

It is recently used in combination with Fuzi (*Radix Aconiti Lateralis Praeparata*) and Huangqi (*Radix Astragali*) to treat pulmonary heart disease and heart failure, which achieves better therapeutic effects.

近年用此配伍附子、黄芪,治肺心病、心力衰竭,有较好疗效。

Usage and Dosage 3-10 g is used in decoction for oral use. 3-6 g is used in the powder.

【用法用量】 水煎服,3～10克。研末服,3～6克。

Xuanfuhua *Flos Inulae*

旋覆花

The source is from the capitulum of *Inula japonica* Thunb., family Compositae. The medicinal material is mainly produced in North China, East China and provinces

为菊科植物旋覆花或欧亚旋覆花的头状花序。主产华北、华东及长江下游各省。

of lower reaches of the Yangtze River, collected in summer and autumn when the bud is open, dried in the sun and the crude one or the one roasted with honey is used.

夏、秋两季花蕾开放时采收,晒干。生用或蜜炙用。

Medicinal Properties Bitter, pungent and salty in flavor, slightly warm in nature and attributive to the spleen, lung, stomach and large intestine meridians.

【药性】 味苦、辛、咸,性微温。归肺、脾、胃、大肠经。

Actions Descend the adverse-rising qi, resolve phlegm and arrest vomiting.

【功效】 降气化痰,降逆止呕。

Application

【临床应用】

1. It is used for phlegm-fluid accumulation in the lung with cough, excessive phlegm, phlegm-retention and sensation of fullness in the chest and hypochondrium. For cough and dyspnea of cold-phlegm type that is companied with superficial syndrome, it is usually combined with Shengjiang (*Rhizoma Zingiberis Recens*), Banxia (*Rhizoma Pinelliae*) and Xixin (*Herba Asari*), such as Jinfucao San (Powder); for sthenia-syndrome of phlegm-heat type manifested as cough and dyspnea, it is usually combined with Jiegeng (*Radix Platycodi*), Sangbaipi (*Cortex Mori Radicis*) and Gualou (*Fructus Trichosanthis*), etc..

1. 用于痰涎壅肺,咳喘痰多,以及痰饮蓄结,胸膈痞闷。用于寒痰咳喘,兼有表证者,常与生姜、半夏、细辛同用,如金沸草散;治痰热咳喘实证,多与桔梗、桑白皮、瓜蒌等配用。

2. For deficiency of spleen-qi and stomach-qi, and adverse ascending of phlegm manifested as vomiting, belching and epigastric fullness, it is usually combined with Daizheshi (*Haematitum*), Banxia (*Rhizoma Pinelliae*), Shengjiang (*Rhizoma Zingiberis Recens*) and Renshen (*Radix Ginseng*), etc., such as Xuanfu Daizhe Tang (Decoction).

2. 用于脾胃气虚,痰浊上逆所致的呕吐,噫气,心下痞满。常配代赭石、半夏、生姜、人参等,如旋覆代赭汤。

Usage and Dosage 3 - 10 g is used in decoction for oral use, which is wrapped with cloth for being decocted.

【用法用量】 水煎服,3~10克。表面有绒毛,须布包煎。

Notes Contraindicated for tuberculosis with cough due to yin deficiency, dry cough due to injury of the body fluids.

【使用注意】 阴虚痨咳,津伤燥咳者禁用。

Pipaye　*Folium Eriobotryae*

枇杷叶

The source is from the leaf of *Eriobotrya japonica* (Thunb.) Lindl., family Rosaceae. The plant is cultivated in most areas of China. The leaf can be collected all year around, dried in the sun, the hair being brushed, and then cut into fine pieces. The crude one or the one roasted with honey is used.

为蔷薇科植物枇杷的叶。中国大部分地区有栽培。全年均可采收,晒干,刷去毛,切丝。生用或蜜炙用。

Medicinal Properties　Bitter in flavor, slightly cold in nature and attributive to the lung and stomach meridians.

【药性】 味苦,性微寒。归肺、胃经。

Actions　Clear away lung-heat, resolve phlegm, relieve cough, lower the adverse-rising qi and arrest vomiting.

【功效】 清肺化痰止咳,降逆止呕。

Application

【临床应用】

1. It is indicated for cough. For cough due to lung-heat, it is usually combined with Sangye (*Folium Mori*), Qianhu (*Radix Peucedani*), etc.; for cough and dyspnea due to dryness-heat, it is combined with Sangbaipi (*Cortex Mori Radicis*), Zhimu (*Rhizoma Anemarrhenae*), and Shashen (*Radix Glehniae*), etc.; for chronic cough due to deficiency of the lung, combined with Ejiao (*Colla Corii Asini*), Baihe (*Bulbus Lilii*) and others that nourish yin and moisten the lung.

1. 用于咳嗽。治肺热咳嗽,常配桑叶、前胡等同用;治燥热咳喘,配伍桑白皮、知母、沙参等;若肺虚久咳,则配阿胶、百合等养阴润肺药同用。

2. For vomiting and nausea caused by stomach-heat, it is usually combined with Jupi (*Pericarpium Citri Tangerinae*), Zhuru (*Caulis Bambusae in Taeniam*), etc..

2. 用于胃热呕吐,呃逆。常配橘皮、竹茹等同用。

Usage and Dosage　5 - 10 g is used in decoction for oral use. The roasted one is suitable for arresting cough and the raw for arresting vomiting.

【用法用量】 水煎服,5～10克。止咳宜炙用,止呕宜生用。

Baibu　*Radix Stemonae*

百　部

The source is from the root tuber of *Stemona sessilifolia* (Miq.) Miq. and *S. japonica* (Bl.) Miq., family Stemonaleae. The medicinal material is mainly

为百部科植物直立百部、蔓生百部或对叶百部的块根。主产于安徽、江苏、湖北、山东

produced in the areas of Anhui, Jiangsu, Hubei, Shandong and others, dug and collected in both spring and autumn, fibrous root being got rid of, boiled in boiling water for a while and then dried in the sun, which is cut into thick pieces. The raw or the one roasted with honey is used.

等地。春、秋两季采挖,除去须根,置沸水中略烫或蒸至无白心,晒干,切厚片。生用或蜜炙用。

Medicinal Properties Bitter and sweet in flavor, slightly warm in nature and attributive to the lung meridians.

【药性】 味甘、苦,性微温。归肺经。

Actions Moisten the lung to arrest cough, and kill worms.

【功效】 润肺止咳,杀虫。

Application

【临床应用】

1. It is indicated for short-term or prolonged cough, whooping cough and cough due to pulmonary tuberculosis. For cough due to wind and cold, it is combined with Jingjie (*Herba Schizonepetae*), Jiegeng (*Radix Platycodi*), etc.; for prolonged cough and deficiency of both qi and yin, combined with Huangqi (*Radix Astragali*), Shashen (*Radix Glehniae*) and Maimendong (*Radix Ophiopogonis*) that can enrich qi, nourish yin and moisten the lung; for whooping cough, it can be used alone or combined with Jingjie (*Herba Schizonepetae*), Jiegeng (*Radix Platycodi*) and Ziwan (*Radix Asteris*); for cough due to pulmonary tuberculosis, combined with Shashen (*Radix Glehniae*), Maimendong (*Radix Ophiopogonis*) and Chuanbeimu (*Bulbus Fritillarae Cirrhosae*), etc.. At present, it is combined with Huangqin (*Radix Scutellariae*) and Danshen (*Radix Salviae Miltiorrhizae*) to treat pulmonary tuberculosis.

1. 用于新久咳嗽,百日咳,肺痨咳嗽。治风寒咳嗽,配荆芥、桔梗等;久咳不已,气阴两虚者,则配黄芪、沙参、麦门冬补气养阴润肺;治百日咳,可单用,也可配荆芥、桔梗、紫菀同用;治肺痨咳嗽,可配沙参、麦门冬、川贝母等。现代配黄芩、丹参,治肺结核,对痰菌转阴及病灶的吸收均有一定疗效。

2. It is indicated for enterobiasis, vaginal trichomoniasis, head louse and scabies. For enterobiasis, it is boiled into thick decoction, with which enema is given to the patients before they sleep; for vaginal trichomoniasis, it can be used alone or combined with Shechuangzi (*Fructus Cnidii*), Kushen (*Radix Sophorae Flavescentis*),

2. 用于蛲虫、阴道滴虫、头虱及疥癣。治蛲虫病,以本品浓煎,睡前保留灌肠;治阴道滴虫,可单用,或配蛇床子、苦参等煎汤坐浴外洗;治头虱、体虱及疥癣,多制成乙醇

etc., which are decocted for hip bath with external washing; for head and bodily louse, and scabies, it is prepared into ethyl alcohol extract or decoction for external application.

液或水煎剂外搽。

Usage and Dosage 5 - 10 g is used in decoction for oral use. Just right amount is for external use. The one roasted with honey is for prolonged and deficient cough.

【用法用量】 水煎服，5～10 克。外用，适量。久咳虚嗽宜蜜炙用。

11 Tranquilizers

第十一章 安神药

Any medicinal herb that calms the mind and has the main action of treating mental disorder is referred to tranquilizers.

They are usually attributive to the heart meridian and mainly indicated for hyperactivity of heart-fire, internal interference of phlegm-heat or heart-qi and heart blood deficiency manifested as irritability, palpitation, insomnia with frequent dreams, infantile convulsion, epilepsy and mania, etc..

They mainly include such medicinal materials as minerals and plant seeds that are used in prescription. The mineral medicines are heavy and lowering in property and have the main action of tranquillizing the mind while the plant seeds are moistening and tonifying in property and have the main action of nourishing the heart and calming the mind.

They should be selected according to causes of disease and pathogenesis, that is, sthenic syndrome should be treated with mineral medicines and asthenic syndrome should be treated with plant seeds. Besides, they must be used in combination accordingly. For example, for hyperactivity of heart-fire, they should be used in combination with medicinal herbs for clearing away heart-frie; for deficiency of yin and blood, those for replenishing the blood and nourishing yin should be combined; and for liver-yang rising, those for calming the liver and suppressing yang should be combined.

Since mineral medicines, if they are used in pill or

凡具有安定神志功效，以治疗神志失常病证为主的药物，称为安神药。

安神药多入心经。主要适用于心火亢盛，痰热内扰或心气虚、心血虚等所致的心神不宁，心悸怔忡，失眠多梦以及惊风、癫痫、癫狂等。

安神药多以矿物药与种子类植物药入药。其中矿物药质重性降，多具重镇安神的作用；种子类药质润性补，多具养心安神作用。

安神药应根据病因病机择用，实证宜选用重镇安神药，虚证宜选用养心安神药。此外，还须作相应的配伍。如心火炽盛者，当与清心火药配伍；阴虚血少者，应与养血补阴药配伍；肝阳上亢者，须与平肝潜阳药配伍。

矿石类药物，如作丸散

powder form, easily damage the stomach-qi, they must be combined with those for nourishing the stomach and strengthening the spleen according to the conditions, and are only taken temporarily. Some of them must be used with caution since they are toxic.

服,易耗伤胃气,须酌情配伍养胃健脾之品,且只宜暂服。部分药物有毒,更须慎用。

Zhusha *Cinnabaris*

朱　砂

It refers to Cinnabar of sulfide type, mainly containing mercuric sulfide. The medicinal material is mainly produced in the areas of Hunan, Sichuan, and Yunnan, etc. and mined at any time. The mineral is refined into powder with water for medication after impurity of stone is removed.

为硫化物类矿物辰砂族辰砂,主要成分含硫化汞。主产于湖南、四川、云南等。随时可采。采得的辰砂矿石击碎后,除去石块杂质,水飞极细,装瓶备用。

Medicinal Properties Sweet in flavor, cold in nature, toxic and attributive to the heart meridian.

【药性】 味甘,性寒。有毒。归心经。

Actions Relieve palpitation and calm the mind, clear away heat and remove toxic materials.

【功效】 镇心安神,清热解毒。

Application

【临床应用】

1. It is used for irritability, restless fever and insomnia due to hyperactivity of heart-fire, it is usually combined with Huanglian (*Rhizoma Coptidis*) and Gancao (*Radix Glycyrrhizae*); for those companied with deficiency of heart-blood, Danggui (*Radix Angelicae Sinensis*) and Dihuang (*Radix Rehmanniae*) are added again; for palpitation due to fear or heart-deficiency, it can be put in pig's heart and cooked for oral use.

1. 用于心火亢盛所致心神不安、烦热、惊悸不眠。多与黄连、甘草配伍;兼有心血虚者,再配当归、地黄;惊恐或心虚所致惊悸怔忡,可将本品入猪心中炖服。

2. It is used for pyocutaneous disease and sore throat. For pyocutaneous disease, it is used together with Xionghuang (*Realgar*), such as Zijin Ding (Troche); for sore throat and aphthae due to heat, used together with Bingpian (*Borneolum Syntheticum*), Pengsha (*Borax*), etc., for external use, such as Bing Peng San (Powder).

2. 用于疮疡肿毒,咽喉肿痛。治疮疡肿毒,可与雄黄配伍,如紫金锭;治热毒咽喉肿痛,口舌生疮,可配冰片、硼砂等外用,如冰硼散。

Usage and Dosage 0.1－0.5 g of the powder is used in pill or powder form. Just right amount is for

【用法用量】 研末,入丸散剂,0.1～0.5克。外用,

external use.

Notes Over dosage and prolonged administration should be avoided to prevent patients from being poisoned by mercury. The medicine is used with caution in cases with incomplete function of the liver and kidneys. It can not be calcined with fire, otherwise mercury can be separated out, which is extremely toxic.

适量。

【使用注意】 内服不宜过量，也不可久服，以防汞蓄积中毒。肝肾功能不全者慎用。忌火煅，火煅析出的水银有剧毒。

Cishi *Magnetitum*

The medicine refers to the magnetic iron ore magnetite, mainly including Fe_3O_4. It is mainly produced in the areas of Hebei, Shandong, and Liaoning, etc. and mined at any time and stored in the dry place. It is broken into pieces or quenched with vinegar and ground into powder for medication.

Medicinal Properties Pungent and salty in flavor, cold in nature and attributive to the liver, heart and kidney meridians.

Actions Tranquilize the mind, calm the liver and suppress the sthenic yang, improve auditory and visual acuity, improve inspiration by invigorating kidney-qi and relieve dyspnea.

Application

1. For deficiency of yin leading to hyperactivity of yang manifested as irritability, palpitation, insomnia, dizziness, headache and epilepsy, usually combined with Zhusha (*Cinnabaris*), Shijueming (*Concha Haliotidis*), Baishaoyao (*Radix Paeoniae Alba*), and Shengdihuang (*Radix Rehmanniae*), etc..

2. For insufficiency of the liver-yin and kidney-yin manifested as tinnitus, deafness, and blurring of vision, etc., it can be combined with Shudihuang (*Radix Rehmanniae Praeparatae*), Shanzhuyu (*Fructus Corni*) and Wuweizi (*Fructus Schisandrae*), etc., such as Erlong Zuoci Wan (Pill); for insufficiency of the liver and

磁　石

为氧化物类矿物尖晶石族磁铁矿的矿石，主含四氧化三铁。主产于河北、山东、辽宁等。随时可采。采得后，置干燥处保存。击碎生用，或醋淬研细用。

【药性】 味辛、咸，性寒。归肝、心、肾经。

【功效】 镇惊安神，平肝潜阳，聪耳明目，纳气平喘。

【临床应用】

1. 用于阴虚阳亢所致的烦躁不宁，心悸，失眠，头晕头痛及癫痫。常与朱砂、石决明、白芍药、生地黄等同用。

2. 用于肝肾阴虚所致的耳鸣、耳聋及目昏等证。可与熟地黄、山茱萸、五味子等配伍，如耳聋左慈丸；治肝肾不足，视力模糊，可与枸杞子、女贞子同用。

kidney with blurring of vision, it can be combined with Gouqizi (*Fructus Lycii*) and Nüzhenzi (*Fructus Ligustri Lucidi*).

3. For shortness of breath due to insufficiency of kidney-qi, it is usually combined with Daizheshi (*Haematitum*), Wuweizi (*Fructus Schisandrae*) and Hutaorou (*Caro Juglamdis*).

3. 用于肾虚不能纳气之虚喘。多与代赭石、五味子、胡桃肉配伍。

Usage and Dosage 10 - 30 g is used in decoction for oral use, which is broken into pieces and decocted early. 1 - 3 g is used in pill and powder form.

【用法用量】 水煎服，10～30 克，打碎先煎。入丸、散，1～3 克。

Notes It can not be used in large amount or prolonged time since it is not easily digested, and used with caution in cases with deficiency of the spleen and stomach.

【使用注意】 口服不易消化，故不可多用。脾胃虚弱者慎用。

Longgu *Os Draconis*

龙　骨

The source is from the fossil of the skeleton of ancient large mammals, such as deer, oxen and elephant types. The medicinal material is mainly produced in the areas of Shanxi, Inner Mongolia Autonomous Region, Gansu, and Hebei, etc., collected all year round and stored in the dry place. It is broken into pieces when it is used and the crude or calcined one is used.

为古代哺乳动物如三趾马、鹿类、牛类、象类等的骨骼化石。主产于山西、内蒙古、甘肃、河北等地。全年可采挖，贮于干燥处。用时打碎，生用或煅用。

Medicinal Properties Sweet and pungent in flavor, slightly cold in nature and attributive to the heart and liver meridians.

【药性】 味甘、涩，性微寒。归心、肝经。

Actions Tranquilize the mind, calm the liver and suppress the hyperactive yang, astringe and invigorate the kidney to preserve essence.

【功效】 镇静安神，平肝潜阳，收敛固涩。

Application

【临床应用】

1. It is used for restlessness, epilepsy and insanity. For restlessness, palpitation, insomnia, poor memory and frequent dreams, it can be combined with Zhusha (*Cinnabaris*), Yuanzhi (*Radix Polygalae*) and Suanzaoren (*Semen Ziziphi Spinosae*), etc.; for epilepsy, convul-

1. 用于神志不安，以及惊痫，癫狂。治心神不安，心悸失眠，健忘多梦，可与朱砂、远志、酸枣仁等配用；治惊痫抽搐，癫狂发作，多与牛黄、胆南

sion and insanity, it is usually combined with Niuhuang (*Calculus Bovis*), Dannanxing (*Arisaema cum Bile*) and others that can resolve phlegm and arrest spasm.

星等化痰止痉药同用。

2. For irritability and dizziness caused by deficiency of yin leading to hyperactivity of yang, it is usually combined with Muli (*Concha Ostreae*), Baishaoyao (*Radix Paeoniae Alba*) and Daizheshi (*Haematitum*), etc., such as Zhengan Xifeng Tang (Decoction).

2. 用于阴虚阳亢所致的烦躁易怒，头晕目眩。常配牡蛎、白芍药、代赭石等同用，如镇肝熄风汤。

3. It is used for syndromes of slippery prolapse. For kidney-deficiency syndrome manifested as emission and spermatorrhea, it is used every time with Muli (*Concha Ostreae*), Shayuanzi (*Semen Astragali Complanati*), and Qianshi (*Semen Euryales*), etc., such as Jinsuo Gujing Wan (Pill); for all kinds of clear leukorrhagia and menorrhagia, combined with Muli (*Concha Ostreae*), Haipiaoxiao (*Os Sepiellae Seu Sepia*) and Shanyao (*Rhizoma Dioscoreae*); for spontaneous perspiration due to superficial asthenia and night sweat due to yin-deficiency, usually combined with Muli (*Concha Ostreae*), Fuxiaomai (*Fructus Tritici Levis*) and Wuweizi (*Fructus Schisandrae*), etc..

3. 用于滑脱诸证。治肾虚遗精，滑精，每与牡蛎、沙苑子、芡实等配伍，如金锁固精丸；治带下清稀及月经过多，配牡蛎、海螵蛸、山药同用；治表虚自汗、阴虚盗汗，常与牡蛎、浮小麦、五味子等配伍。

Besides, the Duanlonggu (*Os Draconis Usta*) that is ground into powder has the action of sucking up moisture and treating skin ulcer disease, so it can be used externally for exudative prurigo and unhealed pyocutaneous disease after evacuation of pus.

此外，煅龙骨研末外用，有吸湿敛疮作用，可用于湿疮痒疹及疮疡溃后久不愈合。

Usage and Dosage 15 - 30 g is used in decotion for oral use, which is broken and then decocted earlier. Just right amount is for external use. The calcined one is used for astringing and invigorating the kidney to preserve essence and the crude one is used for other syndromes.

【用法用量】 水煎服，15～30 克，打碎先煎。外用，适量。收敛固涩煅用，其他生用。

Hupo *Succinum*

琥 珀

The source is from the resin of ancient pines buried in the earth for a long time. The medicinal material is

为古代松科植物的树脂，埋藏地层中经多年转化而成

mainly produced in the areas of Yunnan, Guangxi, Liaoning, and Henan, etc.. It is ground into powder for being used after it is collected and got rid of impurity.

的化石样物质。主产于云南、广西、辽宁、河南等地。采得后去除杂质,研末用。

Medicinal Properties Sweet in flavor, mild in nature and attributive to the heart, liver and bladder meridians.

【药性】 味甘,性平。归心、肝、膀胱经。

Actions Tranquilize the mind, promote blood circulatin to remove blood stasis, promote diuresis and relieve stranguria.

【功效】 定惊安神,活血散瘀,利尿通淋。

Application

【临床应用】

1. It is used for restlessness, convulsion and epilepsy; for palpitation and restlessness, insomnia and frequent dreams, it is combined with Suanzaoren (*Semen Ziziphi Spinosae*), Yejiaoteng (*Caulis Polygoni Multiflori*), and Zhusha (*Cinnabaris*), etc., such as Hupo Dingzhi Wan (Pill); for convulsion and epilepsy, usually combined with Zhusha (*Cinnabaris*), Quanxie (*Scorpio*), etc..

1. 用于心神不安,以及惊风、癫痫。治心悸不安、失眠多梦,可与酸枣仁、夜交藤、朱砂等药配伍,如琥珀定志丸;治惊风癫痫,常与朱砂、全蝎等药同用。

2. It is used for amenorrhea, abdominal mass and pains. For amenorrhea due to blood stasis and qi stagnation, and swelling and pains due to trauma, it should be combined with Danggui (*Radix Angelicae Sinensis*), Ezhu (*Rhizoma Zedoariae*), and Wuyao (*Radix Linderae*), etc.; it is powdered singly and used for scrotum and labial hematoma of woman's vulva or blood stasis in uterine; it is combined with Sanqi (*Radix Notoginseng*), which is ground into powder for oral use to treat coronary heart disease.

2. 用于经闭,癥瘕疼痛等。治血滞气阻之经闭及外伤瘀肿疼痛,配当归、莪术、乌药等;单味为散服可用于阴囊及妇女阴唇血肿或子宫郁血;配三七为末服,还可用于治疗冠心病。

3. For stranguria or retention of urine, especially for bloody stranguria that can be treated effectively with its single form. It is taken with the decoction of Congbai (*Bulbus Cepae*) to treat stranguria of sand and stone types; it is also used together with Jinqiancao (*Herba Lysimachiae*), Bianxu (*Herba Polygoni Avicularis*) and others that can promote diuresis and relieve stranguria to treat stranguria of heat and stone type.

3. 用于淋证或癃闭。尤宜于血淋,单用有效。若用葱白煎汤冲服,可治砂石诸淋;亦可配伍金钱草、萹蓄等利尿通淋之品治热淋、石淋。

Usage and Dosage 1.5 - 3 g of the powder is taken with water. It is not used in decoction.

【用法用量】 研末冲服，1.5～3 克。不入煎剂。

Suanzaoren *Semen Ziziphi Spinosae*

酸枣仁

The source is from the mature seed of *Ziziphus Spinosa* Hu, family Rhamnaceae. The medicinal material is mainly produced in the areas of Hebei, Shaanxi, Liaoning, Shandong, Shanxi, and Henan, etc., collected in the end of autumn and early stage of winter when the fruits are ripe, and dried. The crude or stir-baked one is used.

为鼠李科植物酸枣的成熟种子。主产于河北、陕西、辽宁、山东、山西、河南等地。秋末冬初果实成熟时采收，除去枣肉、核壳，取种子干燥。生用或炒用。

Medicinal Properties Sweet and sour in flavor, mild in nature, and attributive to the heart and liver meridians.

【药性】 味甘，性平。归心、肝经。

Actions Nourish the heart, benefit the liver, tranquilize the mind and stop the excessive perspiration.

【功效】 养心益肝，安神，敛汗。

Application

【临床应用】

1. It is indicated for insomnia and vexation. It is a commonly used medicine to treat restlessness that is caused by various causes, especially by deficient syndrome. For that caused by deficiency of heart-blood and liver-blood, and failure of the heart being nourished, it is usually combined with Danggui (*Radix Angelicae Sinensis*), Baishaoyao (*Radix Paeoniae Alba*) and Heshouwu (*Radix Polygoni Multiflori*), etc.; for vexation and insomnia due to liver-deficiency with heat, combined with Zhimu (*Rhizoma Anemarrhenae*), Fuling (*Poria*), etc., such as Suanzaoren Tang (Decoction); for that due to deficiency of both the heart and spleen, usually combined with Dangshen (*Radix Codonopsis*) and Huangqi (*Radix Astragali*), such as Guipi Tang (Decoction); for that due to insufficiency of the heart and kidney, and yin-deficiency leading to yang-hyperactivity, combined with Shengdihuang (*Radix Rehmanniae*), Xuanshen (*Radix Scrophulariae*) and Baiziren (*Semen Biotae*), etc.,

1. 用于失眠，惊悸怔忡。为治心神不安的常用药，适应于各种原因所致者，尤宜于虚证。心肝血虚，心神失养所致者，多配当归、白芍药、何首乌等同用；肝虚有热之虚烦失眠，与知母、茯苓等同用，如酸枣仁汤；心脾两虚所致者，常与党参、黄芪同用，如归脾汤；属心肾不足，阴虚阳亢所致者，可配生地黄、玄参、柏子仁等同用，如天王补心丹。

such as Tianwang Buxin Dan (Pill).

2. For spontaneous perspiration and night sweating, it is usually combined with Dangshen (*Radix Codonopsis*), Wuweizi (*Fructus Schisandrae*) and Shanzhuyu (*Fructus Corni*).

2. 用于自汗、盗汗。常与党参、五味子、山茱萸同用。

Usage and Dosage 9 - 15 g is used in decoction for oral use. 1.5 - 3 g of the powder is swallowed before sleeping.

【用法用量】 水煎服，9～15克。研末睡前吞服，1.5～3克。

Baiziren *Semen Biotae*

柏子仁

The source is from the seed of *Biota Orientalis* (L.) Endl, family Cupressaceae. The medicinal material is mainly produced in the areas of Shandong, Henan, and Hebei, etc., collected after autumn and dried in the shade after the spermoderm is got rid of. The herbal seed is broken when it is used.

为柏科植物侧柏的种仁。主产山东、河南、河北等地。秋后成熟时采收，除去外壳，阴干。用时打碎。

Medicinal Properties Sweet in flavor, mild in nature, and attributive to the heart, kidney and large intestine meridians.

【药性】 味甘，性平。归心、肾、大肠经。

Actions Nourish the heart and tranquilize the mind, moisten the intestine and relax the bowels.

【功效】 养心安神，润肠通便。

Application

【临床应用】

1. It is indicated for deficiency of heart-qi or insufficiency of heart-yin, and failure of the heart being nourished manifested as vexation, insomnia, convulsion and epilepsy, it is usually combined with Suanzaoren (*Semen Ziziphi Spinosae*), Wuweizi (*Fructus Schisandrae*), and Fuling (*Poria*), etc.; for that companied with night sweating, it is combined with Renshen (*Radix Ginseng*), Muli (*Concha Ostreae*) and Wuweizi (*Fructus Schisandrae*) such as Baiziren Wan (Pill).

1. 用于心气虚或心阴不足，心神失养的虚烦不眠，惊悸怔忡。常与酸枣仁、五味子、茯苓等同用；兼盗汗者，可与人参、牡蛎、五味子同用，如柏子仁丸。

2. It is used for constipation due to dryness of intestine, especially for that due to yin-deficiency and insufficiency of the blood since Baiziren (*Semen Biotae*) is moistening and excessively oily in property. It is usually

2. 用于肠燥便秘。柏子仁质润多油。多用于阴虚血少的肠燥便秘，常与火麻仁、郁李仁同用，如五仁丸。

combined with Huomaren (*Fructus Cannabis*) and Yuliren (*Semen Pruni*), such as Wuren Wan (Pill).

Usage and Dosage 3 - 9 g is used in decoction for oral use.

Notes It is used with caution in cases with loose stool and excessive sputum.

【用法用量】 水煎服，3～9克。

【使用注意】 便溏及多痰者慎用。

Yuanzhi *Radix Polygalae*

远 志

The source is from the root of the perennial herbage *Polygala tenuifolia* Wild., or *P. sibirica* L., family Polygalaceae. The medicinal material is mainly produced in the areas of Shanxi, Shanxi and Henan, etc., dug and collected in spring and autumn, dried in the sun. The crude or roasted one is used.

为远志科植物远志或卵叶远志的根。主产于山西、陕西、河南等省。春、秋两季采挖，晒干。生用或炙用。

Medicinal Properties Pungent and bitter in flavor, slightly warm in nature, and attributive to the lung and heart meridians.

【药性】 味辛、苦，性微温。归肺、心经。

Actions Tranquilize the mind, eliminate phlegm for resuscitation and dissipate the carbuncles.

【功效】 宁心安神，祛痰开窍，消散痈肿。

Application

1. It is used for irritability, palpitation due to fright, insomnia and amnesia, it is usually used together with Renshen (*Radix Ginseng*), Fushen (*Parasita Poriae*) and Shichangpu (*Rhizoma Acori Graminei*), such as Anshen Dingzhi Wan (Pill).

2. For confusion of the mind by phlegm manifested as mental confusion, absentmindedness and epilepsy due to fright, it is usually combined with Shichangpu (*Rhizoma Acori Graminei*), Yujin (*Radix Curcumae*), etc..

3. For cough with excessive phlegm that is difficult to cough out, it is combined with Xingren (*Semen Armeniacae Amarum*), Jiegeng (*Radix Platycodi*), and Gancao (*Radix Glycyrrhizae*), etc..

4. For large carbuncle and pain of the breast, it can be used no matter whether the syndrome is due to cold,

【临床应用】

1. 用于心神不安，惊悸，失眠，健忘。常与人参、茯神、石菖蒲配伍，如安神定志丸。

2. 用于痰阻心窍所致的精神错乱，神志恍惚，惊痫。常与石菖蒲、郁金等同用。

3. 用于咳嗽痰多，质黏难以咯出者，可与杏仁、桔梗、甘草等同用。

4. 用于痈疽肿毒，乳房肿痛。无论寒热虚实均可应用，

heat, asthenia or sthenia. It can be ground into powder that is taken alone with millet wine, or that is mixed for external application.

可单用为末,黄酒送服;也可外用调敷。

Usage and Dosage 3-10 g is used in decoction. Just right amount is for external use.

【用法用量】 水煎服,3~10 克。外用适量。

Notes It is used with caution in patients who suffer from ulcer and gastritis.

【使用注意】 溃疡病及胃炎患者慎用。

Hehuanpi *Cortex Albiziae*

合欢皮

The source is from the bark of *Albizzia julibrissin* Durazz, family Leguminosae. The medicinal material is mainly produced in the provinces of the reaches of the Yangtze River, cut from the tree, dried in the sun and then cut into segments for being used.

为豆科植物合欢的树皮。主产于长江流域各省。夏、秋两季剥取树皮,晒干,切段用。

Medicinal Properties Sweet in flavor, mild in nature, and attributive to the heart and liver meridians.

【药性】 味甘,性平。归心、肝经。

Actions Tranquilize the mind and disperse the depressed qi, activate blood circulation and relieve swelling.

【功效】 安神解郁,活血消肿。

Application

【临床应用】

1. It is used for emotional injury manifested as mental depression, deficient vexation, insomnia and amnesia. It can be used alone or combined with Baiziren (*Semen Biotae*), Longchi (*Dens Draconis*), etc..

1. 用于情志所伤的忿怒忧郁,虚烦不安,健忘失眠。可单用,亦可与柏子仁、龙齿等同用。

2. It is used for trauma and swelling. In the treatment of fracture, it is usually combined with Danggui (*Radix Angelicae Sinensis*), Chuanxiong (*Rhizoma Chuanxiong*) and Xuduan (*Radix Dipsaci*); in the treatment of carbuncle and ulcers, it is usually combined with Pugongying (*Herba Taraxaci*) and Yejuhua (*Flos Chrysanthemi Indici*).

2. 用于跌打骨折及痈肿。治骨折,常与当归、川芎、续断同用;治痈疽疮肿,常与蒲公英、野菊花同用。

Usage and Dosage 10-15 g is used in decoction for oral use.

【用法用量】 水煎服,10~15 克。

Notes The flower or bud of *Albizia julibrissin* Durazz. is used as medicinal herb, which is named Hehuanhua (*Flos Albiziae*). It has similar medicinal properties

【说明】 花或花蕾亦作药用,名合欢花,药性、功效与合欢皮相似,但更长于安神解

and actions to those of Hehuanpi (*Cortex Albiziae*) but is especially effective in tranquilizing the mind and dispersing the depressed qi, and usually used for vexation, insomnia, mental depression, amnesia and frequent dreams.

郁,多用于虚烦不眠,心情抑郁,健忘,多梦。

12 Chinese Medicinal Herbs for Calming the Liver to Stop Endogenous Wind

第十二章 平肝熄风药

Any medicinal herb that has the actions of calming the liver and suppressing the hyperactive yang or calming the liver-wind, and is indicated for syndrome of liver-yang rising or liver-wind stirring is called Chinese medicinal herbs for calming the liver to stop endogenous wind.

具有平肝潜阳或平熄肝风作用，主治肝阳上亢或肝风内动的药物，称为平肝熄风药。

They are mainly attributive to the liver meridian and mostly include animal and mineral medicines such as shell and insect types. They are mainly used for dizziness due to liver-yang rising, and convulsion and epilepsy due to liver-wind stirring inside.

本类药物，主入肝经，多为介类、昆虫等动物药及矿物药，主要用于肝阳上亢，头晕目眩证及肝风内动，抽搐惊痫。

When they are used, one should differently combine them with other medicinal herbs according to the different causes and symptoms. For syndrome of liver-wind stirring inside, which is usually caused by excessive fire-heat and hyperactive liver-yang accompanied by liver-heat, medicinal herbs for clearing away heat, reducing fire and purging liver-heat must be combined. For yin-deficiency with insufficiency of the blood and failure of the liver to nourish resulting in liver-wind stirring inside and liver-yang rising, those for nourishing the kidney and yin or replenishing the blood should be combined. Domination of liver-fire is usually accompanied by restlessness, therefore they should be combined with tranquilizers.

应用平肝熄风药时，应根据不同病因和兼证，予以不同配伍。肝风内动，多由火热炽盛所致；肝阳上亢亦每兼肝热，故须与清热泻火、清泄肝热药同用。阴虚血少，肝失滋养，以致肝风内动与肝阳上亢，则又当与滋肾养阴或补血药同用。肝旺每兼神志不安症状，故又应与安神药同用。

They should be applied distinctively since most of them are a bit on cold or cool side while some of them are a bit on warm and dry side. For chronic convulsion due to

本类药物多偏于寒凉，但也有偏于温燥者，应区别使用。凡脾虚慢惊，非寒凉药所

spleen-deficiency, cold or cool medicinal herbs are not suitable, but for yin-deficiency with insufficiency of the blood, the warm-dry medicinal herbs should be used with caution.

宜;而阴虚血亏者,又当慎用温燥之品。

Shijueming *Concha Haliotidis*

The source is from the shell of *Haliotis diversicolor* Reeve, *H. gigantea* discus Reeve, *H. ovina* chemnitz and others, family Haliotidae. The medicinal materials are distributed over the areas along the sea, caught in summer and autumn and the shells (meat is removed) are cleaned, and then dried in the sun after the impurity is got rid of. The crude or calcined one is used after it is broken.

Medicinal Properties Salty in flavor, cold in nature, and attributive to the liver meridian.

Actions Calm the liver, suppress the hyperactive yang and clear away liver-fire to improve eyesight.

Application

1. For deficiency of liver-yin and kidney-yin and hyperactivity of liver-yang manifested as dizziness and headache, it is every time combined with Shengdihuang (*Radix Rehmanniae*), Baishaoyao (*Radix Paconiae Alba*), and Muli (*Concha Ostreae*), etc.; for hyperactivity of liver-yang with heat, combined with Xiakucao (*Spica Prunellae*), Gouteng (*Ramulus Uncariae cum Uncis*) and Juhua (*Flos Chrysanthemi*).

2. It is an essential medicine for clearing away liver-fire to improve eyesight and used for redness, swelling and pain of the eyes, nebula, and blurring of vision no matter whether they are due to sthenic or asthenic syndromes. For up-flaring of liver-fire manifested as redness, swelling and pain of the eyes, it may be combined with Juemingzi (*Semen Cassiae*), Juhua (*Flos Chrysanthemi*), etc.; for eye disease and nebula due to wind and

石决明

为鲍科动物杂色鲍(光底石决明)或皱纹盘鲍(毛底石决明)、羊鲍、澳洲鲍等的贝壳。分布于沿海地区。夏、秋季捕取,去肉后,洗净贝壳,除去杂质,晒干。打碎生用或煅用。

【药性】 味咸,性寒。归肝经。

【功效】 平肝潜阳,清肝明目。

【临床应用】

1. 用于肝肾阴虚,肝阳上亢所致的眩晕,头痛。每与生地黄、白芍药、牡蛎等配用;如属肝阳亢盛而有热象者,则与夏枯草、钩藤、菊花等同用。

2. 用于目赤肿痛,翳膜遮睛,视物昏糊。为清肝明目之要药,无论实证、虚证均可以运用。治肝火上炎,目赤肿痛,可与决明子、菊花等配伍;治风热目疾,翳膜遮睛,可与密蒙花、谷精草等配伍;肝虚血少,日久目昏,则与菟丝子、

heat, it may be combined with Mimenghua (*Flos Buddlejae*), Gujingcao (*Flos Eriocauli*), etc.; for deficiency of the liver and insufficiency of the blood with dizziness, combined with Tusizi (*Semen Cuscutae*), Shudihuang (*Radix Rehmanniae Praeparata*), etc., such as Shijueming Wan (Pill).

熟地黄等同用,如石决明丸。

Usage and Dosage 15 - 30 g is used in decoction for oral use, which is decocted at first. The crude is used to calm the liver and clear away liver-fire and calcined one is used externally for eye disease.

【用法用量】 水煎服,15～30克,宜先煎。平肝清肝生用,外用点眼宜煅用,水飞。

Muli *Concha Ostreae*

牡 蛎

The source is from the shell of *Ostrea gigas* Thunberg, *O. talienwhanensis* Crosse or *O. rivularis* Gould, family Ostreidae. The medicinal material is produced in the areas along the sea of China, collected in winter and spring and dried in the sun after the shell (meat is removed) is cleaned. The crude or calcined one is used after it is broken.

为牡蛎科动物长牡蛎、大连湾牡蛎或近江牡蛎的贝壳。中国沿海地区均产,冬、春采集,去肉留壳,洗净晒干。捣碎生用,或煅用。

Medicinal Properties Salty in flavor, slightly cold in nature and attributive to the liver and kidney meridians.

【药性】 味咸,性微寒。归肝、肾经。

Actions Calm the liver, suppress the hyperactive yang, soften hardness and disperse the stagnated mass, and astringe, invigorate the kidney to preserve essence.

【功效】 平肝潜阳,软坚散结,收敛固涩。

Application

【临床应用】

1. For hyperactivity of liver-yang manifested as dizziness and tinnitus, it is usually used together with Longgu (*Os Draconis*), Guiban (*Plastrum Testudinis*), and Baishaoyao (*Radix Paeoniae Alba*), etc., such as Zhengan Xifeng Tang (Decoction); for febrile disease injuring the yin and causing endogenous liver wind manifested as convulsion of limbs, usually combined with Guiban (*Plastrum Testudinis*), Biejia (*Carapax Trionycis*), and Dihuang (*Radix Rehmanniae*), etc., such as Da Dingfeng

1. 用于肝阳上亢头晕目眩及耳鸣。常与龙骨、龟版、白芍药等配伍,如镇肝熄风汤;若热病伤阴,肝风内动,四肢抽搐,常配龟版、鳖甲、地黄等药,如大定风珠。

Zhu (Bolus).

2. For stagnation of phlegm and fire manifested as scrofula, subcutaneous nodule and abdominal mass, it is usually used together with Zhebeimu (*Bulbus Fritillariae Thunbergii*) and Xuanshen (*Radix Scrophulariae*), such as Xiaoluo Wan (Bolus). Recently, it is used clinically to treat mass of the hypochondrium, it is usually combined with Danshen (*Radix Salviae Miltiorrhizae*), Zelan (*Herba Lycopi*) and Biejia (*Carapax Trionycis*), etc..

2. 用于痰火郁结之瘰疬，痰核及癥瘕积聚。常与浙贝母、玄参配伍，如消瘰丸。近来临床用以治胁下癥块，常与丹参、泽兰、鳖甲等配伍使用。

3. It is used for all slippery and depletive syndromes. For spontaneous perspiration and night sweat, it may be combined with Huangqi (*Radix Astragali*) and Mahuanggen (*Radix Ephedrae*); for kidney-deficiency syndrome manifested as emission and spermatorrhea, usually combined with Shayuanzi (*Semen Astragali Complanati*) and Qianshi (*Semen Euryales*), such as Jinsuo Gujing Wan (Pill); for metrorrhagia and metrostaxis and abnormal vaginal discharge, combined with Duanlonggu (*Os Draconis Usta*), Haipiaoxiao (*Os Sepiellae seu Sepiae*) and Shanyao (*Rhizoma Dioscoreae*).

3. 用于滑脱诸证。治自汗、盗汗，可与黄芪、麻黄根配伍；治肾虚遗精、滑精，常与沙苑子、芡实同用，如金锁固精丸；治崩漏、带下，则可与煅龙骨、乌贼骨、山药同用。

Besides, it has the action of controlling acid, so it can be used for gastroxynsis and gastric ulcer.

此外，本品尚有制酸作用，可用于胃酸过多、胃溃疡等。

Usage and Dosage 15 - 30 g is used in decoction for oral use, which is decocted earlier. The calcined one is used for astringing, invigorating the kidney to preserve essence and controlling acid and the crude one is used for other symptoms.

【用法用量】 水煎服，15～30 克，先煎。收敛固涩、制酸煅用，余均生用。

Niuhuang *Calculus Bovis*

牛 黄

The source is from the stone in the gallbladder and biliary ducts of *Bos taurus domesticus* Gemelin, family Bovidae. The medicinal material is mainly produced in the areas of Northwest and Northeast China. When a cow is

为牛科动物牛的胆囊或胆管结石。主产于中国西北和东北地区。宰牛时，如发现胆囊、胆管有结石，立即滤去

killed, if one finds the stone in the gallbladder and biliary ducts, one immediately fetches the stone after filtering the bile, the stone being dried in the shade for being used.

胆汁,取出牛黄,阴干,备用。

Medicinal Properties Bitter in flavor, cool in nature and attributive to the liver and heart meridians.

【药性】 味苦,性凉。归肝、心经。

Actions Stop endogenous wind and relieve convulsion, eliminate phlegm for resuscitation, clear away heat to remove toxic materials.

【功效】 熄风止痉,化痰开窍,清热解毒。

Application

【临床应用】

1. For seasonal febrile disease with high fever, coma, spasm and infantile convulsion, it is usually used together with Zhusha (*Cinnabaris*), Quanxie (*Scorpio*), and Gouteng (*Ramulus Uncariae cum Uncis*), etc., such as Niuhuang San (Powder).

1. 用于温热病高热神昏,痉挛抽搐及小儿惊风。常与朱砂、全蝎、钩藤等配伍,如牛黄散。

2. For seasonal febrile disease resulting in heat attacking the pericardium, apoplexy, convulsion and epilepsy, and syndrome of confusion of the mind due to accumulation of phlegm-heat, it is ground singly into powder, which is dissolved in Danzhuli (*Succus Bambusae*) for oral use, or combined with Shexiang (*Moschus artifactus*), Zhizi (*Fructus Gardeniae*) and Huanglian (*Rhizoma Coptidis*), etc., such as Angong Niuhuang Wan (Pill).

2. 用于温热病热入心包、中风、惊风、癫痫等痰热蒙蔽心窍证。单用本品为末,淡竹沥化服即效;或与麝香、栀子、黄连等配伍,如安宫牛黄丸。

3. For heat-toxin syndrome manifested as sore throat and aphthous stomatitis due to heat-toxin accumulation, it is usually combined with Huangqin (*Radix Scutellariae*), Xionghuang (*Realgar*), and Dahuang (*Radix et Rhizoma Rhei*), etc.; if the sore throat is ulcerated, it should be ground together with Zhenzhu (*Margarita*) into powder for external application on the wounded throat, that is, Zhu Huang San (Powder); for large carbuncle, furuncle, breast carcinoma and scrofula, etc., also combined with Shexiang (*Moschus artifactus*), Ruxiang

3. 用于热毒证。热毒壅结之咽喉肿痛,口舌生疮,常与黄芩、雄黄、大黄等同用;若咽喉肿痛并溃烂,可与珍珠为末吹喉,即珠黄散;治痈疽、疔毒、乳岩、瘰疬等,又与麝香、乳香、没药等合用,如犀黄丸。

(*Olibanum*) and Moyao (*Myrrha*), etc., such as Xi Huang Wan (Pill).

Usage and Dosage 0.2-0.5 g is used in pill or powder form. Just right amount is for external use, which is ground into fine powder for application on wounded areas.

【用法用量】 入丸散，0.2～0.5克。外用，适量，研细末敷患处。

Notes It is used with caution in pregnant women.

【使用注意】 孕妇慎用。

Daizheshi *Haematitum*

代赭石

The source is from the red iron of trigonal system, Fe_2O_3 as the chief component. The medicinal material is produced in the areas of Shanxi, Henan, and Shandong, etc., dug out and then cleaned. The crude one or the one prepared with vinegar is broken for being used.

为三方晶系氧化物类矿物赤铁矿的矿石，主要成分含三氧化二铁。产于山西、河南、山东等地。掘出后，洗净。打碎生用，或醋淬后粉碎用。

Medicinal Properties Bitter in flavor, cold in nature and attributive to the liver and heart meridians.

【药性】 味苦，性寒。归肝、心经。

Actions Calm the liver and suppress the hyperactive yang, descend the adverse-rising qi and arrest bleeding.

【功效】 平肝潜阳，降逆，止血。

Application

【临床应用】

1. For hyperactivity of liver-yang manifested as dizziness and headache. It is usually combined with Longgu (*Os Draconis*), Muli (*Concha Ostreae*) and Baishaoyao (*Radix Paeoniae Alba*), such as Zhengan Xifeng Tang (Decoction); for the syndrome with obvious deficiency of liver-yin and kidney-yin, combined with Guiban (*Plastrum Testudinis*), Muli (*Concha Ostreae*), Baishaoyao (*Radix Paeoniae Alba*) and others.

1. 用于肝阳上亢头晕，头痛，目眩。常与龙骨、牡蛎、白芍药同用，如镇肝熄风汤；肝肾阴虚明显者，可与龟版、牡蛎、白芍药等养阴敛肝药同用。

2. It is used for the syndromes of adverse-rising of lung-qi and stomach-qi. The syndrome of adverse-rising of stomach-qi manifested as hiccup and vomiting is treated with it in combination with Xuanfuhua (*Flos Inulae*), Banxia (*Rhizoma Pinelliae*) and Shengjiang (*Rhizoma Zingiberis Recens*), such as Xuanfu Daizhe Tang (Decoction); for deficiency of both the lung and kidney, and ad-

2. 用于肺、胃气逆证。治胃气上逆，呃逆，呕吐，可与旋覆花、半夏、生姜同用，如旋覆代赭汤；治肺肾两虚，气逆喘息，可与人参、山茱萸同用，如参赭镇气汤。

verse-rising of lung-qi with rapid respiration, it is combined with Renshen (*Radix Ginseng*) and Shanzhuyu (*Fructus Corni*), such as Shen Zhe Zhenqi Tang (Decoction).

3. It is used for blood-heat syndrome manifested as haematemesis, epistaxis, and metrorrhagia and metrostaxis. For haematemesis and epistaxis, it may be combined with Baishaoyao (*Radix Paeoniae Alba*), Zhuru (*Caulis Bambusae in Taeniam*), and Niubangzi (*Fructus Arctii*), etc., such as Hanjiang Tang (Decoction); for prolonged metrorrhagia and metrostaxis with dizziness, combined with Yuyuliang (*Limonitum*), Chishizhi (*Halloystium Rubrum*) and Wulingzhi (*Faeces Trogopyerorum*), etc., such as Zhenling Dan (Pill).

3. 用于血热吐血、衄血及崩漏等。治吐血、衄血,可与白芍药、竹茹、牛蒡子等配伍,如寒降汤;若崩漏日久,头晕眼花者,配禹余粮、赤石脂、五灵脂等,共奏固涩及祛瘀生新之效,如镇灵丹。

Usage and Dosage 10-30 g is used in decoction for oral use, which is broken and decocted early. Or may be used in pill or powder form. The crude one is used for lowering adverse-rising of qi and calming the liver and the calcined one for arresting bleeding.

【用法用量】 水煎服,10～30克,打碎先煎。或入丸、散。降逆、平肝宜生用,止血宜煅用。

Notes It is used in pregnant women with caution.

【使用注意】 孕妇慎用。

Lingyangjiao *Cornu Saigae Tataricae*

羚羊角

The source is from the horn of *Saiga tatarica* L., family Bovidae. The medicinal material is mainly produced in the areas of Xinjiang, Qinghai and others of China. The animal is caught all year round. After capture of the animal, the horn is cut, and when it is used, it can be prepared as juice, slices or powder.

为牛科动物赛加羚羊的角。主产于新疆、青海等地。全年均可捕捉,捕得后切取角,用时磨汁、锉末或镑为薄片。

Medicinal Properties Bitter in flavor, cold in nature and attributive to the liver and heart meridians.

【药性】 味咸,性寒。归肝、心经。

Actions Calm the liver and stop endogenous wind, clear away heat and remove toxic materials, clear away liver-fire to improve eyesight.

【功效】 平肝熄风,清热解毒,清肝明目。

Application

【临床应用】

1. It is indicated for liver-wind stirring inside manifested as convulsion, and is an essential medicine to treat

1. 用于肝风内动,惊痫抽搐。为治疗肝风内动的要药,

syndrome of liver-wind stirring inside and most suitable for overabundance of heat bringing about convulsion. For seasonal febrile disease with overabundance of heat that results in wind syndrome manifested as high fever, coma and convulsion of extremities, it is used in combination with Gouteng (*Ramulus Uncariae cum Uncis*), Juhua (*Flos Chrysanthemi*) and Shengdihuang (*Radix Rehmanniae*), that is Lingyang Gouteng Tang (Decoction); for epilepsy due to phlegm-heat and palpitation due to fright, combined with Gouteng (*Ramulus Uncariae cum Uncis*), Yujin (*Radix Curcumae*) and Zhusha (*Cinnabaris*).

最适宜于热极生风。用治温热病热邪亢盛,盛极动风,症见壮热神昏,四肢抽搐,配钩藤、菊花、鲜生地黄,即羚羊钩藤汤;治痰热癫痫、惊悸,则与钩藤、郁金、朱砂同用。

2. For seasonal febrile disease with high fever, delirium, mania and eruption, it is combined with Shigao (*Gypsum Fibrosum*), Niuhuang (*Calculus Bovis*), etc., such as Zixue Dan (Pill).

2. 用于温热病高热谵语,躁狂,发斑。可与石膏、牛黄等配伍同用,如紫雪丹。

3. It is used for dizziness due to hyperactivity of liver-yang or headache and redness of eyes due to up-rising of liver-fire. For the former, it is combined with Juhua (*Flos Chrysanthemi*) and Shijueming (*Concha Haliotidis*); for the latter, combined with Huangqin (*Radix Scutellariae*), Longdan (*Radix Gentianae*), etc., such as Lingyangjiao San (Powder).

3. 用于肝阳上亢的头晕目眩或肝火上炎之头痛,目赤。前者可与菊花、石决明同用;后者则配黄芩、龙胆等,如羚羊角散。

Usage and Dosage 1-3 g is decocted alone for two hours, the decoction being taken after mixing it with other decoction. It is also pounded into juice or ground into powder, 0.3-0.5 g being suitable use.

【用法用量】 水煎服,宜另煎汁冲服,1～3克,单煎2小时。亦可磨汁或锉末服,0.3～0.5克。

Gouteng *Ramulus Uncariae cum Uncis*

钩 藤

The source is from the hooked vine of *Uncaria rhynchophylla* (Miq.) Jacks., family Rubiaceae. The medicinal material is mainly produced in the provinces of Hunan, Fujian and Guangdong, collected in spring and autumn, dried in the sun and cut into segments. The crude is used.

为茜草科植物钩藤及其同属多种植物的带钩茎枝。主产于湖南、福建、广东等省。春、秋两季采收带钩的茎枝,晒干,切段。生用。

Medicinal Properties Sweet in flavor, slightly cold in nature and attributive to the liver, heart and pericardium meridians.

【药性】 味甘，性微寒。归肝、心包经。

Actions Stop endogenous wind to relieve convulsion, and clear away liver-heat and calm the liver.

【功效】 熄风止痉，清热平肝。

Application

【临床应用】

1. It is used for liver-wind stirring inside with convulsion. For infantile convulsion, high fever and coma, it is combined with Tianma (*Rhizoma Gastrodiae*), Shijueming (*Concha Haliotidis*), and Quanxie (*Scorpio*), such as Gouteng Yin (Decoction); for seasonal febrile disease with overabundance of heat bringing about wind syndrome, it is combined with Lingyangjiao (*Cornu Saigae Tataricae*), Longdan (*Radix Gentianae*), and Juhua (*Flos Chrysanthemi*), etc.; for convulsion and cry of epilepsy, used with Tianzhuhuang (*Concertio Silicea Bambusae*), Chantui (*Periostracum Cicadae*) and Huanglian (*Rhizoma Coptidis*), etc., such as Gouteng Yinzi (Decoction).

1. 用于肝风内动，惊痫抽搐。治小儿惊风，壮热神昏，与天麻、石决明、全蝎等配伍，即钩藤饮；治温热病热极动风，可与羚羊角、龙胆、菊花等同用；治痫证抽搐，啼叫，可与天竺黄、蝉蜕、黄连等同用，如钩藤饮子。

2. For liver-meridian heat syndrome manifested as distention of head, headache and redness of eyes or hyperactivity of liver-yang with dizziness, it is usually combined with Xiakucao (*Spica Prunellae*), Huangqin (*Radix Scutellariae*), Juhua (*Flos Chrysanthemis*) and Shijueming (*Concha Haliotidis*), etc. so as to clear away heat and calm the liver.

2. 用于肝经有热，头胀头痛，目赤或肝阳上亢、头晕目眩等证。常配夏枯草、黄芩、菊花、石决明等，以清热平肝。

Besides, it has good effect of lowering the blood pressure, so it can be used to treat hypertension.

此外，本品有良好的降血压功效，可用治高血压病。

Notes 3 - 12 g is used in decoction for oral use, but it is not suitable to be decocted for a long time.

【用法用量】 水煎服，3～12克，不宜久煎。

Tianma *Rhizoma Gastrodiae*

天　麻

The source is from the tuber of *Gastrodia elata* BI., family Orchidaceae. The medicinal material is mainly produced in the areas of Sichuan, Yunnan and Guizhou,

为兰科寄生植物天麻的块茎。主产于四川、云南、贵州等地。冬、春两季出芽和茎

etc., dug and collected in winter and spring when the plant buds or the stem is dried, boiled with water or steamed and dried on mild fire after the cortex is removed. When used, it is soaked and cut into slices.

枯时采挖。除去菌丝及外皮，洗净煮透或蒸熟，微火烤干。用时润透切片。

Medicinal Properties Sweet in flavor, mild in nature and attributive to the liver meridian.

【药性】 味甘，性平。归肝经。

Actions Stop endogenous wind to arrest convulsion, calm the liver and suppress yang.

【功效】 熄风止痉，平肝潜阳。

Application

【临床应用】

1. It is used for syndromes of liver-wind stirring inside with convulsion and so on. For acute infantile convulsion, it is usually combined with Gouteng (*Ramulus Uncariae cum Uncis*), Lingyangjiao (*Cornu Saigae Tataricae*), and Quanxie (*Scorpio*), etc., that is, Gouteng Yinzi (Decoction); for chronic infantile convulsion of spleen-deficiency type with slightly moving of hands and feet, it is combined with Renshen (*Radix Ginseng*), Baizhu (*Rhizoma Atractylodis Macrocephalae*), and Baijiangcan (*Bombyx Batryticatus*), etc., such as Xingpi Wan (Pill); for the treatment of tetanus, epilepsy and opisthotonos, combined with Tiannanxing (*Rhizoma Arisaematis*), Baifuzi (*Rhizoma Typhonii*) and Fangfeng (*Radix Saposhnikoviae*), etc., such as Yuzhen San (Powder).

1. 用于肝风内动，惊痫抽搐等证。治小儿急惊风，多配钩藤、羚羊角、全蝎等，即钩藤饮子；治小儿脾虚慢惊风，手足微动，则配人参、白术、白僵蚕等品，如醒脾丸；配天南星、白附子、防风等，即玉真散，可治破伤风痉挛抽搐、角弓反张。

2. It is used for dizziness and headache due to hyperactivity of liver-yang, and is an essential herb of treating dizziness. For that due to hyperactivity of liver-yang, it is usually combined with Gouteng (*Ramulus Uncariae cum Uncis*), Huangqin (*Radix Scutellariae*), and Niuxi (*Radix Achyranthis Bidenatatae*), etc.; for that due to up-attacking of wind-phlegm, combined with Banxia (*Rhizoma Pinelliae*), Baizhu (*Rhizoma Atractylodis Macrocephalae*) and Fuling (*Poria*), etc., that is Banxia Baizhu Tianma Tang (Decoction).

2. 用于肝阳上亢所致的眩晕、头痛等证。为治眩晕之要药。肝阳上亢所致者，常与钩藤、黄芩、牛膝等配用；属风痰上扰者，则须与半夏、白术、茯苓同用，即半夏白术天麻汤。

Besides, it can also expel wind and dampness, and alleviate obstructive pain, and so it is used for obstructive pain, numbness of the extremities and unsmooth movement of hands and feet, etc., it is usually combined with Qinjiao (*Radix Gentianae Macrophyllae*), Qianghuo (*Rhizoma et Radix Notopterygii*), Niuxi (*Radix Achyranthis Bidenatatae*) and Sangjisheng (*Ramulus Taxilli*).

此外，还能祛风湿，止痹痛，用于风湿痹痛及肢体麻木、手足不遂等证。多与秦艽、羌活、牛膝、桑寄生等同用。

Usage and Dosage 3－10 g is used in decoction for oral use. 1—1.5 g of the powder is swallowed.

【用法用量】 水煎服，3～10克。研末吞服，1～1.5克。

Quanxie *Scorpio*

全　蝎

The source is from the whole body of *Buthus martensii* Karsch, family Buthidae. The medicinal material is produced in all parts of China and mostly in the north areas of Yangtze River, is caught in spring and autumn, killed by boiling water or boiled with salt after being grasped, and then dried in the sun.

为全蝎科昆虫东亚钳蝎的干燥体。产中国各地，长江以北地区较多。春、秋均可捕捉。捕得后，投入沸水中烫死或加盐煮，晒干。

Medicinal Properties Pungent in flavor, mild in nature, toxic, and attributive to the liver meridian.

【药性】 味辛，性平。有毒。归肝经。

Actions Stop endogenous wind to relieve convulsion, eliminate toxic materials and disperse the lumps, and dredge the meridian and alleviate pain.

【功效】 熄风止痉，解毒散结，通络止痛。

Application

1. For spasm and convulsion, it is often used in clinic together with Wugong (*Scolopendra*), which are ground together into powder that is called Zhijing San (Powder). For acute infantile convulsion, combined with Tianma (*Rhizoma Gastrodiae*), Gouteng (*Ramulus Uncariae cum Uncis*), and Lingyangjiao (*Cornu Saigae Tataricae*), etc.; for chronic infantile convulsion due to spleen deficiency, usually combined with Dangshen (*Radix Codonopsis*), Baizhu (*Rhizoma Atractylodis Macrocephalae*) and Tianma (*Rhizoma Gastrodiae*), etc.; for

【临床应用】

1. 用于痉挛抽搐。与蜈蚣共研细末，即止痉散，临床常用。如治小儿急惊风，可配天麻、钩藤、羚羊角等；脾虚慢惊，则常配党参、白术、天麻等；治中风口眼歪斜，常与白附子、白僵蚕同用，即牵正散；治破伤风，角弓反张，又多与天南星、蝉蜕配伍。

apoplexy with distortion of the face, usually used together with Baifuzi (*Rhizoma Typhonii*) and Baijiangcan (*Bombyx Batryticatus*), that is Qianzheng San (Powder); for tetanus and opisthotonos, usually yet combined with Tiannanxing (*Rhizom Arisaematis*) and Chantui (*Periostracum Cicadae*).

2. For pyocutaneous disease, scrofula and subcutaneous nodes, Quanxie (*Scorpio*) in combination with Zhizi (*Fructus Gardeniae*) is fried in sesame oil and then prepared with yellow wax into medicinal extract for applying on the wounded areas.

2. 用于疮疡肿毒，瘰疬结核。常用麻油煎全蝎、栀子，加黄蜡为膏，敷于患处。

3. For intractable headache and migraine and pain of Bi-syndrome due to wind and dampness, it is ground alone into powder for being swallowed; it is also used together with Wugong (*Scolopendra*) and Baijiangcan (*Bombyx Batryticatus*).

3. 用于顽固性偏正头痛，风湿痹痛。单味研末吞服即能奏效；亦可配伍蜈蚣、白僵蚕同用。

Usage and Dosage 2 - 5 g is used in decoction for oral use. 0.6 - 1 g of the powder is swallowed. Just right amount is for external use.

【用法用量】 水煎服，2～5克。研末吞服，0.6～1克。外用，适量。

Notes It is toxic, so the dosage can not be over large and used with caution in the cases with wind syndrome due to blood-deficiency.

【使用注意】 本品有毒，用量不可过大。血虚生风者慎用。

Wugong *Scolopendra*

蜈蚣

The source is from the dried whole body of *Scolopendra subspinipes* mutilans L., Koch., family Scolopendrae. The insect is produced in all parts of China, and caught in spring, dried in the sun or dried after being scalded by boiled water. The crude or roasted one is used.

为蜈蚣科昆虫少棘巨蜈蚣的干燥体。全国各地均产，春季捕捉。捕后用长竹片贯插头尾，晒干；或用沸水烫过，干燥。生用或炙用。

Medicinal Properties Pungent in flavor, warm in nature, toxic and attributive to the liver meridian.

【药性】 味辛，性温。有毒。归肝经。

Actions Stop endogenous wind to relieve convulsion, eliminate toxic materials and disperse lumps, and dredge meridian and alleviate pain.

【功效】 熄风止痉，解毒散结，通络止痛。

Application

1. It is used for acute and chronic convulsion and tetanus. Its action is similar to that of Quanxie (*Scorpio*), so the two medicines arc often combined with each other to treat convulsion of hands and feet and opisthotonos.

2. It is used for pyocutaneous disease and ulcerative scrofula. It is combined with Xionghuang (*Realgar*) for external application to treat malignant sores; it is ground with tea leaf into fine powder for external application to treat scrofula and pyocutaneous disease. Besides, it is also used to treat poisonous snake bite.

3. In treating intractable spasm and pain of the head, and pain of Bi-syndrome due to wind and dampness, it is usually used together with Quanxie (*Scorpio*), Tianma (*Rhizoma Gastrodiae*), Baijiangcan (*Bombyx Batryticatus*) and Chuanxiong (*Rhizoma Chuanxiong*), etc..

Usage and Dosage 3 - 5 g is used in decoction; its powder of 0.6 - 1 g is swallowed or applied externally with a proper amount of powder or oil mixture.

Notes With its poisonous nature, the dosage adopted should be small, and contraindicated for the pregnant women.

【临床应用】

1. 用于急慢惊风，破伤风。功效与全蝎相似，治手足抽搐，角弓反张，两药常相须为用。

2. 用于疮疡肿毒，瘰疬溃烂。外敷治肿毒恶疮，与雄黄配伍；治瘰疬溃烂，与茶叶共为细末外敷。此外，还可治疗毒蛇咬伤。

3. 用于顽固性头部抽掣疼痛，风湿痹痛。多与全蝎、天麻、白僵蚕、川芎等同用。

【用法用量】 水煎服，3～5克。研末吞服，0.6～1克，外用，适量，研末或油调敷患处。

【使用注意】 本品有毒，用量不可过大。孕妇忌用。

Dilong *Lumbricus*

The source is from the dry body with the organs removed of *Pheretima aspergillum* (Perrier) or the whole body of *Allolobophora caliginosa* (Savigny) trapezoids (Ant. Duges), family Megascolecidae. The former sort is mainly seen in Guangdong and Guangxi, called Guangdilong, and the latter three kinds are seen everywhere, called Tudilong. They are caught in spring and summer, dried in the sun for use. The crude or fresh one can be used.

地 龙

为巨蚓科环节动物参环毛蚓、通俗环毛蚓、威廉环毛蚓或栉盲环毛蚓的干燥全体。前一种，主产于广东、广西，称广地龙；后三者，各地均产，称土地龙。夏、秋季捕捉，晒干。生用或鲜用。

Medicinal Properties Salty in flavor, cold in nature, and attributive to the liver, spleen and bladder meridians.

【药性】 味咸,性寒。归肝、脾、膀胱经。

Actions Clear away heat and stop endogenous wind, relieve asthma, dredge meridians and promote diuresis.

【功效】 清热熄风,平喘,通络,利尿。

Application

【临床应用】

1. It is applied for high fever with convulsion and spasm. For seasonal febrile disease manifested as coma, delirium, spasm and convulsion, it is usually used together with Gouteng(*Ramulus Uncariae cum Uncis*), Baijiangcan (*Bombyx Batryticatus*), and others with action of calming the liver and stop endogenous wind. In the case of epilepsy and depressive and manic syndromes, it can be mixed with salt for drinking.

1. 用于壮热惊痫、抽搐。治温热病热极生风神昏谵语、痉挛抽搐,多与钩藤、白僵蚕等平肝熄风药同用。治癫狂、癫痫,可同食盐共化为水饮服。

2. It is applied for heat in the lung with bronchial asthma. It can be used singly or together with Mahuang (*Herba Ephedrae*), Xingren (*Semen Pruni Armeniacae*) and Shigao (*Gypsum Fibrosum*),etc., or made for acupoint-injection or muscular injection.

2. 用于肺热哮喘、痰鸣息粗。可单用,或配伍麻黄、杏仁、石膏等同用,也可以制成注射液穴位或肌内注射。

3. It is applied for Bi-syndrome of heat-type with reddish, swelling, feverish and painful joints, unsmooth movement of joints, and sequela of wind stroke. In the case of Bi-syndrome of heat-type, it is usually used together with Sangzhi (*Ramulus Mori*), Rendongteng (*Caulis Lonicerae*) and Chishaoyao (*Radix Paeoniae Rubra*), etc.; in Bi-syndrome of cold-damp-type with stiffness of extremities, used with Chuanwu (*Radix Aconiti*) and Caowu (*Radix Aconiti Kusnezoffii*); in the treatment of blocked meridians due to deficiency of qi and stagnation of the blood after apoplexy manifested as numbness of the extremities and hemiplegia, used with Huangqi (*Radix Astragali*), Danggui (*Radix Angelicae Sinensis*) and Honghua (*Flos Carthami*), etc., such as

3. 用于热痹关节红肿热痛、屈伸不利及中风后遗症。治热痹,常与桑枝、忍冬藤、赤芍药等配伍;与川乌、草乌配伍,还可以治寒湿痹痛,肢体屈伸不利;中风后气虚血滞、经络不利,症见肢体麻木,半身不遂,可配黄芪、当归、红花等治疗,如补阳还五汤。

Buyang Huanwu Tang (Decoction).

4. It is applied for heat-syndrome of the bladder with dysuria or retention of urine. In the case of dysuria, it is used together with Cheqianzi (*Semen Plantaginis*), Mutong (*Caulis Akebia*), etc.; for retention of urine, smashed Dilong (*Lumbricus*) being soaked in water, from which the thick decoction is taken for oral use.

4. 用于热结膀胱,小便不利,或尿闭不通。治小便不利,可配伍车前子、木通等;治尿闭,以本品捣烂,浸水,滤取浓汁饮服有效。

In addition, it is also effective for mumps, chronic ulcer of lower limbs, and burns with external application of its extract when live Dilong is put into sugar.

此外,如取活体的白糖浸出液,涂敷痄腮、慢性下肢溃疡、烫伤,有一定疗效。

Usage and Dosage 5 - 9 g is used in decoction for oral use; 10 - 20 g of the fresh; or 1 - 2 g of the ground powder for drinking; external application with proper amount.

【用法用量】 水煎服,5～9 克;鲜品10～20 克。研末服,1～2 克。外用,适量。

Baijiangcan *Bombyx Batryticatus*

白僵蚕

The source is from the larva of *Bombyx mori* L. (silkworm) before its spinning of silk infected by *Beauveria* (Bals.) Vuill. The medicinal material is mainly produced in Zhejiang, Jiangsu and Sichuan, etc.. The crude or stir-baked one is used for medication.

为蚕蛾科昆虫家蚕的幼虫在未吐丝前,因感染白僵菌而发病致死的僵化虫体。主产于浙江、江苏、四川等地。晒干。生用或炒用。

Medicinal Properties Salty and pungent in flavor, mild in nature, and attributive to the liver, and lung meridians.

【药性】 味咸、辛,性平。归肝、肺经。

Actions Stop endogenous wind to relieve convulsion, expel wind and relieve pain, eliminate mass by detoxification.

【功效】 熄风止痉,祛风止痛,解毒散结。

Application

【临床应用】

1. It is applied for convulsion due to liver-wind stirring inside, or for that induced by hyperstagnation of phlegm-heat. It is usually used together with Quanxie (*Scorpio*), Tianma (*Rhizoma Gastrodiae*) and Dannanxing (*Arisaema cum Bile*), such as Qianzheng San (Powder). In the case with chronic diarrhea or chronic infantile convulsion due to deficiency of the spleen, it

1. 用于肝风内动或痰热壅盛所致的抽搐惊痫。常与全蝎、天麻、胆南星同用,如牵正散;若脾虚久泻,慢惊抽搐,又当配党参、白术、天麻等;治中风口眼歪斜,面部肌肉抽动,则配伍全蝎、白附子。

should be used together with Dangshen (*Radix Salviae Miltiorrhizae*), Baizhu (*Rhizoma Atractylodis Macrocephalae*) and Tianma (*Rhizoma Gastrodiae*), etc.; for apoplexy with distortion of the face, used together with Quanxie (*Scorpio*), Baifuzi (*Rhizoma Typhonii*).

2. It is applied for upper attack of wind-heat or liver-heat manifested as headache, reddish eyes, or sore throat. In the case with headache due to wind-heat or epiphora induced by wind, it is used together with Sangye (*Folium Mori*), Muzei (*Herba Equiseti Hiemalis*), etc., such as Baijiangcan San (Powder); for sore throat or hoarse voice, it can be combined with Jiegeng (*Radix Platycodi*), Fangfeng (*Radix Saposhnikoviae*) and Gancao (*Radix Glycyrrhizae*).

2. 用于风热上攻或肝热上炎所致的头痛目赤，咽喉肿痛。治风热头痛，迎风流泪，可配桑叶、木贼等，如白僵蚕散；治咽喉肿痛，声音嘶哑，可与桔梗、防风、甘草同用。

3. It is applied for subcutaneous nodule and scrofula, or syndrome with furuncle and erysipelas, it is usually combined with Zhebeimu (*Bulbus Fritillariae Thunbergii*), Xiakucao (*Spica Prunellae*) and Lianqiao (*Fructus Forsythiae*), etc..

3. 用于瘰疬痰核、疔肿丹毒等。常与浙贝母、夏枯草、连翘等同用。

In addition, It has the action of expelling wind and relieving itching, so it can be used for itching due to rubella.

此外，本品尚有祛风止痒作用，可用于风疹瘙痒。

Usage and Dosage 5 - 15 g is used in decoction for oral use, 10 - 20 g of the fresh is used and 1 - 2 g of the powder for drinking.

【用法用量】 水煎服，5～15 克，鲜品 10～20 克。研末服，1～2 克。

13 Chinese Resuscitative Medicines

第十三章 开窍药

The medicines with the main action of regaining conciousness which are used for sthenia-syndome of coma are known as Chinese resuscitative medicines. Since this sort of medicines have a strong aromatic and running nature, they are also called aromatic resuscitative medicines.

They are pungent in nature with aroma, and enter the heart meridian. They function as medicine for opening orifices and regaining conciousness. They are mainly used for such internal obstruction sthenia-syndromes as pathogenic heat attacking the pericardium due to warm febrile disease, or for sudden coma and delirium caused by stagnation of phlegm-turbidity, or sudden syncope in process of convulsion, wind stroke, etc..

Unconciousness, which is seen both in sthenia-syndrome of coma and in collapse syndrome, should be clearly differentiated of its nature. Sthenia-syndrome of coma caused by pathogenic factors obstructing inside is manifested as clenched teeth, tight fist, loud voice, hoarse breath and forceful pulse, whereas collapse syndrome due to exhausted healthy qi manifests opening mouth, loose fist, low and weak breath, sweating and cold extremities, or feeble and faint pulse. They can only be suitable for sthenia-syndrome of coma and not for the collapse type of unconsciousness which should be treated through supplementing deficiency. Meanwhile, sthenia-syndrome of coma includes heat and cold type. The syndrome of cold type shows bluish complexion and cold body, white tongue coating and slow pulse, etc. while syndrome of heat type

凡以开窍醒神为主要作用,用于治疗闭证神昏的药物,称为开窍药。因本类药物均具有较强的辛香走窜之性,故又称为芳香开窍药。

开窍药味辛,气芳香,皆入心经。具有通关开窍,苏醒神志的作用。主要适用于外感温热病热陷心包或痰浊蒙蔽心窍所致的神昏谵语,以及惊痫、中风等疾病过程中出现的卒然昏厥等内闭实证。

神志昏迷,不仅见于闭证,也可见于脱证,必须明确鉴别病变性质:闭证为实邪内闭,症见口噤握拳,声壮息粗,脉象有力;脱证为正气虚脱,症见口开手撒,声息低弱,汗出肢冷,脉微欲绝。开窍药只可用于闭证,而脱证治当补虚固脱,决非本类药所宜。另外,闭证又有寒热之分,寒闭多见面青身凉、苔白脉迟等症;热闭多见面赤身热、苔黄脉数等症。治疗时,寒闭者当用性温开窍药,且须配温里祛寒行气之品;热闭者当用性凉

is usually manifested as reddish complexion and general fever, yellowish tongue coating and rapid pulse, etc.. In treatment, medicines with warm nature and action of regaining resuscitation should be used in cold type, what's more, combined with herbs for warming the interior and dispersing cold; for heat type, medicines with cold nature and action of regaining resuscitation should be used and be combined with herbs for clearing away heat and eliminating toxic materials.

开窍药，而且应配清热解毒之品。

Chinese medicines for regaining resuscitation are used in emergent cases for the purpose of alleviating symptoms, and are prohibited from taking for long term to avoid damage to primordial qi. In addition, for their aromatic nature, most of them should be avoided in decoction, but used in pill or powder.

开窍药为救急、治标之品，只宜暂用，不宜久服，以免耗泄元气。此外，开窍药性味辛香，其有效成分容易散失，一般不入煎剂，只入丸散。

Shexiang *Moschus*

麝 香

It is a dry substance secreted by a gland in the subumbilical sac of the male musk deer. It is mainly produced in provinces of Sichuan, Tibet, Yunnan, Shaanxi, and Inner Mongolia of China, etc.. For the wild, it's mostly hunted in winter, and cut of the musk gland for musk; while the tamed one, the musk is taken by operation. The musk should be dried in shade, and stored in the closed and light-proof container.

为鹿科动物雄性林麝、马麝或原麝脐下香囊中的干燥分泌物。主产于四川、西藏、云南、陕西、内蒙等地。野生者，多于冬季猎捕，割取香囊，取出麝香；人工养殖者一般均用手术取香。阴干，贮于密闭、避光容器中备用。

Medicinal Properties Pungent in flavor, warm in nature and attributive to the heart and spleen meridians.

【药性】 味辛，性温。归心、脾经。

Actions Regain consciousness, activate the blood, disperse stasis, arrest pain and induce abortion.

【功效】 开窍醒神，活血散结，止痛，催产。

Application

【临床应用】

1. It is used for coma, delirium, stroke and convulsion due to seasonal febrile diseases in which pathogenic heat attacks the pericardium. For coma of heat type, it's often prescribed along with Xijiao (*Cornu Rhinocerotis*) and Niuhuang (*Calculus Bovis*), etc., such as Zhibao

1. 用于温热病热入心包之神昏痉厥，中风痰厥及惊痫。属热闭者，常与犀角、牛黄等同用，如至宝丹、安宫牛黄丸；属寒闭者，常与苏合香、

Dan (Bolus) and Angong Niuhuang Wan (*Pill*); for coma of cold type, combined with Suhexiang (*Styrax Liquidus*), Dingxiang (*Flos Caryophylli*), and Tanxiang (*Lignum Santali*), etc., such as Suhexiang Wan (Pill).

丁香、檀香等同用，如苏合香丸。

2. It is applied for pyocutaneous disease or sore throat. It can be used orally or externally. For the former, it is usually used together with Xionghuang (*Realgar*), Ruxiang (*Olibanum*), etc., such as Xingxiao Wan (Pill); for the latter, it is used together with Niuhuang (*Calculus Bovis*), Xionghuang (*Realgar*), and Bingpian (*Borneolum Syntheticum*), such as Liushen Wan (Pill).

2. 用于疮疡肿毒，咽喉肿痛。内服、外用均可，前者常与雄黄、乳香等同用，如醒消丸；后者常与牛黄、雄黄、冰片同用，如六神丸。

3. It is applied for angina pectoris, trauma and Bi-syndrome with pain. For pain in the chest and abdomen, it is used together with Muxiang (*Radix Aucklandiae*) and Taoren (*Semen Persicae*); for trauma and swollen pain due to blood stasis, used together with Sumu (*Lignum Sappan*), Moyao (*Myrrha*), etc..

3. 用于心腹暴痛，跌打瘀痛及痹证疼痛。治心腹疼痛，可配木香、桃仁；治跌打损伤，瘀血肿痛，可配苏木、没药等。

4. For abdominal mass, amenorrhea, dead fetus or retention of placenta, it is used together with Sanleng (*Rhizoma Sparganii*), Ezhu (*Rhizoma Zedoariae*), and Rougui (*Cortex Cinnamomi*), etc..

4. 用于癥瘕，经闭，胎死腹中或胞衣不下。常与三棱、莪术、肉桂等同用。

Usage and Dosage 0.06 - 0.1 g is used in powder or pill, not in decoction, and proper amount is for external application.

【用法用量】 研末，入丸、散，0.06～0.1克，不入煎剂。外用，适量。

Notes Contraindicated for Pregnant women.

【使用注意】 孕妇忌用。

Bingpian　*Borneolum Syntheticum*

冰片

The source is from *Dryobalanops aromatic* Gaertn. f., family Dipterocarpceae, or crystals from evaporated trunk. When the medicinal material is made from leaf of *Artemisia argyi* levl. et Vant., family Compositae., it is called resin of *Artemisia argyi* Levl. et Vant. It is mostly synthesized from camphor and turpentine oil, called synthetic one. The finished product should be stored in cool place and in closed container. It is ground

为龙脑香科植物龙脑香的树脂的加工品或树干经蒸馏冷却而得的结晶，称为“龙脑冰片”或“梅片”。由菊科植物艾纳香叶的升华物经加工而成，称“艾片”。现多以松节油、樟脑等为原料，经化学方法合成，称“机制冰片”或“机

into powder in application.

片”。成品贮于阴凉处，密闭。研粉用。

Medicinal Properties Pungent and bitter in flavor, slightly cold in nature, and attributive to the heart, spleen and lung meridians.

【药性】 辛、苦，微寒。归心、脾、肺经。

Actions Regain conciousness; clear away heat and alleviate pain.

【功效】 开窍醒神，清热止痛。

Application

【临床应用】

1. It is applied for wind stroke due to stagnation of phlegm and coma. With its cold nature, it is suitable for the sthenic syndrome of coma of heat type and mostly used together with Shexiang (*Moschus*, artificial), such as Angong Niuhuang Wan (Pill), Zhibao Dan (Bolus), etc..

1. 用于中风痰厥，神昏惊厥等证。性寒，故宜于热闭证，常与麝香相须配伍，如安宫牛黄丸、至宝丹等。

2. It is applied for sore throat, aphthae, reddish swollen and painful eyes, or ulcer. In the case of sore throat, it is used together with Pengsha (*Borax*), Zhusha (*Cinnabaris*), and Xuanmingfen (*Natrii Sulfas Exsiccatus*), etc., such as Bing Peng San (Powder); in the case of reddish swollen and painful eyes, with Huanglian (*Rhizoma Coptidis*), Luganshi (*Calamina*), such as in Buoyun San (Powder). In addition, it is found in many prescriptions for the purpose of clearing away heat and promoting tissue regeneration.

2. 用于咽喉肿痛，口舌生疮，目赤肿痛及疮疡。治咽喉肿痛，可配硼砂、朱砂、玄明粉，即冰硼散；治目赤肿痛可配黄连、炉甘石，如拨云散。此外，许多清热、生肌的复方中，都配有本品。

Usage and Dosage 0.03 - 0.1 g is used in pill or powder and not in decoction. Proper amount is for external application .

【用法用量】 入丸、散，0.03～0.1克，不入煎剂。外用，适量。

Notes It is used in pregnant women with caution.

【使用注意】 孕妇慎用。

Shichangpu *Rhizoma Acori Graminei*

石菖蒲

The source is from Rhizoma of *Acorus gramineus* Soland., family Araceae, mainly produced in the areas of Sichuan, Zhejiang and Jiangsu, etc.. The medicinal material is harvested in autumn and winter, processed by removing fibrous root and cleaning, and dried in the sun. The crude or fresh one can be used.

为天南星科植物石菖蒲的根茎。主产于四川、浙江、江苏等地。秋冬采挖后除去须根，洗净。晒干生用或鲜用。

Medicinal Properties Pungent in flavor, warm in nature, and attributive to the heart and stomach meridians.

【药性】 味辛,性温。归心、胃经。

Actions Regain consciousness and tranquilize the mind, eliminate dampness and harmonize the stomach.

【功效】 开窍宁神,化湿和胃。

Application

【临床应用】

1. It is applied for coma of sthenia type due to the accumulation of dampness or phlegm, or epilepsy. For the former , it is usually used together with Yujin (*Radix Curcumae*), Banxia (*Rhizoma Pinelliae*), etc., such as in Changpu Yujin Tang (Decoction). For epilepsy and dementia, the ground powder is taken with the soup of pig heart. α-Asarone, the active component of it, is extracted for use as well.

1. 用于湿浊蒙蔽清窍所致的神志昏乱及癫痫。前者常与郁金、半夏等同用,如菖蒲郁金汤。治癫证、痴呆,可用本品研末,猪心汤送服。也可从中提取有效成分 α-细辛醚使用。

2. For amnesia, palpitation, insomnia, or tinnitus, it is usually used together with Yuanzhi (*Radix Polygalae*), Fuling (*Poria*), Renshen (*Radix Ginseng*) and Longchi (*Dens Draconis*), such as Anshen Dingzhi Wan (Pill).

2. 用于心气不足,心悸,失眠,健忘,耳鸣。常与远志、茯苓、人参、龙齿配用,如安神定志丸。

3. For stagnation of dampness in the spleen and stomach manifested as fullness of the chest and stomach and poor appetite, it is used together with Jupi (*Pericarpium Citri Tangerinae*), Houpo (*Cortex Magnoliae Officinalis*), and Banxia (*Rhizoma Pinelliae*). It is combined with Huanglian (*Rhizoma Coptidis*) and Fuling (*Poria*), etc. to compose a prescription of Kaijin San (Powder) to treat dysentery and tenesmus with inability to take food.

3. 用于湿阻脾胃之胸闷腹胀、食少纳呆。可与橘皮、厚朴、半夏等配用。与黄连、茯苓等组成开噤散,能治痢疾里急后重,水食不进。

Usage and Dosage 3 - 10 g is used in decoction. It is unsuitable for decocting for a long time.

【用法用量】 水煎服,3～10 克。不宜久煎。

14 Restoratives

第十四章 补益药

All medicinal herbs for replenishing qi, blood, nourishing yin and yang, improving the functions of internal organs and body immunity, and relieving the various kinds of symptoms of weakness are defined as restoratives, also known as restoratives for reinforcing asthenia or tonics.

Though they complicatedly manifest themselves in clinic, basically, deficiency syndromes are summarized as deficiency of qi, yang, blood, or yin. So correspondingly, restoratives are classified into four categories: restoratives for invigorating qi, reinforcing yang, nourishing yin, and nourishing blood. There are interdependence relationships to exist among qi, blood, yin and yang, so deficiency of yang is often accompanied by deficiency of qi that is inclined to resulting in deficiency of yang, deficiency of qi and deficiency of yang both indicating a hypofunctioning state of human body; deficiency of yin is mostly accompanied by deficiency of blood that will easily lead to deficiency of yin, these two deficiencies indicating a consumption of essence, blood and body fluids. In this way, Chinese medicinal herbs for tonifying qi, yang, blood and yin are usually used according to the mutual promotion principle. In a case with deficiency of both qi and blood, or both yin and yang, the restoratives for nourishing both qi and blood, or both yin and yang should be used simultaneously.

Restoratives do not fit for the case with incompletely expelled pathogenic factors, and unshortage of healthy qi so as to prevent pathogenic factors from being removed

凡能补益人体气血阴阳不足，改善脏腑功能，提高抗病能力，消除各种虚弱证候的药物，称为补益药，亦称为补虚药或补养药。

虚证临床表现非常复杂，但概括起来有气虚、阳虚、血虚、阴虚之分。根据其作用和适应范围，补益药也相应分为补气、补阳、补血、补阴四类。由于人体的气血阴阳有着相互依存的关系，阳虚多兼有气虚，气虚也易导致阳虚，气虚和阳虚表示人体生理功能不足；阴虚多兼有血虚，血虚也易导致阴虚，血虚和阴虚表示人体精血津液的损耗。因此，补气和补阳、补血和补阴药常相须为用。如果气血不足、阴阳俱虚的证候同时出现，又当气血双补或阴阳并补。

补益药不宜用于实邪未尽而正气不虚者，以免影响邪气的驱除而加重病情，但若病

but make the disease severe. However, in a case with deficiency of healthy qi and uncleared pathogenic factors, the choice of restoratives is recommendable for the purpose of strengthening the body resistance against disease.

邪未清而正气已虚的,可于祛邪药中酌加补益药,以增强抗病能力,扶正祛邪。

Restoratives are usually taken in a long course, and are difficult to digest, so they are often combined with some herbs with actions of strengthening the stomach and spleen to achieve a better effect. They should be used strictly instead of loosely in case some other symptoms arise.

补益药一般服药时间较久,且某些药物有碍消化,故常配伍健脾胃药物,以加强疗效。补益药虽可补虚,但不可滥用,以防变生他证。

14. 1 Restoratives for invigorating qi

第一节　补气药

Restoratives for invigorating qi, which are mainly sweet in flavor and warm in nature, can tonify qi of both zangfu and general body to strengthen the functional activity of the body and are mainly used for symptoms due to qi deficiency, particularly those due to deficiency of spleen-qi manifested as weakness, poor appetite, loose stool, emaciation, edema and prolapse of anus, and those due to deficiency of lung-qi manifested as no desire to talk, low voice, shortness of breath, spontaneous sweating, or dyspnea in moving.

补气药性味以甘、温为主,能补脏腑及一身之气,增强机体的活动功能,主要适用于气虚证,尤其适用于脾气虚之神倦乏力,食欲不振,大便溏泻,脘腹胀满,浮肿,脱肛,以及肺气虚之少气懒言、语音低微、气短自汗、动则气喘等证。

As vigorous qi can benefit the production of the blood, and qi governs the blood, they are also used for blood-deficiency and bleeding syndrome due to qi deficiency.

因为气旺可以生血,气能统摄血液,所以,补气药还常用于血虚证及气虚出血证。

When taking qi tonics, one tends to feel fullness in the chest and poor appetite as well. This is due to the blocked qi in body, so they are usually prescribed together with a small amount of Chinese medicinal herbs for stimulating the circulation of qi and strengthening the stomach.

服用补气药容易壅气而出现胸膈胀满、食欲不振等证,可少量配伍行气健胃之品。

Renshen *Radix Ginseng*

人　参

The source is from the root of *Panax ginseng* C. A.

为五加科植物人参的根。

Mey. , family Araliceae. The medicinal material is mainly produced in Jilin, Liaoning and Heilongjiang provinces, etc.. Among them, the product from Fusong county of Jilin province is the best in quality. The wild ginseng is called "Mountainous Ginseng" while the cultivated one is called " Garden Ginseng" which is usually harvested in the autumn and processed in different ways: dried in the sunlight, steamed, or stir-baked with sugar. According to different processing methods, they are named as: sunlight-dried ginseng, red ginseng and sugar ginseng respectively. The wild ginseng is dried plainly in the sunlight without any processing, called "dried wild ginseng". Its head is usually removed and it is sliced for use.

主产于吉林、辽宁、黑龙江等地。以吉林抚松县产者质佳。野生者称为"山参",栽培者称为"园参"。园参一般在秋季采挖,晒干或烘干,称"生晒参";蒸制后干燥,称"红参"(大力参);经糖汁浸渍晒干,称"糖参"(白参);细根称"参须"。山参经晒干,称"生晒山参"。入药去芦头切片用。

Medicinal Properties Sweet and slightly bitter in flavor, warm in nature, and attributive to the spleen, lung and heart meridians.

【药性】 味甘、微苦,性平。归脾、肺、心经。

Actions Invigorate renal qi, strengthen qi of the spleen and lung, promote production of the body fluids to quench thirst, and calm the mind to promote intelligence.

【功效】 大补元气,补脾肺气,生津止渴,安神益智。

Application

【临床应用】

1. For collapse syndrome due to qi-deficiency manifested as shortness of breath, fatigue, feeble pulse, extreme weakness after severe disease, prolonged illness, heavy blood loss or severe vomiting, it is recommended to stew a thick decoction of single ginseng in large amount, which is called Dushen Tang (Decoction); for yang depletion such as qi collapse with sweating and cold extremities, it is used together with Fuzi (*Radix Aconiti Lateralis Praeparata*), named Shen Fu Tang (Decoction).

1. 用于气虚欲脱证。大病、久病或大出血、大吐泻后气短神疲、脉微欲绝、虚极欲脱之证,可单用人参大量煎浓汁服,即独参汤;如气脱兼汗出肢冷等亡阳之象者,可与附子同用,名参附汤。

2. It is applied for deficiency of the spleen manifested as fatigue, poor appetite, fullness in upper abdomen, or diarrhea and qi deficiency with weakness caused by various factors; it is usually used together with Baizhu (*Rhizoma Atractylodis Macrocephalae*), Fuling (*Po-*

2. 用于脾虚证。脾气不足之倦怠乏力、食欲不振、上腹痞满、泄泻等及各种原因所致的气虚体弱之证,常与白术、茯苓、炙甘草同用,即四君

ria), Zhigancao (*Radix Glycyrrhizae*, honey-fried), named Sijunzi Tang (*Decoction*).

子汤。

3. It is applied for deficiency of lung-qi manifested as shortness of breath, weakness, feeble pulse and spontaneous perspiration, and usually used with Hutaorou (*Caro Juglandis*), Wuweizi (*Fructus Schisandrae*), and Gejie (*Gecko*), etc., such as Renshen Hutao Tang (Decoction) and Renshen Gejie San (Powder). In the case with chronic cough and bloody sputum due to consumptive disease, it is used together with Ziwan (*Radix Asteris*), Zhimu (*Rhizoma Anemarrhenae*) and Ejiao (*Colla Corii Asini*), etc., such as Ziwan Tang (Decoction).

3. 用于肺气亏虚之咳喘,气短无力,脉虚自汗。多与胡桃肉、五味子、蛤蚧等同用,如人参胡桃汤、人参蛤蚧散。若虚劳咳嗽痰中带血,可与紫菀、知母、阿胶等同用,如紫菀汤。

4. It is applied for diabetes with thirst due to consumption of the body fluids. For febrile disease with consumption of both qi and the body fluids manifested as excessive sweating, shortness of breath, or weak and thin pulse; it is usually used together with Maimendong (*Radix Ophiopogonis*), Wuweizi (*Fructus Schisandrae*), such as Shengmai San (Powder). Now its injection is used in clinic for emergency treatment. For diabetes with thirst and frequent micturition, it is used together with Shengdihuang (*Radix Rehmanniae*), Xuanshen (*Radix Scrophulariae*), Maimendong (*Radix Ophiopogonis*) and Tianhuafen (*Radix Trichosanthis*).

4. 用于津伤口渴,消渴证。热病气津两伤之口渴、汗多、气短、脉虚微细之证,常与麦门冬、五味子配伍,如生脉散。现多制成注射剂用于抢救休克。消渴病口渴多尿,常与生地黄、玄参、麦门冬、天花粉等同用。

5. It is applied for deficiency of qi and blood resulting in failure of the heart to nourish manifested as palpitation, amnesia, insomnia or weakness; and used together with Danggui (*Radix Angelicae Sinensis*), Suanzaoren (*Semen Ziziphi Spinosae*) and Guiyuanrou (*Arillus Longan*) because of its action of replenishing heart-qi and soothing the mind, such as Guipi Tang (Decoction).

5. 用于气血不足,心神失养之心神不安,失眠多梦,惊悸健忘,身倦乏力。人参又能补心气,安心神,常与当归、酸枣仁、桂圆肉等配伍,如归脾汤。

6. It is applied for deficiency of both qi and blood, or syndrome of blood deficiency. In the case of deficiency of both qi and blood, it is used together with Shudihuang

6. 用于气血两虚或血虚证。气血两虚,常与熟地黄同用,如两仪膏。血虚证,可与

(*Radix Rehmanniae Praeparata*), such as Liangyi Gao (Soft extract). In the case of blood deficiency, it can be used together with blood tonics such as Danggui (*Radix Angelicae Sinensis*).

当归等补血药同用。

In addition, it is also recommended to treat impotence due to kidney deficiency in combination with some yang invigorating tonics. For susceptibility to pathogenic factors from weakness, it is used together with some other herbs to invigorate the body resistance to disease, and to promote healthy qi and eliminate the pathogenic factors.

此外，以本品配伍补阳药，可用于肾虚阳痿；在治体虚外感或体虚不耐攻下方中配用本品，可增强抗病能力，扶正祛邪。

Usage and Dosage 5 -10 g is used in decoction. It should be decocted individually on the mild fire, and mixed with decoction of other herbs when drinking. Or the ground powder of 1 -2 g is swallowed. It amounts to 15 -30 g that is used in decoction for a syndrome of collapse, which is taken in several times.

【用量用法】 水煎服，5～10 克，入汤剂宜文火另煎，将煎液兑入其他药液中服。或研末吞服，1～2 克。如挽救虚脱，应增量至 15～30 克煎汁，分次服用。

Notes Contraindicated for the sthenia and heat syndrome without deficiency of healthy qi. It is incompatible with Lilu (*Rhizoma et Radix Veratri*), Wulingzhi (*Faeces Trogopterorum*), and Zaojia (*Fructus Gleditsiae*). Turnip and tea should be avoided in the course of treatment in case they affect its tonic effect.

【使用注意】 实证、热证而正气不虚者忌服。不宜与藜芦、五灵脂、皂荚同用。服药期间不宜吃萝卜、喝茶，以免影响补力。

Dangshen *Radix Codonopsis*

党 参

The medicinal material is from the root of *Codonopsis pilosula* (Franch.) Nannf., and other several species of the same catalogue, family Campanulaceae. It is classified into the wild and cultivated one according to sources, and mostly produced in Shanxi, Shaanxi and Gansu, and harvested in autumn, dried and cut into segments. It is used crudely.

为桔梗科植物党参、素花党参或川党参的根。野生者习称野台党，栽培者习称潞党参。主产于山西、陕西、甘肃。秋季采挖。晒干，切段。生用。

Medicinal Properties Sweet in flavor, warm in nature, and attributive to the spleen and lung meridians.

【药性】 味甘，性平。归脾、肺经。

Actions Invigorate the stomach and spleen, and

【功效】 补中益气，生津

benefit qi, promote the production of the body fluids and nourish the blood.

养血。

Application

【临床应用】

1. It is suitable for deficiency of the spleen with fatigue, loss of appetite, loose stool and syndrome with deficiency of qi and weakness due to various causes. It is usually used together with Baizhu (*Rhizoma Atractylodis Macrocephalae*), Fuling (*Poria*) and Gancao (*Radix Glycyrrhizae*).

1. 用于脾虚倦怠乏力、食少便溏及各种原因所致的气虚体弱之证。常与白术、茯苓、甘草同用。

2. It is suitable for insufficiency of lung-qi with shortness of breath, cough, or low voice. It is usually used together with Huangqi (*Radix Astragali*), Wuweizi (*Fructus Schisandrae*), such as Bufei Tang (Decoction).

2. 用于肺气亏虚之气短咳喘，言语无力，声音低弱。常与黄芪、五味子同用，如补肺汤。

3. It is used for febrile diseases resulting in consumption of both qi and the body fluids with shortness of breath and thirst. It is usually used together with Maimendong (*Radix Ophiopogonis*), Wuweizi (*Fructus Schisandrae*), etc..

3. 用于热病气津两伤，气短口渴。多配伍麦门冬、五味子等同用。

4. It is suitable for dizziness due to deficiency of blood or sallow complexion or edema of face. It is usually used with Danggui (*Radix Angelicae Sinensis*), Shudihuang (*Radix Rehmanniae Praeparata*), Baishaoyao (*Radix Paeoniae Alba*) and Jixueteng (*Caulis Spatholobi*).

4. 用于血虚头晕，或面黄浮肿。可与当归、熟地黄、白芍药、鸡血藤等同用。

In addition, it can be combined with diaphoretics and purgatives and used in the case with weakness and exogenous affection or constipation due to deficiency of healthy qi.

此外，本品亦可配入解表、攻下药中，用于体虚外感及便秘而正气虚者。

Usage and Dosage 10 -30 g is used in decoction, or in pill.

【用法用量】 水煎服，10～30克；或入丸散剂。

Notes Contraindicated for heat-syndrome, syndrome of deficiency of yin and hyperactivity of yang. It is incompatible with Lilu (*Rhizoma et Radix Veratri*).

【使用注意】 热证及阴虚阳亢证不宜用。反藜芦。

Explanation As its action is similar to Renshen (*Radix Ginseng*), it can be used as substitute for Renshen (*Radix Ginseng*), but it is unsuitable for collapse syndrome due to deficiency of qi because of its weaker action of qi tonifying.

【说明】 党参作用类似人参,一般病证可代人参用,但补气力弱,气虚欲脱者不宜。

Xiyangshen *Radix Panacis Quinquefolii*

西洋参

The source is from the root of *Panax Quinquefolium*, L. family Campanulaceae. The medicinal material mainly grows in U. S. A., Canada, and France and cultivated in China as well, and in autumn the roots with 3 - 6 year's growth are harvested. After it is processed by being peeled and smoked with Liuhuang (*Sulfur*) and then dried, it is called as "peeled Xiyangshen", and used crudely with sliced pieces.

为五加科植物西洋参的根。主产于美国、加拿大及法国,中国亦有栽培。秋季采挖生长3~6年的根,除去分枝、须尾,晒干。喷水湿润,去外皮,再用硫黄熏之,晒干后,称"光西洋参";挖起后即连皮晒干或烘干者,称"原皮西洋参"。切片。生用。

Medicinal Properties Sweet and slightly bitter in flavor, cold in nature, and attributive to the heart, lung and kidney meridians.

【药性】 味甘、微苦,性寒。归心、肺、肾经。

Actions Supplement qi and nourish yin, clear away fire and promote the production of the body fluids.

【功效】 补气养阴,清火生津。

Application

【临床应用】

1. It is applied for exuberant fire due to deficiency of yin manifested as cough with dyspnea and bloody sputum. It is usually combined with Zhimu (*Rhizoma Anemarrhenae*), Chuanbeimu (*Bulbus Fritillariae Cirrhosae*) and Ejiao (*Colla Corii Asini*), etc..

1. 用于阴虚火旺,喘咳痰血。常与知母、川贝母、阿胶等同用。

2. For febrile diseases causing damage to both qi and yin with manifestations of dysphoria, fatigue and thirst, it can be decocted singly; or used together with Shengdihuang (*Radix Rehmanniae*) and Xianshihu (*Herba Dendrobii*, fresh), etc., and others that can nourish yin, clear away heat and promote the production of the body fluids.

2. 用于热病气阴两伤,烦倦,口渴。单用水煎有效,也常与生地黄、鲜石斛等养阴清热生津药同用。

Usage and Dosage 3 - 6 g is decocted and mixed

【用法用量】 另煎兑服,

with other medicines after being decocted separatedly.

Notes Contraindicated for coldness and dampness in the stomach due to deficiency and weakness of middle energizer yang. It is incompatible with Lilu (*Rhizoma et Radix Veratri*).

Huangqi *Radix Astragali*

The source is from the root of *Astragalus membranaceus* (Fisch.) Bunge var. *mongholicus* (Bunge) Hsiao, and *A. membranaceus* (Fisch.) Bunge, family Leguminosae. It mainly grows in Inner Mongolia, Shanxi, Gansu and Heilongjiang, etc., harvested in spring and autumn, sliced and dried with removal of head and fine roots. It is used crudely or roasted with honey for use.

Medicinal Properties Sweet in flavor, slightly warm in nature, and attributive to the spleen and lung meridians.

Actions Replenish qi to invigorate yang; benefit the lung to strengthen the body; promote diuresis and relieve edema; relieve skin infection and promote tissue regeneration.

Application

1. It is used for the syndrome with qi-deficiency of the spleen and lung, and visceroptosis with hyposplenic qi manifested as fatigue and weakness due to prolonged illness, it is used together with Renshen (*Radix Ginseng*), such as Shen Qi Gao (Soft extract); for that accompanied by deficiency of yang manifested as chill, fatigue and polyhidrosis, it is used with Fuzi (*Radix Aconiti Lateralis Praeparata*), such as Qi Fu Gao (Soft extract). For deficiency of both qi and blood, it is used together with Danggui (*Radix Angelicae Sinensis*). For deficiency of spleen-qi manifested as poor appetite, loose stool or diarrhea, it is used together with Baizhu (*Rhizoma Atractylodis Macrocephalae*), such as Qi Zhu Gao (Soft extract).

3～6克。

【使用注意】 中阳衰微，胃有寒湿者忌服。反藜芦。

黄 芪

为豆科植物蒙古黄芪或膜荚黄芪的根。主产于内蒙古、山西、甘肃、黑龙江等地。春、秋两季采挖，除掉须根及根头。切片，晒干。生用或蜜炙用。

【药性】 味甘，性微温。归脾、肺经。

【功效】 补气升阳，益肺固表，利水消肿，托毒生肌。

【临床应用】

1. 用于脾肺气虚及中气下陷证。病后气虚体弱，倦怠乏力，常与人参配伍，如参芪膏；兼阳虚而见畏寒，体倦多汗者，可与附子同用，如芪附膏；气虚血亏，可与当归同用；脾气虚弱，食少便溏或泄泻者，可与白术同用，如芪术膏；脾阳不升，中气下陷，内脏下垂，子宫脱垂，久泻脱肛，可与人参、白术、升麻、柴胡等配伍，如补中益气汤；若气虚不能摄血之便血、崩漏等，又可

For descending of spleen-yang, visceroptosis with hyposplenic qi, prolaps of uterus, and prolaps of rectum due to chronic diarrhea, it is used with Renshen (*Radix Ginseng*), Baizhu (*Rhizoma Atractylodis Macrocephalae*), Shengma (*Rhizoma Cimicifugae*), and Chaihu (*Radix Bupleuri*), etc., such as Buzhong Yiqi Tang (Decoction). For deficiency of qi resulting in inability to govern the blood manifested as bloody stool and metrorrhagia and metrostaxis, it may be used together with Renshen (*Radix Ginseng*), Suanzaoren (*Semen Ziziphi Spinosae*) and Guiyuanrou (*Arillus Longan*), etc., such as Guipi Tang (Decoction).

与人参、酸枣仁、桂圆肉等配伍，如归脾汤。

2. It is applied for cough due to lung deficiency, superficies-asthenia with profuse sweating, or night sweating. For deficiency of lung qi with cough or shortness of breath or dyspnea, it is frequently used with Ziwan (*Radix Asteris*), Wuweizi (*Fructus Schisandrae*), etc.; for superficies-asthenia with profuse sweating and suspectility to common cold, it is used with Baizhu (*Rhizoma Atractylodis Macrocephalae*) and Fangfeng (*Radix Saposhnikoviae*), such as Yupingfeng San (Powder); for night sweating, it can be used with Shengdihuang (*Radix Rehmannia*), Huangbai (*Cortex Phellodendri*), etc., such as Danggui Liuhuang Tang (Decoction).

2. 用于肺虚咳喘，肌表不固之自汗、盗汗。治肺气虚弱，咳喘气短，常与紫菀、五味子等同用；治体虚多汗，容易感冒，常与白术、防风同用，如玉屏风散；盗汗可与生地黄、黄柏等同用，如当归六黄汤。

3. It is applied for maltransformation of water and dampness due to deficiency of qi with facial edema, oliguria or palpitation, and dyspnea. And it is used together every time with Fangji (*Radix Stephaniae Tetrandrae*), Baizhu (*Rhizoma Atractylodis Macrocephalae*), etc., such as Fangji Huangqi Tang (Decoction). It is remarkably effective for edema from chronic nephritis with presence of protein in urine for a long time.

3. 用于气虚水湿失运之面目浮肿，小便短少，心悸，气促。每与防己、白术等同用，如防己黄芪汤；对慢性肾炎浮肿，尿中蛋白长期不消者，用之有良好疗效。

4. It is applied for unruptured carbuncle or ruptured but unhealed one due to deficiency of qi and blood. For

4. 用于气血不足之痈疽不溃或溃久不敛。治痈疽久

unruptured carbuncle, it is often used together with Danggui (*Radix Angelicae Sinensis*), Zaojiaoci (*Spina Gleditsiae*), etc., such as Tounong San (Powder). For ruptured carbuncle with watery pus and no tendency to healing, it can be used with Danggui (*Radix Angelicae Sinensis*), Renshen (*Radix Ginseng*), and Rougui (*Cortex Cinnamomi*), etc., such as Shiquang Dabu Tang (Decoction).

不溃,常与当归、皂角刺等同用,如透脓散;溃久脓水清稀,久不收口,可与当归、人参、肉桂等配伍,如十全大补汤。

5. For numbness of limbs and hemiplegia due to deficiency of qi and stagnation of blood, it is often used with Guizhi (*Ramulus Cinnamomi*), Baishaoyao (*Radix Paeoniae Alba*), etc., such as Huangqi Guizhi Wuwu Tang (Decoction); or used with Danggui (*Radix Angelicae Sinensis*), Honghua (*Flos Carthami*) and Taoren (*Semen Persicae*), etc., such as Buyang Huanwu Tang (Decoction).

5. 用于气虚血滞之肢体麻木及中风后半身不遂。常与桂枝、白芍药等同用,如黄芪桂枝五物汤;也与当归、红花、桃仁等配伍,如补阳还五汤。

In addition, it is also used for treating diabetes in combination with Shengdihuang (*Radix Rehmannia*), Maimendong (*Radix Ophiopogonis*), Tianhuafen (*Radix Trichosanthis*), and Shanyao (*Rhizoma Dioscoreae*), etc..

此外,还可与生地黄、麦门冬、天花粉、山药等配伍,用治消渴。

Usage and Dosage Decoction: 10 -15 g or up to 30 -60 g is used crudely in general; but honey-roasted one is selected for the purpose of replenishing qi and invigorating yang.

【用法用量】 水煎服,10~15克,大剂量可用至30~60克。补气升阳宜炙用,其他宜生用。

Notes Contraindicated in the case with superficial-sthenia syndrome with excessive pathogenic factors, stagnation of qi and dampness, indigestion, hyperactivity of yang due to deficient yin, onset of carbuncle at the early stage or one ruptured but unhealed for a long time with excessive heat-toxin.

【使用注意】 表实邪盛,气滞湿阻,食积内停,阴虚阳亢,痈疽初起或溃久热毒尚盛者,均不宜用。

Baizhu *Rhizoma Atractylodis Macrocephalae*

白 术

The source is from the Rhizome of *Atractylodes macrocephala* Koidz, family Compositae. The medicinal

为菊科植物白术的根茎。主产于浙江、湖北、湖南、江西

material is mainly produced in Zhejiang, Hubei, Hunan, and Jiangxi, etc. and now mostly cultivated. It is harvested in winter and processed by slicing and drying. The crude or stir-baked with bran or earth into burnt colour is used for application.

等地，现多栽培。冬季采挖，切片，晒干。生用或麸炒、土炒、炒焦用。

Medicinal Properties Bitter and sweet in flavor, warm in nature, and attributive to the spleen and stomach meridians.

【药性】 味苦、甘，性温。归脾、胃经。

Actions Invigorate the spleen and benefit qi, eliminate dampness and promote diuresis, stop sweating and soothe the fetus.

【功效】 补气健脾，燥湿利水，止汗，安胎。

Application

1. For deficiency of spleen-qi and stomach-qi with failure of the spleen to transport and transform manifested as poor appetite, loose stools, fullness of epigastric abdomen, or fatigue, it is used every time with Renshen (*Radix Ginseng*), Fuling (*Poria*) and Gancao (*Radix Glycyrrhizae*), such as Sijunzi Tang (Decoction). In the case with severe deficiency and coldness manifested as cold abdominal pain or loose stool, it is used together with Dangshen (*Radix Codonopsis*), Ganjiang (*Rhizoma Zingiberis*), etc., such as Lizhong Tang (Decoction). For deficiency of the spleen with stagnated food in the stomach manifested as poor appetite or fullness in the epigastric abdomen, it is used together with Zhishi (*Fructus Aurantii Immaturus*), that is Zhi Zhu Wan (Pill).

2. It is applied for edema due to deficiency of the spleen and retention of phlegm. In the case with retention of phlegm manifested as fullness in the chest or vertigo, it is used together with Guizhi (*Ramulus Cinnamomi*), Fuling (*Poria*), Zhigancao (*Radix Glycyrrhizae*, honey-fried) to form a prescription named Ling Gui Zhu Gan Tang (Decoction). In the case with general edema and dysuria, it is used together with Fuling (*Poria*), Zexie

【临床应用】

1. 用于脾胃气虚，运化无力所致的食少便溏，脘腹胀满，倦怠无力。每与人参、茯苓、甘草同用，如四君子汤。若虚寒较重，见脘腹冷痛、大便泄泻者，可配党参、干姜等，如理中汤；若脾虚饮食积滞，食欲不振，脘腹痞满，又可与枳实配伍，即枳术丸。

2. 用于脾虚水湿、痰饮内停。痰饮停聚，胸胁满闷，头眩者，可与桂枝、茯苓、炙甘草同用，名苓桂术甘汤；全身水肿，小便不利，则可与茯苓、泽泻、桂枝等或附子、干姜同用，如五苓散、真武汤。

(*Rhizoma Alismatis*) and Guizhi (*Ramulus Cinnamomi*), etc., or Fuzi (*Radix Aconiti Lateralis Praeparata*), Ganjiang (*Rhizoma Zingiberis*), such as Wuling San (Powder), Zhenwu Tang (Decoction).

3. For spontaneous sweating due to deficiency of the spleen and qi, and superficies-asthenia, it is used together with Huangqi (*Radix Astragali*), Fangfeng (*Radix Saposhnikoviae*), Fuxiaomai (*Fructus Tritici Levis*).

3. 用于脾虚气弱,肌表不固之自汗。可与黄芪、防风、浮小麦同用。

4. For threatened abortion due to deficiency of splenogastric qi, it is used together with Zisuye (*Folium Perillae*), Sharen (*Fructus Amomi*).

4. 用于中气不足,胎动不安。常与紫苏叶、砂仁同用。

In addition, it is not only used for loose stool, but also, with its large dosage(over 30 g) and crude form, for constipation due to weakness of spleen-qi and dysfunctioning in transporting and transforming. It can be singly decocted into thick decoction, or can be used in combination with Maziren (*Semen Ricini*) and Zisuzi (*Semen Perillae*).

此外,白术不仅可以治大便溏泻,大量(30 克以上)生用也可以治疗脾气虚弱,运化无力的便秘。单味浓煎内服有效,也可以配麻子仁、紫苏子同用。

Usage and Dosage 5-15 g is used in decoction or pill. It should be used crudely for the purpose of drying dampness and promoting diuresis; or used with one that is stir-baked with bran for nourishing qi and strengthening the spleen; or used the one that is stir-baked with earth or over-stir-baked into burnt-colour for strengthening the spleen and stopping diarrhea.

【用法用量】 5～15 克,水煎服或入丸散。燥湿利水宜生用,补气健脾宜麸炒用,健脾止泻宜土炒或炒焦用。

Explanation Both Baizhu (*Rhizoma Atractylodis Macrocephalae*) and Cangzhu (*Rhizoma Atractylodis*) are from family Compositae and meanwhile with the same actions of strengthening the spleen and drying dampness and treating dysfunction of transporting and transforming and stagnation of watery dampness due to deficiency of the spleen. However, Baizhu (*Rhizoma Atractylodis Macrocephalae*) is good at nourishing the spleen and usually used for syndrome of watery dampness due to deficiency

【说明】 白术、苍术均为菊科植物,都能健脾燥湿,同治脾虚运化功能失常,水湿内停之证。白术长于补脾,多用于因脾虚导致的水湿证;另可治脾胃气虚证,以及表虚自汗,胎动不安。苍术以燥湿见长,有泄水开郁之功,适用于湿邪困脾的实证;又能发汗解

of the spleen. It is also fit for deficiency of spleen-qi and stomach-qi, and spontaneous sweating due to superficial deficiency and threatened abortion. Cangzhu (*Rhizoma Atractylodis*) is exclusively for drying dampness and is used for excess syndrome due to dampness stagnated in the spleen. It can promote sweating, so it can also be indicated for superficial syndrome of wind-cold-damp type and can bright the eyes to treat night blindness.

表胜湿，用于风寒湿表证；还能明目，主治夜盲症。

Shanyao *Rhizoma Dioscoreae*

山 药

The source is from rhizome of *Dioscorea Opposite* Thunb., family Dioscoreaceae. The medicinal material is produced in Hebei, Shanxi, and Shandong, with the best from Xinxiang county of Henan Province, and harvested in winter and processed in a procedure of washing, peeling, steaming with sulphur, drying, softening and slicing. The crude or stir-baked with bran can be used.

为薯蓣科植物薯蓣的根茎。以河南新乡地区产者最佳，称“怀山药”。河北、山西、山东亦产。冬季采挖，洗净，刮去粗皮，用硫黄熏过，晒干，或再浸软，加工搓成圆柱状，磨光，切片。生用或麸炒用。

Medicinal Properties Sweet in flavor, mild in nature, and attributive to the spleen, lung and kidney meridians.

【药性】 味甘，性平。归脾、肺、肾经。

Actions Invigorate the spleen and stomach; promote production of the body fluids and benefit the lung, invigorate the kidney and preserve the essence.

【功效】 补脾养胃，生津益肺，补肾涩精。

Application

【临床应用】

1. For deficiency of the spleen and stomach with poor appetite, fatigue or loose stools and diarrhea, it is often used together with Renshen (*Radix Ginseng*), Baizhu (*Rhizoma Atractylodis Macrocephalae*) and Fuling (*Poria*), etc., such as Shen Ling Baizhu San (Powder).

1. 用于脾胃虚弱，食少体倦或便溏、泄泻。常与人参、白术、茯苓等同用，如参苓白术散。

2. For dyspnea and cough due to deficiency of the lung, it is frequently used together with Dangshen (*Radix Codonopsis*), Maimendong (*Radix Ophiopogonis*) and Wuweizi (*Fructus Schisandrae*), etc..

2. 用于肺虚喘咳。常与党参、麦门冬、五味子等同用。

3. It is applied for kidney-deficiency with emission, frequent micturition or leucorrhagia. In the case of emis-

3. 用于肾虚遗精，带下，尿频。肾虚遗精，可与熟地

sion due to deficiency of the kidney, it is used together with Shudihuang (*Radix Rehmanniae Praeparata*), Shanzhuyu (*Fructus Corni*), etc., such as Liuwei Dihuang Wan (Pill). For frequent micturition and enuresis, it is used together with Yizhiren (*Fructus Alpiniae Oxyphyllae*), Wuyao (*Radix Linderae*), etc., such as Suoquan Wan (Pill). For leucorrhagia due to deficiency of the spleen with dampness, it is usually combined with Dangshen (*Radix Codonopsis*), Baizhu (*Rhizoma Atractylodis Macrocephalae*), Cheqianzi (*Semen Plantaginis*); that with damp-heat, used with Huangbai (*Cortex Phellodendri*), etc.. It should be used together with Shudihuang (*Radix Rehmanniae Praeparata*), Shanzhuyu (*Fructus Corni*), and Tusizi (*Semen Cuscutae*), etc., in a case with deficient kidney and inability to preserve the essence.

黄、山茱萸等同用,如六味地黄丸。尿频,遗尿,可与益智仁、乌药等配伍,如缩泉丸。妇女带下过多,属脾虚有湿者,常配伍党参、白术、车前子等;有湿热者,应与黄柏等配伍;肾虚不固者,可与熟地黄、山茱萸、菟丝子等同用。

4. It is applied for diabetes or consumption of the body fluids due to deficiency of yin accompanied by dysphoric fever or thirst. For the light diabetes, it is recommended that 250 g is decocted as a substitute for tea everyday for a long course; or else, to be used together with Huangqi (*Radix Astragali*), Gegen (*Radix Puerariae*), Tianhuafen (*Radix Trichosanthis*), and Zhimu (*Rhizoma Anemarrhenae*), etc., such as Yuye Tang (Decoction). For thirst due to consumption of the body fluids, it is used with Maimendong (*Radix Ophiopogonis*), Yuzhu (*Rhizoma Polygonati Odorati*), etc..

4. 用于消渴或阴虚津亏,烦热口渴。治消渴轻症,可每日用250克,煎水代茶,长期服用;也可与黄芪、葛根、天花粉、知母等配伍,如玉液汤。治津亏口渴,可与麦门冬、玉竹等同用。

Usage and Dosage 15–30 g or up to 60–250 g is used in decoction; or 6–10 g of the powder. It's better to use the crude product for the purpose of nourishing yin and promoting the production of the body fluids, and to use the stir-baked one with bran for strengthening the spleen and stopping diarrhea.

【用量用法】 水煎服,15~30克,大剂量可用至60~250克;研末服,6~10克。养阴生津宜生用,健脾止泻宜麸炒用。

Notes Contraindicated for the case with excessive

【使用注意】 湿盛中满

dampness in the stomach or with stagnation.

或有积滞者不宜用。

Gancao *Radix Glycyrrhizae*

甘 草

The source is from the root of *Glycyrrhiza uraleusis* Fisch. Or *G. grabra* L., family Leguminosae. The medicinal material is mainly produced in Inner Mongolia, Shanxi, Gansu and Xinjiang of China, etc., and harvested in autumn. It is applied crudely or roasted with honey for use after being processed by removing the root, slicing and drying.

为豆科植物甘草、光果甘草、胀果甘草的根及根茎。主产于内蒙古、山西、甘肃、新疆等地。秋季采挖,除去残根及须根,切片晒干。生用或蜜炙用。

Medicinal Properties Sweet in flavor, mild in nature, and attributive to the heart, lung, spleen and stomach meridians.

【药性】 味甘,性平。归心、肺、脾、胃经。

Actions Enrich qi and invigorate the stomach and spleen, moisten the lung and resolve phlegm, clear away heat and toxin, relieve spasm and alleviate pain.

【功效】 益气补中,润肺化痰,清热解毒,缓急止痛。

Application

【临床应用】

1. It is used for syndromes of deficiency of heart-qi and spleen-qi. In the case with deficiency of heart-qi manifested as palpitation, spontaneous sweating and knotted or slow-regular-intermittent pulse, Zhigancao (*Radix Glycyrrhizae*, honey-fried) is mainly used together with Renshen (*Radix Ginseng*), Maimendong (*Radix Trichosanthis*), Guizhi (*Ramulus Cinnamomi*) and Ejiao (*Colla Corii Asini*), etc., such as Zhigancao Tang (Decoction); in the case due to deficiency of the spleen with fatigue, poor appetite or loose stool, it is used with Dangshen (*Radix Codonopsis*), Baizhu (*Rhizoma Atractylodis Macrocephalae*), etc., such as Sijunzi Tang (Decoction).

1. 用于心气虚及脾气虚证。治心气虚弱,心悸,自汗,脉结代者,以炙甘草为主,配人参、麦门冬、桂枝、阿胶等,如炙甘草汤;治脾虚倦怠乏力,食少便溏,常作为党参、白术等的辅助药物,如四君子汤。

2. It is applied for cough and dyspnea. As it has the action of moistening the lung and resolving phlegm, it is indicated for many kinds or syndromes of cough and dyspnea. For a cough due to wind-heat, it is used together with Jiegeng (*Radix Platycodi*), Qianhu (*Radix Peuce-*

2. 用于咳嗽气喘。本品既能润肺,又能化痰,所以适用于多种咳喘证。风热咳嗽,与桔梗、前胡、桑叶等同用;风寒咳嗽,配麻黄、杏仁,如三拗

dani), and Sangye (*Folium Mori*), etc.; for that due to wind-cold, with Mahuang (*Herba Ephedrae*), Xingren (*Semen Pruni Armeniacae*), such as San'ao Tang (Decoction); for that due to lung-heat, with Shengshigao (*Gypsum Fibrosum*), Mahuang (*Herba Ephedrae*), Xingren (*Semen Pruni Armeniacae*), etc., such as Ma Xing Shi Gan Tang (Decoction); for that due to stagnation of damp-phlegm, used with Banxia (*Rhizoma Pinelliae*), Fuling (*Poria*), etc..

汤;肺热咳喘,可与生石膏、麻黄、杏仁同用,即麻杏石甘汤;湿痰咳喘,则配半夏、茯苓等。

3. It is applied for pyocutaneous disease, sore throat or drug and food poisoning. For pyocutaneous disease, it is used with Jinyinhua (*Flos Lonicerae*), Lianqiao (*Fructus Forsythiae*) etc.; for sore throat, used with Jiegeng (*Radix Platycodi*), such as Jiegeng Tang (Decoction). For drug and food poisoning, thick decoction of Gancao (*Radix Glycyrrhizae*) should be given frequently, or combined with Lüdou (*Semen Phaseoli Radiati*) and Fangfeng (*Radix Saposhnikoviae*), which are decocted for oral use when there is no particularly effective medicine for detoxification.

3. 用于疮疡肿毒、咽喉肿痛及药物、食物中毒。治疮疡肿毒,可与金银花、连翘等同用;咽喉肿痛,常与桔梗同用,如桔梗汤;药物、食物中毒,在无特殊解毒药时,可以生甘草浓煎频服,也可与绿豆或防风同用,水煎服。

4. It is applied for spasm or pain of epigastric abdomen and limbs. In treating pain of epigastric abdomen, it is used with Guizhi (*Ramulus Cinnamomi*), Baishaoyao (*Radix Paeoniae Alba*), and Yitang (*Saccharum cum Malto*), etc., such as Xiao Jianzhong Tang (Decoction); for spasm and pain of limbs, used with Baishaoyao (*Radix Paeoniae Alba*), such as Shaoyao Gancao Tang (Decoction).

4. 用于脘腹及四肢拘挛疼痛。脘腹疼痛,常与桂枝、白芍药、饴糖等同用,如小建中汤;四肢拘挛疼痛,常配白芍药同用,如芍药甘草汤。

In addition, Gancao (*Radix Glycyrrhizae*) in a prescription exerts an effect on decreasing or moderating medicinal side-effects or toxicity and regulating actions of all other herbs.

此外,复方中用甘草,可以减低或缓和药物的偏性或毒性,并起调和诸药的作用。

Usage and Dosage 2 -10 g or up to 10 -30 g is used in decoction when used as a dominant herb. It fits to

【用法用量】 水煎服,2～10 克,作主药可用至 10～

be used crudely in the prescription for clearing or purging while the honey-roasted Gancao (*Radix Glycyrrhizae*) is used in the one for tonifying and nourishing.

30克。入清泻药中宜生用，入补益药中宜蜜炙用。

Notes Contraindicated for the case with fullness of epigastric abdomen, vomiting or edema due to excessive dampness. And it should be avoided using for a long course and in large amount to prevent a case from having edema. Also, it is incompatible with Daji (*Radix Euphorbiae Pekinensis*), Gansui(*Radix Euphorbiae Kansui*) and Yuanhua (*Flos Genkwa*).

【使用注意】 湿盛胀满、呕吐、水肿者忌服。久服、大量服易引起水肿。反大戟、甘遂、芫花。

Fengmi *Mel*

蜂 蜜

It refers to the honey made by bees (*Apis cerma* Fabricius and *A. mellifera* L., family Apidae). It is available all over China, collected from spring to autumn.

为蜜蜂科昆虫中华蜜蜂或意大利蜂所酿成的蜜。中国各地均产。春至秋季采收，过滤后用。

Medicinal Properties Sweet in flavor, mild in nature, and attributive to the lung, spleen and large intestine meridians.

【药性】 味甘，性平。归肺脾、大肠经。

Actions Nourish the stomach and spleen, alleviate pain and moisten the intestine.

【功效】 补中缓急，润燥。

Application

1. For epigastric abdominal pain due to deficiency of the spleen and stomach, it is usually used together with Shaoyao (*Radix Paeoniae Alba*), Gancao (*Radix Glycyrrhizae*), etc., which can play a synergistic role. In TCM, many pills and soft extracts are shaped with the help of honey and some medicinal herbs are processed by being roasted with honey, which are all related to its actions of nourishing and moderating nature of other herbs.

2. It is applied for dry cough due to deficiency of the lung and constipation due to dry intestine. For dryness of the lung with cough and hemoptysis, it is usually used with Renshen (*Radix Ginseng*), Shengdihuang (*Radix Rehmanniae*), etc., such as Qiongyu Gao (Soft ex-

【临床应用】

1. 用于中虚脘腹疼痛，常与芍药、甘草等配伍，协同取效。许多滋补丸剂、膏剂常用蜂蜜作为赋形剂，不少中药用蜜炙法，都与其具有补益和缓和药性的作用有关。

2. 用于肺虚燥咳及肠燥便秘。治肺虚燥咳，干咳咯血，常配人参、生地黄等，如琼玉膏；治肠燥便秘，单用30～60克冲服，或与当归、胡麻仁、

tract); for constipation due to dry intestine, a drink with 30 - 60 g is suggested everyday, or used with Danggui (*Radix Angelicae Sinensis*), Humaren (*Semen Sesami*), Heshouwu (*Radix Polygoni Multiflori*), etc..

何首乌等配伍。

Besides, it is also recommendable for detoxifying medicinal herbs such as Wutou (*Radix Aconiti*), or applying externally on ruptured but unhealed pyocutaneous disease, or burns from water and fire, etc..

此外,还用于解乌头类中药的毒性。外用还可以治疮疡久不收口及水火烫伤等。

Usage and Dosage 15 - 30 g is used in decoction or drinking. A proper amount is used to help make pills, extracts or suppository.

【用法用量】 水煎服或冲服,15～30 克。制丸剂、膏剂或栓剂等,随方适量。

Notes Be cautious in the case with fullness in the epigastric abdomen due to stagnation of dampness, stagnation of phlegm due to damp-heat, loose stool, or diarrhea.

【使用注意】 湿阻中满、湿热痰滞、便溏或泄泻者宜慎用。

14. 2 Restoratives for reinforcing yang

第二节 补阳药

This category of herbs is mostly sweet, salty or pungent in flavor, and warm or hot in nature, with the action of warming and nourishing yang of the body. As kidney-yang is the master of yang qi all over the body, the nourishing of the kidney-yang is to warm all other organs so as to get rid of or improve all syndromes of yang-deficiency all over the body simultaneously. In this way, they focus on nourishing and tonifying kidney-yang. They are fit for deficiency of kidney-yang manifested as cold extremities, backache, lack of sexual desire, impotence, emission, sterility, frequent micturition, or enuresis; and failure of the kidney to receive qi due to deficiency of kidney-yang manifested as chronic cough and dyspnea; and failure of the spleen to warm and transport due to deficiency of kidney-yang marked by cold abdominal pain and morning diarrhea; and deficiency of body essence due to deficiency of

本类药物性味多甘温或咸温或辛热,能温补人体之阳气。因肾阳为一身阳气之本。肾阳之虚得补,就能温煦其他脏腑,从而消除或改善全身的阳虚诸证。故补阳药以温补肾阳为主。适用于肾阳不足的畏寒肢冷,腰膝酸软,性欲淡漠,阳痿,早泄,宫冷不孕,尿频遗尿;肾阳虚而不能纳气的慢性咳嗽喘促,肾阳衰、脾失温运的腹中冷痛,黎明泄泻;肾阳虚精髓亦虚的眩晕耳鸣,须发早白,筋骨疲软,小儿发育不良,囟门不合,齿迟,行迟等证。

kidney-yang manifested as dizziness, tinnitus, early whitening of hair, flaccidity of extremities or maldevelopment, delayed walking, delayed teeth eruption and closure of fontanel in infants, etc..

They are mostly warm and dry in nature, which tends to flourish fire and hurt yin, so it's unfit for the case with hyperactive fire due to deficiency of yin.

补阳药性多温燥,易助火伤阴,故阴虚火旺者不宜使用。

Lurong *Cornu Cervi Pantotrichum*

鹿 茸

The source is from the horn of male beast of *Cervus Nippon* Temminck or *C. elaphus* L. family Cerrridaae. The producing areas are in Northeast, Northwest, Inner Mongolia, Xinjiang and mountainous areas of Southwest in China. The medicinal material is cut in summer and autumn, dried after being processed, and used in the form of slices or powder.

为鹿科动物梅花鹿或马鹿的雄鹿未骨化密生茸毛的幼角。产于中国东北、西北和内蒙、新疆及西南山区。夏秋锯取鹿茸,经加工后阴干或烘干,切片或研粉用。

Medicinal Properties Sweet and salty in flavor, warm in nature, and attributive to the liver and kidney meridians.

【药性】 味甘、咸,性温。归肝、肾经。

Actions Nourish kidney-yang, promote the production of the essence and blood, strengthen tendons and bones.

【功效】 补肾阳,益精血,强筋骨。

Application

【临床应用】

1. It is applied for deficiency of kidney-yang or deficiency of the essence and blood manifested as chill, cold limbs, impotence, emission, sterility due to uterine cold, frequent micturition, dizziness, tinnitus, or fatigue. It can be ground into powder and used alone, or used together with Renshen (*Radix Ginseng*), Shudihuang (*Radix Rehmanniae Praeparata*), etc., such as Shen Rong Guben Wan (Pill).

1. 用于肾阳不足,精血亏虚之畏寒肢冷,阳痿滑精,宫冷不孕,小便频数,腰膝酸痛,头晕耳鸣,精神倦怠。可单用研末服,或与人参、熟地黄等配伍,如参茸固本丸。

2. For deficiency of the liver and kidney manifested as flaccidity of extremities, or maldevelopment, delayed walking, delayed teeth eruption and delayed closure of fontanel in infants, it is often used with Shudihuang

2. 用于肝肾不足,筋骨无力及小儿发育不良、行迟、齿迟、囟门不合等,常与熟地黄、山药、山茱萸等配伍,如加

(*Radix Rehmanniae Praeparata*), Shanyao (*Rhizoma Dioscoreae*), and Shanzhuyu (*Fructus Corni*), etc., such as Jiawei Dihuang Wan (Pill).

味地黄丸。

3. It is applied for deficiency and coldness of thoroughfare and conception vessels in women manifested as metrorrhagia and metrostasis and leucorrhagia due to weakness of belt vessel. For the former, it is used with Ejiao (*Colla Corii Asini*), Wuzeigu (*Os Sepiellae seu Sepiae*), etc., such as Lurong San (Powder); for the latter, used with Gouji (*Rhizoma Cibotii*), Bailian (*Herba Polygalae Japonica*).

3. 用于妇女冲任虚寒之崩漏、带脉不固之带下增多。前者可与阿胶、乌贼骨等同用,如鹿茸散;后者可与狗脊、白蔹配伍。

Besides, it is useful for treating unhealed skin lesions.

此外,阴疽内陷不起,溃久不敛用之,有温补托疮之效。

Usage and Dosage 1-3 g of its powder is for drinking; or in a pill or powder.

【用法用量】 研末吞服,1～3 克,或入丸、散剂。

Notes Contraindicated in the case with deficiency of yin and hyperactivity of yang, blood-heat, hyperpyrexia of the stomach, cough due to phlegm-heat, or febrile disease due to exogenous pathogenic factors. The amount used in the course should start gradually from small to large.

【使用注意】 阴虚阳亢,血热,胃火亢盛,痰热咳嗽及外感热病忌服。运用时应从小量开始,逐渐加量。

Bajitian *Radix Morindae Officinalis*

巴戟天

The source is from the root of *Morinda officinalis* How, family Rubiceae. The medicinal material is mainly produced in Guangdong, Guangxi, and Fujian, etc., available all year round. The one after being dried, steamed, and its wood centre removed is named as Bajirou. It is cut into fragments and dried, used crudely or soaked in a salty solution.

为茜草科植物巴戟天的根。主产于广东、广西、福建等地。全年均可采挖。晒干,再经蒸透,除去木心者,称"巴戟肉"。切段,干燥。生用或盐水炙用。

Medicinal Properties Sweet and pungent in flavor, slightly warm in nature, and attributive to the kidney and liver meridians.

【药性】 味甘、辛,性微温。归肾、肝经。

Actions Nourish kidney-yang, strengthen tendons

【功效】 补肾阳,强筋

and bones, and eliminate wind and dampness.

骨，祛风湿。

Application

【临床应用】

1. It is applied for deficiency of kidney-yang manifested as impotence, sterility, irregular menstruation, or cold pain in lower abdomen. In the case of impotence and sterility, it is used with Renshen (*Radix Ginseng*), Shanyao (*Rhizoma Dioscoreae*), and Roucongrong (*Herba Cistanchis*), etc.; for cold pain in lower abdomen or irregular menstruation, used with Gaoliangjiang (*Rhizoma Alpiniae Officinarum*), Rougui (*Cortex Cinnamomi*), Wuzhuyu (*Fructus Evodiae*), etc., such as Baji Wan (Pill).

1. 用于肾阳不足的阳痿，不孕，月经不调，少腹冷痛。治阳痿、不孕，常配人参、山药、肉苁蓉等；治少腹冷痛，月经不调，常与高良姜、肉桂、吴茱萸等同用，如巴戟丸。

2. For deficiency of kidney-yang accompanied by lumbago or fatigue, it is used with Bixie (*Rhizoma Dioscoreae*), Duzhong (*Cortex Eucommiae*), etc., such as Jingang Wan (Pill).

2. 用于肾阳虚兼有风湿之腰膝疼痛或软弱无力。可与萆薢、杜仲等同用，如金刚丸。

Usage and Dosage 3 - 9 g is used in decoction.

【用法用量】 水煎服，3～9克。

Notes It is not suitable for the case with deficiency of yin causing hyperactivity of yang or for that with damp-heat.

【作用注意】 阴虚火旺及有湿热者不宜用。

Yinyanghuo *Herba Epimedii*

淫羊藿

The source is from the branch and leaf of *Epimedium sagittatum* (Sieb. et Zucc.) Maxim. or *E. brevicornum* Maxim., *Epimedium pubescens* Maxim., wushan *Epimedium*, and *Epimedium Koreanum* Nakai. family Berberidaceae. The medicinal material is mostly produced in Shaanxi, Sichuan, Hubei, Shanxi, and Guangxi, etc., harvested in spring and autumn in bloom, and dried after removal of stem and other undesired part. It is used crudely or roasted with sheep fat.

为小檗科植物淫羊藿、箭叶淫羊藿、柔毛淫羊藿、巫山淫羊藿或朝鲜淫羊藿的地上部分。主产于陕西、四川、湖北、山西、广西等地。夏、秋茎叶茂盛时采割，除去梗及杂质，干燥。生用或用羊脂油炙用。

Medicinal Properties Pungent and sweet in flavor, warm in nature, and attributive to the liver and kidney meridians.

【药性】 味辛、甘，性温。归肝、肾经。

Actions Invigorate the kidney and strengthen yang, eliminate wind and dampness.

【功效】 补肾壮阳,祛风除湿。

Application

【临床应用】

1. For impotence due to deficiency of the kidney manifested as soreness of the waist and knees, frequent micturition, or sterility, it can be soaked alone in spirit for drinking, or used with Shudihuang (*Radix Rehmanniae Praeparata*), Shanzhuyu (*Fructus Corni*), Xianmao (*Rhizoma Curculignis*), and Gouqizi (*Fructus Lycii*), etc..

1. 用于肾虚阳痿,腰膝无力,尿频及妇女不孕。可单用浸酒服,或与熟地黄、山茱萸、仙茅、枸杞子等同用。

2. For Bi-syndrome of wind-cold-dampness type with spasm and numbness of extremities, etc., it is used together with Weilingxian (*Radix Clematidis*), Cang'erzi (*Fructus Xanthii*), etc., such as Xianlingpi San (Powder).

2. 用于风寒湿痹、筋骨拘挛、手足麻木等。可与威灵仙、苍耳子等同用,如仙灵脾(淫羊藿)散。

In addition, it is used with Xianmao (*Rhizoma Curculignis*), Bajitian (*Radix Morindae Officinalis*), etc., named as Erxian Tang (Decoction); and is effective for climacteric hypertention; also applied for cough and asthma due to deficiency of yang in the combination with Buguzhi (*Fructus Psoraleae*), Hutaorou (*Juglandis Regiae*), and Wuweizi (*Fructus Schisandrae*), etc..

此外,与仙茅、巴戟天等同用,名二仙汤,用于更年期高血压病。配伍补骨脂、胡桃肉、五味子等,还用于阳虚喘咳。

Usage and Dosage 3-9 g is used in decoction; or soaked in spirit for drinking; or decocted into extract or in pills and powder.

【用量用法】 水煎服,3～9克;亦可浸酒、熬膏或入丸散。

Roucongrong *Herba Cistanchis*

肉苁蓉

The source is from the fleshy stem of *Cistauche deserticola* Y. C. Ma, family Orobanchaceae. The medicinal material is mostly produced in Inner Mongolia, Xinjiang, and Qinghai of China, etc., and is dug out in spring when there is no bud coming out, then cleaned and cut into thick pieces. It is used crudely or soaked in spirit.

为列当科植物肉苁蓉带鳞片的肉质茎。主产于内蒙古、新疆、青海等地。春季苗未出土或刚出土时采挖,除去花序,干燥,切厚片。生用或酒制用。

Medicinal Properties Sweet and salty in flavor, warm in nature, and attributive to the kidney and large

【药性】 味甘、咸,性温。归肾、大肠经。

intestine meridians.

Actions Invigorate kidney-yang, supplement the essence and blood, moisten the intestine and relax bowels.

【功效】 补肾阳,益精血,润肠通便。

Application

【临床应用】

1. It is applied for the deficiency of kidney-yang and insufficiency of the blood and essence manifested as impotence, sterility, soreness of waist and knees, or flaccidity of tendons and bones. For impotence, it is combined with Shudihuang (*Radix Rehmanniae Praeparata*), Tusizi (*Semen Cuscutae*), and Wuweizi (*Fructus Schisandrae*), etc., such as Roucongrou Wan (Pill); for sterility, usually with Lujiaojiao (*Colla Cornus Cervi*), Danggui (*Radix Angelicae Sinensis*), Ziheche (*Placenta Hominis*), etc.; for soreness of waist and knees, or flaccidity of tendons and bones, with Bajitian (*Radix Morindae Officinalis*), Bixie (*Rhizoma Dioscoreae*), and Duzhong (*Cortex Eucommiae*), etc., such as Jingang Wan (Pill).

1. 用于肾阳不足,精血亏虚的阳痿,不孕,腰膝酸软,筋骨无力。治阳痿,常配熟地黄、菟丝子、五味子等,如肉苁蓉丸;治宫冷不孕,常配鹿角胶、当归、紫河车等;治腰膝酸软,筋骨无力,常配巴戟天、萆薢、杜仲等,如金刚丸。

2. For constipation due to dryness of the intestine, particularly in the aged with deficiency of kidney-yang and insufficiency of the blood and essence, it is usually combined with Danggui (*Radix Angelicae Sinensis*), Zhike (*Fructus Aurantii*), etc., such as Jichuan Jian (Decoction).

2. 用于肠燥便秘。对老人肾阳不足,精血亏虚者尤宜。常配当归、枳壳等同用,如济川煎。

Usage and Dosage 10 -15 g is used in decoction.

【用法用量】 水煎服,10~15克。

Notes Contraindicated in the case with hyperactive fire due to deficiency of yin, or loose stool and also in the case with damp-heat in the intestine or stomach.

【使用注意】 阴虚火旺及大便溏泄者忌用。肠胃有湿热者亦不宜用。

Yizhiren *Fructus Alpiniae Oxyphyllae*

益智仁

The source is from ripe fruit of *Alpinia oxyphylla* wliq., family Zingiberaceae. The medicinal material is mostly produced in Hainan, Guangdong, and Guangxi,

为姜科植物益智的成熟果实。主产海南、广东、广西等地。夏、秋间果实由绿变红

etc., and harvested in autumn when the fruit turns reddish from green, and then dried and taken out of the seeds. It is used crudely or stir-baked with a salty solution, and ground for use.

时采收。晒干,去壳取仁。生用或盐水炒用,用时捣碎。

Medicinal Properties Pungent in flavor, warm in nature, and attributive to the kidney and spleen meridians.

【药性】 味辛,性温。归肾、脾经。

Actions Warm the kidney to preserve the essence and decrease micturition, warm the spleen to stop diarrhea and check saliva.

【功效】 暖肾固精缩尿,温脾止泻摄唾。

Application

【临床应用】

1. It is used for deficiency of kidney-yang manifested as nocturnal emission, spermatorrhea, enuresis or frequent micturition because of its actions of nourishing the kidney and invigorating yang, astringing and solidifying the essence, and stopping frequent micturition. For nocturnal emission, it is used with Buguzhi (*Fructus Psoraleae*), Longgu (*Os Draconis*), and Jinyingzi (*Fructus Rosae Laevigatae*), etc.; for enuresis or nocturia, it is made in pills in combination with Shanyao (*Rhizoma Dioscoreae*), Wuyao (*Radix Linderae*), such as Suoquan Wan (Pill).

1.用于肾阳不足,遗精,滑精,遗尿,尿频。能补肾助阳,且性兼收涩,善于固精缩尿。治遗精,可配补骨脂、龙骨、金樱子等;治遗尿或夜尿频多,可与山药、乌药为丸服,如缩泉丸。

2. It is applied for diarrhea, cold pain in abdomen or salivation due to spleen-stomach cold deficiency. For diarrhea due to weakness and cold in the spleen and stomach, it is usually used together with Baizhu (*Rhizoma Atractylodis Macrocephalae*), Ganjiang (*Rhizoma Zingiberis*), etc.; for salivation, used together with Dangshen (*Radix Codonopsis*), Baizhu (*Rhizoma Atractylodis Macrocephalae*), and Jupi (*Pericarpium Citri Tangerinae*), etc..

2.用于中寒泄泻,腹中冷痛,口多涎唾。治脾胃虚寒泄泻,常配白术、干姜等;治口多涎唾或小儿流涎不禁,可配党参、白术、橘皮等。

Usage and Dosage 3 -10 g is used in decoction.

【用法用量】 水煎服,3~10克。

Buguzhi *Fructus Psoraleae*

The source is from the fruits of *Psoalea corylifolia* L., family Leguminosae. The medicinal material is mainly produced in Henan, Sichuan, etc., harvested in autumn and dried for use. It is used crudely or stir-baked with a salty solution.

Medicinal Properties Pungent and bitter in flavor, warm in nature, and attributive to the kidney and spleen meridians.

Actions Invigorate the kidney and strengthen yang, arrest nocturnal seminal emission and reduce urination with astringent drugs, and warm the spleen and stop diarrhea.

Application

1. It is applied for deficiency of kidney-yang manifested as impotence, emission, cold pain of waist and knees, frequent micturition or enuresis. For cold pain of waist and knees, it is usually used together with Duzhong (*Cortex Eucommiae*), Hutaorou (*Juglandis Regiae*), such as Qing'e Wan (Pill); for emission and impotence, with Tusizi (*Semen Cuscutae*), Hutaorou (*Juglandis Regiae*), etc., such as Buguzhi Wan (Pill); for frequent micturition and enuresis, with Xiaohuixiang (*Fructus Foeniculi*), such as Puoguzhi Wan (Pill), that is, Buguzhi Wan (Pill).

2. For deficiency of spleen-kidney-yang manifested as chronic diarrhea, it is used together with Roudoukou (*Semen Myristicae*), Wuweizi (*Fructus Schisandrae*), Wuzhuyu (*Fructus Evodiae*), such as Sishen Wan (Pill).

In addition, it can also be made into tincture for external application to treat vitiligo and alopecia areata.

Usage and Dosage 5 - 10 g is used in decoction; or in pill or powder.

Notes Contraindicated for hyperactivity of fire due

补骨脂

为豆科植物补骨脂的成熟果实。主产于河南、四川等地。秋季采收，晒干。生用或盐水炒用。

【药性】 味辛、苦，性温。归肾、脾经。

【功效】 补肾壮阳，固精缩尿，温脾止泻。

【临床应用】

1. 用于肾阳虚弱，阳痿遗精，腰膝冷痛，尿频遗尿。治腰膝冷痛，常与杜仲、胡桃肉配伍，即青娥丸；治阳痿遗精，常与菟丝子、胡桃肉等同用，如补骨脂丸；治尿频遗尿，又可与小茴香配伍，如破故纸(补骨脂)丸。

2. 用于脾肾阳虚，慢性泄泻。常与肉豆蔻、五味子、吴茱萸配伍，如四神丸。

此外，还可以制成酊剂外用，治白癜风及斑秃。

【用量用法】 水煎服，5～10克。或入丸散。

【使用注意】 阴虚火旺

to deficiency of yin, or for constipation.

及大便秘结者忌服。

Tusizi *Semen Cuscutae*

菟丝子

The source is from the ripe seeds of *Cuscuta chinensis* Lam., family Convolvulaceae. The medicinal material is produced in most parts of China, collected in autumn when the fruits are ripe in autumn. The seeds are threshed after dried in the sun, the impurity being removed. It is used crudely or used by roasting with a salt solution.

为旋花科植物菟丝子的成熟种子。中国大部分地区均产。秋季果实成熟时采收植株,晒干,打下种子,除去杂质。生用或盐水炙用。

Medicinal Properties Sweet in flavor, warm in nature, and attributive to the liver and kidney meridians.

【药性】 味甘,性温。归肝、肾、脾经。

Actions Invigorate the kidney and supplement the essence, nourish the liver and improve eyesight, stop diarrhea, soothe the fetus.

【功效】 补肾固精,养肝明目,止泻,安胎。

Application

【临床应用】

1. It is applied for deficiency of the kidney manifested as lumbago, impotence, emission, enuresis, or leucorrhagia because of its action of nourishing both kidney-yin and kidney-yang and that of arresting seminal emission and reducing urination with astringent drugs and stopping leucorrhagia. For sore in waist and knees, it is usually used together with Duzhong (*Cortex Eucommiae*); for impotence or emission, with Gouqizi (*Fructus Lycii*), Wuweizi (*Fructus Schisandrae*), and Fupenzi (*Fructus Rubi*), etc., such as Wuzi Yanzong Wan (Pill); for frequent micturition, with Sangpiaoxiao (*Ootheca Mantidis*), Lurong (*Cornu Cervi Pantotrichum*), and Wuweizi (*Fructus Schisandrae*), etc.; for leucorrhagia, turbid urine, with Fuling (*Poria*), Lianzi (*Semen Nelumbinis*), and Qianshi (*Semen Euryales*), etc., such as Fuling Wan (Pill).

1. 用于肾虚腰痛,阳痿遗精,尿频,带下。既补肾阳,又补肾阴,且有固精、缩尿、止带之效。治腰膝酸痛,常配杜仲;治阳痿、遗精,常配枸杞子、五味子、覆盆子等,如五子衍宗丸,治小便不禁,常配桑螵蛸、鹿茸、五味子等;治带下、尿浊,则可配茯苓、莲子、芡实等,如茯苓丸。

2. It is applied for insufficiency of the kidney and liver and malnutrition of eyes with manifestations of blurred vision and weakness of eyesight; usually used together with Shudihuang (*Radix Rehmanniae Praeparata*),

2. 用于肝肾不足,目失所养的目昏目暗,视力减退。常配熟地黄、枸杞子、车前子等,如驻景丸。

Gouqizi (*Fructus Lycii*), and Cheqianzi (*Semen Plantaginis*), etc., such as Zhujing Wan (Pill).

3. It is applied for diarrhea due to deficiency of both the spleen and kidney with its action of warming the kidney and nourishing the spleen to stop diarrhea, used together with Renshen (*Radix Ginseng*), Baizhu (*Rhizoma Atractylodis Macrocephalae*), and Buguzhi (*Fructus Psoraleae*), etc..

3. 用于脾肾两虚泄泻。能温肾补脾而止虚泻，可配人参、白术、补骨脂等同用。

4. It is applied for insufficiency of the liver and kidney resulting in threatened abortion with its action of nourishing the liver and kidney to soothe the fetus, usually used together with Chuanxuduan (*Radix Dipsaci*), Sangjisheng (*Herba Taxilli*) and Ejiao (*Colla Corii Asini*), such as Shoutai Wan (Pill).

4. 用于肝肾不足的胎动不安。有补肝肾，安胎之效。常与川续断、桑寄生、阿胶配伍应用，如寿胎丸。

In addition, Tusizi (*Semen Cuscutae*) also has the action of treating diabetes due to deficiency of the kidney. It is ground singly into powder for oral use or used together with Tianhuafen (*Radix Trichosanthis*), Wuweizi (*Fructus Schisandrae*), and Lurong (*Cornu Cervi Pantotrichum*), etc..

此外，菟丝子还能治肾虚消渴。单味研末服，或与天花粉、五味子、鹿茸等配伍。

Usage and Dosage 6 -12 g is used in decoction.

【用法用量】 水煎服，6～12 克。

Dongchongxiacao *Cordyceps*

冬虫夏草

The source is from the compound of the stroma formed by *Cordyceps sinensis* (Berk.) Sacc. Parasitized on the larva of *Hepialus armoricanus* Oberthru and the larva. The medicinal material is produced in Sichuan, Qinghai, and Tibet of China, etc., and dug out at early summer when the stroma has not dispersed yet. And it is processed by drying it in the sun to 60%- 70% dry, removing impurity, and then drying in the sun or drying in low temperature. It can be used crudely.

为麦角菌科真菌冬虫夏草寄生在蝙蝠蛾科昆虫幼虫的子座及幼虫尸体的复合体。产于四川、青海、西藏等地，初夏子座出土，孢子未发散时挖取。晒至 6～7 成干，除去杂质，晒干或低温干燥。生用。

Medicinal Properties Sweet in flavor, slightly warm in nature, and attributive to the lung and kidney

【药性】 味甘，性微温。归肺、肾经。

meridians.

Actions Invigorate the kidney and nourish the lung, strengthen yang and body essence, relive cough and dyspnea.

【功效】 益肾补肺,壮阳益精,平喘止嗽。

Application

【临床应用】

1. It is applied for deficiency of kidney-yang with impotence or lumbago. With its unique feature of warm but not dry in nature, both invigorating the kidney and strengthening yang, and supplementing the essence, it is frequently adopted as medicinal herbs for supplementing deficiency. For deficiency of the kidney with impotence or emission, it is used together with Bajitian (*Radix Morindae Officinalis*) and Tusizi (*Semen Cuscutae*); for deficiency of the kidney with soreness in waist and knees, with Duzhong (*Cortex Eucommiae*), etc..

1. 用于肾阳虚阳痿,腰痛。温而不燥,既能补肾壮阳,又能益精,为补虚常用药。治肾虚阳痿,遗精,可单用浸酒服,亦可配巴戟天、菟丝子同用;治肾虚腰膝酸痛,常配杜仲等同用。

2. It is applied for deficiency of the lung or deficiency of both the lung and kidney with chronic cough, dyspnea, or cough with blood-tinged sputum. For chronic cough with blood-tinged sputum, it is used together with Shashen (*Radix Adenophorae*), Ejiao (*Colla Corii Asini*), and Chuanbeimu (*Bulbus Fritillariae Cirrhosae*), etc.; for dyspnea or palpitation, with Renshen (*Radix Ginseng*), Hutaorou (*Juglandis Regiae*), etc..

2. 用于肺虚或肺肾两虚的久咳虚喘,劳嗽痰血。治劳嗽痰血,常配沙参、阿胶、川贝母等;治虚喘短气,常配人参、胡桃肉等。

In addition, it is also used for weakness after disease, spontaneous sweating or chillness, etc., and stewed with chicken, duck or pork, etc., which has a remarkable nutritious effect.

此外,本品还可用于病后体虚、自汗畏寒等,可以与鸡、鸭、猪肉等炖食,有良好的滋补功效。

Usage and Dosage 5-10 g is used in decoction; or in pills; or stewed with chicken, duck, or pork.

【用量用法】 水煎服,5~10克;亦可入丸散,或与鸡、鸭、猪肉等炖服。

Notes Contraindicated in the case with pathogenic factors attacking the exterior.

【使用注意】 有表邪者忌服。

Duzhong *Cortex Eucommiae*

杜 仲

The source is from the bark of *Eucommia ulmoides*

为杜仲科植物杜仲的树

Oliv., family Eucommiaceae. The medicinal material is produced in the areas of Sichuan, Yunnan, Guizhou, and Hubei, etc.. The tree is barked from April to May, and the bark is scraped and dried in the sun, then cut into segments and used crudely or stir-baked with a salt solution for medication.

皮。产于四川、云南、贵州、湖北等地。4～6月剥取,刮去粗皮,晒干。切块生用或盐水炙用。

Medicinal Properties Sweet in flavor, warm in nature and attributive to the liver and kidney meridians.

【药性】 味甘,性温。归肝、肾经。

Actions Invigorate the liver and kidney, strengthen the tendons and bones, and soothe the fetus.

【功效】 补肝肾,强筋骨,安胎。

Application

【临床应用】

1. It is indicated for deficiency of the liver and kidney manifested as cold sensation and soreness of the loins and knees, weakness of tendons and bones, and impotence and frequent micturition. For the former, it is usually used together with Buguzhi (*Fructus Psoraleae*), etc., such as Qing'e Wan (Bolus); for the latter, used together with Shanzhuyu (*Fructus Corni*), Tusizi (*Semen Cuscutae*), and Fupenzi (*Fructus Rubi*), etc..

1. 用于肝肾不足,腰膝冷痛,筋骨无力及阳痿、尿频。前者常与补骨脂等配伍,如青娥丸;后者可与山茱萸、菟丝子、覆盆子等同用。

2. For threatened abortion, vaginal bleeding or habitual miscarriage, it is usually combined with Xuduan (*Radix Dipsaci*) and Zaorou (*Caro Jujube*), such as Duzhong Wan (Bolus), or combined with others that invigorate the kidney to arrest excessive menstruation, such as Tusizi (*Semen Cuscutae*) and Ejiao (*Colla Corii Asini*).

2. 用于妊娠胎动不安,阴道流血,或习惯性流产。常与续断、枣肉配伍,如杜仲丸。或与其他补肾固经药如菟丝子、阿胶同用。

In addition, it can be used for hypertension which is accompanied by deficiency of the kidney, it can be combined with Juhua (*Flos Chrysanthemi*), Niuxi (*Radix Achyranthis Bidentatae*), and Xiakucao (*Spica Prunellae*), etc..

此外,还可用于高血压病而有肾虚见症者,可与菊花、牛膝、夏枯草等配伍。

Usage and Dosage 10 –15 g is used in decoction for oral use. The one stir-baked with salt water is more effective than the raw.

【用量用法】 水煎服,10～15克。盐水炒用疗效较生用为佳。

Shayuanzi *Semen Astragali Complanati* 沙苑子

The source is from the ripe seed of the herbage *Astragalus complanatus* R. Br, family Leguminosae. The plants are mainly produced in the areas of Shanxi, Shaanxi, etc., cut and collected at the end of autumn and the early stage of winter, dried in the sun, and then threshed and the seeds are got in. The seeds can be used crudely or stir-baked with a salt solution for medication.

为豆科植物扁茎黄芪的成熟种子。产于山西、陕西等地。秋末冬初采割植株，晒干，打下种子。生用或盐水炒用。

Medicinal Properties Sweet in flavor, warm in nature and attributive to the liver and kidney meridians.

【药性】 味甘，性温。归肝、肾经。

Actions Invigorate the kidney to arrest spontaneous emission and nourish the liver to improve vision.

【功效】 补肾固精，养肝明目。

Application

【临床应用】

1. It is indicated for deficiency of the kidney manifested as impotence, emission, premature ejaculation, dripping discharge of urine, excessive leucorrhea and soreness of loins since it can tonify kidney-yang, benefit kidney-yin, arrest spontaneous emission and decrease the frequency of micturition. In treating impotence, emission, frequent micturition and leucorrhea, it is usually used together with Longgu (*Os Draconis*), Lianxu (*Stamen Nelumbinis*), and Qianshi (*Semen Euryales*), etc., such as Jinsuo Gujing Wan (Bolus); in treating soreness of loins due to deficiency of the kidney, it can be pounded singly into powder for oral use, or also combined with Shudihuang (*Radix Rehmanniae Praeparata*) and Duzhong (*Cortex Eucommiae*).

1. 用于肾虚阳痿、遗精早泄、小便遗沥、白带过多及腰痛等。能补肾阳，益肾阴，固精缩尿。治阳痿遗精，尿频带下，常配龙骨、莲须、芡实等同用，如金锁固精丸；治肾虚腰痛，可单用本品研末服，也可配熟地黄、杜仲同用。

2. It has the action of nourishing the liver and kidney to improve vision, so it can be used for insufficiency of the kidney manifested as dizziness and blurred vision, it is usually combined with Gouqizi (*Fructus Lycii*), Tusizi (*Semen Cuscutae*), and Juhua (*Flos Chrysanthemi*), etc..

2. 用于肝肾不足的眩晕，目暗，视物不明。有补养肝肾以明目之效，常配枸杞子、菟丝子、菊花等同用。

Usage and Dosage 10 - 15 g is used in decoction

【用法用量】 水煎服，

for oral use.

10～15克。

14.3 Restoratives for nourishing the blood

第三节 补血药

This kind of restoratives can invigorate the liver, nourish the heart and benefit the spleen to promote the production of the blood. They are indicated for various blood deficiency syndromes such as pale or sallow complexion, excessive leucorrhea, pale lips and whitish nails, dizziness, palpitation, delayed and scanty menstruation with pale flow and sometimes amenorrhea. Some of them yet have yin tonifying action, so they are also indicated for yin-deficiency syndrome.

本类药物能补肝养心益脾，并以此滋生血液，适用于面色萎黄，唇舌爪甲苍白，头晕眼花，心慌心悸，以及妇女月经后期，量少，色淡，甚至经闭等各种血虚证。某些药物还具有补阴作用，适用于阴虚证。

They are unusually rich and tend to obstruct the digestive functions of the stomach and supporting dampness, thus they are contraindicated in conditions of deficiency of the spleen and stomach with poor appetite and loose stool, or with superficial pathogenic factors.

补血药滋腻碍胃，助湿恋邪，凡脾胃虚弱，食少纳呆，大便溏泄，表邪未尽者应忌用。

Danggui *Radix Angelicae Sinensis*

当归

The source is from the root of *Angelica sinensis* (Oliv.) Diels, family Umbelliferae. The medicinal material is mainly produced in the areas of Gansu, Shaanxi, etc., and that produced in Min County of Gansu is the best in quality. The root is dug at the end of autumn, whose fibrous root is removed, dried with mild fire, cut into pieces and used crudely or stir-baked with wine for medication.

为伞形科植物当归的根。主产于甘肃、陕西等地。以产于甘肃岷县的当归质量最好。秋末采挖后除去须根，用微火熏干，切片。生用或酒炒用。

Medicinal Properties Sweet and pungent in flavor, warm in nature and attributive to the liver, heart and spleen meridians.

【药性】 味甘、辛，性温。归肝、心、脾经。

Actions Nourish the blood, promote blood circulation, relieve pain and moisten the intestine.

【功效】 补血，活血，止痛，润肠。

Application

1. It is indicated for blood deficiency syndromes such as sallow complexion, pale lips, dizziness, palpitation and whitish nails, it is usually used together with Huangqi (*Radix Astragali*), such as Buxue Tang (Decoction).

2. It is used for irregular menstruation, amenorrhea and dysmenorrhea. For those due to blood deficiency, it is used together with Shudihuang (*Radix Rehmanniae Praeparata*), Baishaoyao (*Radix Paeoniae Alba*), and Ejiao (*Colla Corii Asini*), etc., such as Siwu Tang (Decoction) and Jiao'ai Tang (Decoction); for those due to blood stasis, used together with Chuanxiong (*Rhizoma Ligustici*), Chishaoyao (*Radix Paeoniae Rubra*), Taoren (*Semen Persicae*), and Honghua (*Fructus Carthami*), etc., such as Tao Hong Siwu Tang (Decoction); for those accompanied by depression of liver-qi resulting in stagnation of qi, combined with Xiangfu (*Rhizoma Cyperi*), Chaihu (*Radix Bupleuri*), and Yujin (*Radix Curcumae*), etc., as well, such as Xuanyu Tongjing Tang (Decoction).

3. It is used for various pains due to blood stasis or Bi-syndrome with pain due to wind-damp. For pains due to blood stasis in limbs, it may be combined with Danshen (*Radix Salviae Miltiorrhizae*), Ruxiang (*Olibanum*), and Moyao (*Myrrha*), etc., such as Huoluo Xiaoling Dan (Bolus); for swelling and pains due to trauma, usually combined with Dahuang (*Radix et Rhizoma Rhei*), Taoren (*Semen Persicae*), and Honghua (*Flos Carthami*), etc., such as Fuyuan Huoxue Tang (Decoction); for pains in shoulder and arms due to wind-dampness, usually combined with Qianghuo (*Rhizoma et Notopterygii*), Fangfeng (*Radix Saposhnikoviae*), and Jianghuang (*Rhizoma Curcumae Longae*), etc., such as Juanbi Tang (Decoction). It is also used together with Guizhi

【临床应用】

1. 用于血虚面色萎黄，唇舌色淡，头晕心悸，指(趾)甲苍白。常与黄芪同用，如当归补血汤。

2. 用于月经不调，经闭，痛经。因血虚而致者，配熟地黄、白芍药、阿胶等，如四物汤、胶艾汤；因瘀血而致者，常配川芎、赤芍药、桃仁、红花等，如桃红四物汤；若兼肝郁气滞者，又当配香附、柴胡、郁金等，如宣郁通经汤。

3. 用于各种瘀血疼痛及风湿痹痛。肢体瘀血作痛，可配丹参、乳香、没药等，如活络效灵丹；跌打损伤，瘀肿疼痛，常配大黄、桃仁、红花等，如复元活血汤；治风湿肩臂疼痛，多配羌活、防风、姜黄等，如蠲痹汤。与桂枝、白芍药、生姜同用，还可用治中焦虚寒腹痛。

(*Ramulus Cinnamorni*), Baishaoyao (*Radix Paeoniae Alba*) and Shengjiang (*Rhizoma Zingiberis Recens*) in treating abdominal pain due to deficiency and cold of the middle-energizer.

4. It is used for large carbuncle and pyocutaneous disease. For the early stage of those with redness, swelling and pain, it is combined with Jinyinhua (*Flos Lonicerae*), Chishaoyao (*Radix Paeoniae Rubra*), and Tianhuafen (*Radix Trichosanthis*), etc., such as Xianfang Huoming Yin (Decoction); for the middle age of that with pus before rupture, it should be combined with Zaojiaoci (*Spina Gleditsiae*), Huangqi (*Radix Astragali*), and Shudihuang (*Radix Rehmanniae Praeparata*), etc., such as Tounong San (Powder); for that unhealed after rupture due to deficiency of qi and blood, and with running pus, it is usually combined with Renshen (*Radix Ginseng*), Huangqi (*Radix Astragali*), and Shudihuang (*Radix Rehmanniae Praeparata*), etc., such as Shiquan Dabu Tang (Decoction).

4．用于痈疽疮疡。初起红肿疼痛而尚未化脓者，与金银花、赤芍药、天花粉等配伍，如仙方活命饮；中期脓成未溃者，应与皂角刺、黄芪等配用，如透脓散；若溃后因气血不足，脓水不尽，久不收口者，常配人参、黄芪、熟地黄等，如十全大补汤。

5. It is used in patients with constipation due to blood deficiency and dryness of the intestine, especially for those with weakness due to prolonged illness, the aged and women with postpartum blood deficiency and constipation due to insufficiency of the body fluids, it is usually combined with Shengheshouwu (*Radix Polygoni Multiflori*, unprepared), Huomaren (*Fructus Cannabis*), Roucongrong (*Herba Cistanchis*), etc..

5．用于血虚肠燥便秘。尤其适宜于久病体虚、老年人及产后血虚津亏便秘，常配生何首乌、火麻仁、肉苁蓉等同用。

In addition, 5% of Danggui Injection is injected in the acupoints such as Feishu (BL 13) and Tanzhong (CV 17) to treat chronic bronchitis.

此外，还可以用5%当归注射液注入肺俞、膻中等穴位，治疗慢性支气管炎。

Usage and Dosage 5-15 g is used in decoction for oral use. The crude one is generally used, but the one stir-baked with wine is used to promote blood circulation and dredge meridians.

【用法用量】 水煎服，5～15克。一般生用；活血通经，酒炒用。

Notes Contraindicated in the cases with domination of dampness and fullness in the middle energizer and diarrhea.

【使用注意】湿盛中满，大便溏泻者忌服。

Shudihuang *Radix Rehmanniae Praeparata*

熟地黄

The source is from the root of *Rehmannia glutinosa* Libosch., family Scrophulariaceae. The medicinal material is mainly produced in the areas of Henan, Hebei, and Inner Mongolia, etc.. After dried, it is prepared by steaming with wine, Sharen (*Fructus Amomi*) and Jupi (*Pericarpium Citri Tangerinae*), and drying itself repeatedly until it becomes black internally and externally, has the quality of softness and stickiness. It is cut into slices for medication.

为玄参科植物地黄的根，经加工炮制而成。主产于河南、河北、内蒙古等地。生地黄干燥后，以黄酒、砂仁、橘皮为辅料，经反复蒸晒，至内外色黑、质地柔软粘腻为度。切片用。

Medicinal Properties Sweet in flavor, slightly warm in nature and attributive to the liver and kidney meridians.

【药性】味甘，性微温。归肝、肾经。

Actions Enrich the blood and nourish yin, and supplement the essence.

【功效】养血滋阴，补精益髓。

Application

【临床应用】

1. It is indicated for blood deficiency manifested as sallow complexion, dizziness, palpitation, irregular menstruation and metrorrhagia and metrostaxis, it is usually combined with Danggui (*Radix Angelicae Sinensis*), Baishaoyao (*Radix Paeoniae Alba*), Chuanxiong (*Rhizoma Chuanxiong*), etc., such as Siwu Tang (Decoction).

1. 用于血虚萎黄、眩晕、心悸、失眠、月经不调、崩漏等。常与当归、白芍药、川芎等同用，如四物汤。

2. For deficiency of liver-yin and kidney-yin manifested as hectic fever, night sweat, emission and diabetes, it is usually used together with Shanyao (*Rhizoma Dioscoreae*), Shanzhuyu (*Fructus Corni*), etc., such as Liuwei Dihuang Wan (Bolus). For insufficiency of kidney-yin resulting in preponderant deficiency-fire with low fever and obvious night sweat, used together with Zhimu (*Rhizoma Anemarrhenae*), Huangbai (*Cortex Phellodendri*), Guiban (*Plastrum Testudinis*) and others that

2. 用于肝肾阴虚所致的潮热、盗汗、遗精、消渴等。常与山药、山茱萸等同用，如六味地黄丸。如肾阴不足，虚火偏旺，低热、盗汗明显者，还可配滋阴清火之知母、黄柏、龟版等，如大补阴丸。

can nourish yin to clear fire, such as Da Buyin Wan (Bolus).

3. For insufficiency of the essence and blood resulting in soreness of loins and knees, dizziness, tinnitus, deafness, poor vision, premature whitening of hair, etc., it is usually used with Heshouwu (*Radix Polygoni Multiflori*), Nüzhenzi (*Fructus Ligustri Lucidi*), Hanliancao (*Herba Ecliptae*), and Shanzhuyu (*Fructus Corni*), etc..

3. 用于精血亏虚而致的腰膝酸软、眩晕耳鸣、耳聋、视物不清、须发早白等。常与何首乌、女贞子、旱莲草、山茱萸等同用。

Usage and Dosage 10 -15 g is used in decoction for oral use.

【用量用法】 水煎服，10～15 克。

Notes It is sticky and rich in property and tends to obstruct digestion, therefore, it is not suitable for cases with excessive sputum, fullness in the epigastric region, poor appetite and loose stool.

【使用注意】 本品性质黏腻，有碍消化，故凡气滞痰多、脘腹胀满、食少便溏者均不宜服用。

Explanation Shengdihuang (*Radix Rehmanniae*) and Shudihuang (*Radix Rehmanniae Praeparata*) are different in processing, so their actions are also different. Shengdihuang (*Radix Rehmanniae*) is effective in clearing away heat and cooling the blood, promoting the production of the body fluids, and mostly used in treating seasonal febrile disease resulting in heat invading yingfen and xuefen, general fever and eruption, bleeding due to blood-heat, thirst and constipation due to consumption of the body fluids caused by yin-deficiency. Whereas the nature of Shudihuang (*Radix Rehmanniae Praeparata*) is warm that is changed from the cold nature of Shengdihuang (*Radix Rehmanniae*) so that Shudihuang (*Radix Rehmanniae Praeparata*) is effective in enriching the blood and nourishing yin, it is usually used in treating syndromes of deficiency of yin and the blood, and insufficiency of essence.

【说明】 生、熟地黄由于加工方法不同，其功效和适用症也有区别，生地黄长于清热凉血生津，多用治温热病热入营血，身热发斑；血热出血以及阴虚津伤之口渴、便秘。熟地黄药性由凉转温，长于补血滋阴，多用治阴血虚及精亏证。

Heshouwu *Radix Polygoni Multiflori*

何首乌

The source is from the root tuber of *Polygonum*

为蓼科植物何首乌的块

multiflorum Thunb., family Polygonaceae. The medicinal material is produced in all parts of China, dug and collected in both winter and autumn, and then cleaned, cut into slices and dried in the sun. That prepared by drying is known as crude sample, and that prepared by steaming again and again with the juice of black soya beans into dark brown as prepared sample.

根。中国各地均有产。秋、冬两季采挖后，洗净，切厚片，干燥，称为生何首乌；将生何首乌用黑豆汁拌匀，反复蒸至内外均呈棕褐色，晒干，称制何首乌。

Medicinal Properties The prepared sample is sweet and astringent in flavor, warm in nature and attributive to the liver and kidney meridians while the crude sample is sweet and bitter in flavor, mild in nature and attributive to the heart and liver meridians.

【药性】 制何首乌味甘、涩，性温。归肝、肾经。生首乌味甘、苦，性平。归心、肝经。

Actions The prepared sample benefits the essence and blood, invigorate the kidney to make hair black; the crude sample prevents recurrence of malaria, eliminates toxic materials and moistens the intestine to relax the bowels.

【功效】 制何首乌补益精血，固肾乌须；生首乌截疟解毒，润肠通便。

Application

1. It is indicated for insufficiency of the essence and blood manifested as dizziness, insomnia, premature whitening of hair, soreness of waist and flaccid feet, seminal emission, etc.. For sallow complexion and insomnia, it can be used together with Shudihuang (*Radix Rehmanniae Praeparata*), Danggui (*Radix Angelicae Sinensis*) and Suanzaoren (*Semen Ziziphi Spinosae*); for insufficiency of the liver and kidney essence, usually combined with Danggui (*Radix Angelicae Sinensis*), Gouqizi (*Fructus Lycii*), and Tusizi (*Semen Cuscutae*), etc., such as Qibao Meiran Dan (Bolus). Recently, it is combined with Danshen (*Radix Salviae Miltiorrhizae*), Sangjisheng (*Ramulus Taxilli*), etc., to treat hyperlipemia, hypertension and coronary heart disease.

2. For deficiency of both qi and blood and constant upset of malaria, the crude sample is combined with Ren-

【临床应用】

1. 用于精血亏虚之头晕眼花、失眠健忘、须发早白、腰酸脚软、遗精滑泄等。血虚面色萎黄，失眠健忘，与熟地黄、当归、酸枣仁配伍；肝肾精亏证，常与当归、枸杞子、菟丝子等同用，如七宝美髯丹。配丹参、桑寄生等，近来用治疗高血脂症、高血压、冠心病。

2. 用于气血两虚，久疟不止。以生何首乌配人参、当

shen (*Radix Ginseng*), Danggui (*Radix Angelicae Sinensis*), and Jupi (*Pericarpium Citri Tangerinae*), etc., such as Heren Yin(Decoction).

归、橘皮等同用,如何人饮。

3. For carbuncle, it is combined with Jinyinhua (*Flos Lonicerae*), Lianqiao (*Fructus Forsythiae*), and Pugongying (*Herba Taxaxaci*), etc.; for scrofula, combined with Xiakucao (*Spica Prunellae*), Zhebeimu (*Bulbus Fritillariae Thunbergii*), and Xuanshen (*Radix Scrophulariae*), etc.. In treating itching of skin, skin disease and rash, the crude sample can be used together with Aiye (*Folium Artemisiae Argyi*), which are decocted for washing.

3. 用于疮肿,瘰疬。前者可与金银花、连翘、蒲公英等同用,后者可与夏枯草、浙贝母、玄参等同用。若治皮肤瘙痒、疮疹等,可用生何首乌与艾叶煎汤外洗。

4. For dryness of the intestine and constipation due to blood deficiency, the crude sample is also used together with Danggui (*Radix Angelicae Sinensis*), Huomaren (*Fructus Cannabis*), etc..

4. 用于血虚肠燥便秘。也用生何首乌与当归、火麻仁等同用。

Usage and Dosage 6-12 g is used in decoction for oral use. For enriching the essence and blood, the prepared sample should be used; for preventing recurrence of malaria, eliminating toxic materials and moistening the intestine, the crude sample should be used.

【用量用法】 水煎服,6~12克。补益精血当用制何首乌;截疟、解毒、润肠宜用生首乌。

Notes It is not suitable for diarrhea or for cases with severer dampness-phlegm.

【使用注意】 大便溏泻及湿痰较重者不宜服用。

Baishaoyao *Radix Paeoniae Alba*

白芍药

The source is from the root of *Paeonia Lactiflora* Pall., family Ranunculaceae. The medicinal material is mainly produced in the areas of Zhejiang, Anhui, and Sichuan, etc.. After the root is dug and collected in summer and autumn, and cleaned, the head, thin root and external peel must be got rid of. The clean root is dried in the sun after it is slightly boiled in boiling water, then cut into slices. The crude or stir-baked one or the one stir-baked with wine can be used.

为毛茛科植物芍药的根。主产于浙江、安徽、四川等地,均系栽培。夏秋采挖后洗净,除去头尾和细根、外皮,沸水略煮后晒干,切片。生用、炒用或酒炒用。

Medicinal Properties Bitter and sour in flavor,

【药性】 味苦、酸,性微

slightly cold in nature and attributive to the liver and spleen meridians.

寒。归肝、脾经。

Actions Enrich the blood and regulate menstruation, astringe yin and arrest sweating, calm the liver and arrest pain.

【功效】 养血调经,敛阴止汗,平肝止痛。

Application

【临床应用】

1. It is used for blood deficiency manifested as irregular menstruation, dysmenorrhea and metrorrhagia and metrostaxis, it is usually combined with Danggui (*Radix Angelicae Sinensis*), Chuanxiong (*Rhizoma Chuanxiong*), and Shudihuang (*Rhizoma Rehmanniae Praeparata*), etc., such as Siwu Tang (Decoction).

1. 用于血虚月经不调,痛经,崩漏。常与当归、川芎、熟地黄等同用,如四物汤。

2. It is used for spontaneous perspiration due to low body resistance and imbalance between yingqi and weiqi, and night sweat due to yin deficiency. For the former, it is usually combined with Guizhi (*Ramulus Cinnamomi*); for the latter, combined with Shengdihuang (*Radix Rehmanniae*), Muli (*Concha Ostreae*), and Fuxiaomai (*Fructus Tritici Levis*), etc..

2. 用于营卫不和的表虚自汗及阴虚盗汗。前者常与桂枝配伍;后者与生地黄、牡蛎、浮小麦等同用。

3. It is used for insufficiency of liver-yin and disharmony of liver-qi manifested as pains in the chest and hypochondrium, muscular spasm and pain of extremities. For pain in the hypochondrium due to stagnation of liver-qi, it is usually combined with Chaihu (*Radix Bupleuri*), Xiangfu (*Rhizoma Cyperi*), etc., such as Chaihu Shugan San (Powder); for pain and spasm in the epigastrium and extremities, combined with Gancao (*Radix Glycyrrhizae*), such as Shaoyao Gancao Tang (Decoction); for incoordination between the liver and spleen with abdominal pain and diarrhea, combined with Baizhu (*Rhizoma Atractylodis Macrocephalae*), Jupi (*Pericarpium Citri Tangerinae*) and Fangfeng (*Radix Saposhnikoviae*) to form a formula, that is Tongxie Yaofang (Decoction); for dysentery and abdominal pain, combined with Muxiang

3. 用于肝阴不足,肝气不和,胁肋脘腹疼痛,或四肢拘挛作痛。如治肝郁胁痛,常配柴胡、香附等,如柴胡疏肝散;治脘腹、手足挛急作痛,可与甘草配用,如芍药甘草汤;治肝脾不调,腹痛泄泻,可配白术、橘皮、防风,即痛泻要方;治痢疾腹痛,可与木香、槟榔、黄连等同用。

(*Radix Aucklandiae*), Binglang (*Semen Arecae*), and Huanglian (*Rhizoma Coptidis*), etc..

4. For dizziness due to hyperactivity of liver-yang, it is usually combined with Shengdihuang (*Radix Rehmanniae*), Niuxi (*Radix Achyranthis Bidentatae*), and Daizheshi (*Haematitum*), etc., such as Jianling Tang (Decoction).

4. 用于肝阳上亢的头痛眩晕。常与生地黄、牛膝、代赭石等同用,如建瓴汤。

Usage and Dosage 5 -15 g is used in decoction for oral use, and the large dosage that can be used is 15 - 30 g. The crude is usually used for astringing yin, calming the liver and treating dysentery; the stir-baked one for smoothing the liver and arresting pain, and the one stir-baked with wine can decrease its cold nature.

【用法用量】 水煎服,5~15克,大剂量可用至15~30克。敛阴、平肝、治痢多生用;柔肝止痛多炒用。酒炒可减其寒性。

Notes It is incompatible with Lilu (*Rhizoma et Radix Veratri*).

【使用注意】 反藜芦。

Explanation It is from the same source as Chishaoyao (*Radix Paeoniae Rubra*) of the medicinal herbs that can clear away heat, but it is cultivated and must be boiled when prepared; whereas Chishaoyao (*Radix Paeoniae Rubra*) is wild and the crude one is used for medication. Their effects are very different, therefore, they must be distinguished when they are used.

【说明】 本品与清热药中赤芍药来源为同种植物,但此为栽培品,加工时要用水煮;而赤芍药为野生品,入药生用。两者功效相差很大,应用时要注意区别。

Ejiao *Colla Corii Asini*

阿 胶

The source is from donkey hide stewed and concentrated as gelatinous mass of *Equus asinus* L., family Equidae. The medicinal material is mainly produced in the areas of Shandong, Zhejiang, and Jiangsu, etc.. The one produced in Dong'e County of Shandong Province is the most famous. It is used crudely, pounded into pieces or stir-baked with powder of clam, cattail pollen, and talc into pearl of Ejiao.

为马科动物驴的皮,经漂泡去毛后煎煮浓缩而成的胶块。主产于山东、浙江、江苏等地。以山东东阿县的产品最著名。原药生用,捣成碎块,或用蛤粉、蒲黄粉、滑石粉炒成阿胶珠用。

Medicinal Properties Sweet in flavor, mild in nature and attributive to the lung, liver and kidney meridians.

【药性】 味甘,性平。归肺、肝、肾经。

Actions Enrich the blood and stop bleeding, nourish yin and moisten dryness.

【功效】 补血止血,滋阴润燥。

Application

【临床应用】

1. For blood-deficiency with sallow complexion, dizziness and palpitation, it is usually combined with Shudihuang (*Rhizoma Rehmanniae Praeparata*), Danggui (*Radix Angelicae Sinensis*), Huangqi (*Radix Astragali*), and Dangshen (*Haematitum*), etc..

1. 用于血虚面色萎黄,眩晕心悸。常与熟地黄、当归、黄芪、党参等同用。

2. For various bleeding syndromes, especially for bleeding accompanied by insufficiency of yin and blood, it can be melted alone for oral use or combined with other medicinal herbs according to morbid conditions. For instance, in treating hematemesis and hemoptysis, it can be combined with Maimendong (*Radix Ophiopogonis*) and Shengdihuang (*Radix Rehmanniae*); in treating hemafecia due to deficiency of spleen-yang and stomach-yang, usually combined with Baizhu (*Rhizoma Atractylodis Macrocephalae*) and Fuzi (*Radix Aconiti Praeparata*), such as Huangtu Tang (Decoction); in treating metrorrhagia and metrostaxis, excessive menstruation, bleeding during pregnancy and endless bleeding after miscarriage, usually combined with Shengdihuang (*Radix Rehmanniae*), Baishaoyao (*Radix Paeoniae Alba*) and Aiye (*Folium Artemisiae Argyi*), such as Jiao Ai Tang (*Decoction*).

2. 用于多种出血证。对出血而兼阴血亏虚者最为适宜。可单用本品烊化服,或根据病情配伍他药。如治吐血、咯血,可配麦门冬、生地黄;治脾胃阳虚便血,常配白术、附子,如黄土汤;治妇女崩漏,月经过多,妊娠下血,小产后下血不止,常配生地黄、白芍药、艾叶,如胶艾汤。

3. For vexation and insomnia due to yin-deficiency, usually combined with Huanglian (*Rhizoma Coptidis*), Baishaoyao (*Radix Paeoniae Alba*), and Jizihuang (*Vitellus Galli*), etc., such as Huanglian Ejiao Tang (Decoction).

3. 用于阴虚心烦失眠。常与黄连、白芍药、鸡子黄等同用,如黄连阿胶汤。

4. For cough and dyspnea due to asthenia of viscera or dry cough due to yin-deficiency, it is usually combined with Shashen (*Radix Adenophorae*), Maimendong (*Radix Ophiopogonis*), Sangye (*Folium Mori*), and

4. 用于虚劳喘咳或阴虚燥咳。常与沙参、麦门冬、桑叶、杏仁等同用。

Xingren (*Semen Armeniacae Amarum*), etc..

Usage and Dosage It is melted and taken after mixing it with water, or dissolved in boiling water or millet wine; the dosage is 5 -10 g. For enriching blood and nourishing yin, the crude is used; for stopping bleeding, the one stir-baked with cattail pollen is suitable to be used; for moistening the lung, the one stir-baked with clam powder is suitable.

【用法用量】 烊化冲服,或用开水、黄酒化服:5～10克,补血、滋阴可原药生用;止血宜蒲黄炒;润肺止咳宜蛤粉炒。

Notes It is rich in property and obstructs digestion, therefore, it is not suitable for deficiency of the spleen and stomach with poor appetite, abdominal distention and loose stool.

【使用注意】 本品性质粘腻,有碍消化,故脾胃虚弱、不思饮食、腹胀便溏者不宜用。

14. 4 Restoratives for nourishing yin

第四节 补阴药

This kind of restoratives are mostly sweet and cold or salty and cold, can aid in nourishing the yin, regenerate the body fluids and moisten dryness. They are indicated for dry cough with less sputum, dry mouth and tongue; a red tongue with less coating, dry throat and thirst due to insufficiency of stomach-yin; dry eyes, blurred vision, dizziness and tinnitus due to deficiency of liver-yin; sore and weak waist and knees, seminal emission and night sweat due to deficiency of kidney-yin.

本类药物大都甘寒,或咸寒,能滋养阴液,生津润燥。适用于肺阴不足之干咳少痰、口干舌燥;胃阴不足之舌红少苔、咽干口渴;肝阴不足之两目昏涩、头晕耳鸣;肾阴不足之腰膝酸软、遗精盗汗等。

Beishashen *Radix Glehniae*

北沙参

The source is from the root of *Glehnia littoralis* Fr. Schmidt *ex* Miq., family Umbelliferae. The medicinal material is mainly produced in the areas of Shandong, Hebei, Liaoning, and Jiangsu, etc., dug and collected in summer and autumn, and then cleaned, the fibrous root being got rid of, scalded by boiling water, surface with cork being removed and then cut into segments, dried in the sun, or after being cleaned, it can be directly dried in

为伞形科植物珊瑚菜的根。主产于山东、河北、辽宁、江苏等地。夏秋采挖后洗净,除去须根,开水烫后剥去外皮,切片成切段,晒干。或洗净直接晒干。

the sun.

Medicinal Properties Sweat in flavor, slightly cold in nature and attributive to the lung and stomach meridians.

【药性】 味甘,性微寒。归肺、胃经。

Actions Nourish yin, clear away lung-heat, replenish the stomach and regenerate the body fluids.

【功效】 养阴清肺,益胃生津。

Application

【临床应用】

1. For dry cough due to lung-heat or chronic cough due to asthenia of viscera with dry throat and hoarse voice, it is usually combined with Maimendong (*Radix Ophiopogonis*), Yuzhu (*Rhizoma Polygonati Odorati*), and Sangye (*Folium Mori*), etc., to treat the former, such as Shashen Maidong Tang (Decoction), and with Zhimu (*Rhizoma Anemarrhenae*), Maimendong (*Radix Ophiopogonis*), and Tianhuafen (*Radix Trichosanthis*), etc., to treat the latter.

1. 用于肺热燥咳或劳嗽久咳、咽干音哑。前者常与麦门冬、玉竹、桑叶等配伍,如沙参麦冬汤;后者多与知母、麦门冬、天花粉等同用。

2. For deficiency of stomach-yin or consumption of the body fluids due to heat with dry tongue and thirst, poor appetite, or dull pain in epigastric region, epigastric upset, and retching, etc., it is usually combined with Shengdihuang (*Radix Rehmanniae*), Maimendong (*Radix Ophiopogonis*), etc., such as Yiwei Tang (Decoction); if the body fluids are consumed seriously with dark red tongue and less fluid, it can be used together with Shengdihuang (*Radix Rehmanniae*), Xianshihu (*Herba Dendrobii*, fresh), etc..

2. 用于胃阴虚或热伤津液、舌干口渴、食欲不振等或见胃脘隐痛、嘈杂、干呕。常与生地黄、麦门冬等同用,如益胃汤;若津伤较重,舌绛少津者,可与鲜生地黄,鲜石斛等同用。

Usage and Dosage 10 -15 g is used in decoction for oral use.

【用法用量】 水煎服,10~15克。

Notes It is incompatible with Lilu (*Rhizoma et Radix Veratri*).

【使用注意】 反藜芦。

Explanation In addition, there is another medicinal herb, Nanshashen (*Radix Adenophorae*) that consists of the root of *Adenophora tetraphylla* (Thunb.) Fisch. and *Adenophora stricta* Miq. Shashen, family Campanu-

【说明】 另有南沙参,为桔梗科植物轮叶沙参或杏叶沙参的根,功效与北沙参类似,养阴作用较弱,但兼有化

laceae. Its action is similar to that of Beishashen (*Radix Glehniae*), the action of nourishing yin being weaker, but is companied with that of resolving phlegm, so it can be used for cough due to dry phlegm or cough with sputum due to deficiency of lung-yin.

痰作用,可用于燥痰咳嗽,或肺阴虚挟痰咳嗽。

Maimendong *Radix Ophiopogonis*

麦门冬

The source is from the root tuber of *Ophiopogon japonicus* (Thunb.) Ker. Gawl., family Liliaceae. The medicinal material is produced in all parts of China. It is dug and collected in summer, the fibrous roots being removed, cleaned, dried and used crudely.

为百合科植物麦门冬的块根。中国各地均产,夏季采挖,除去须根,洗净,晒干。生用。

Medicinal Properties Sweet and slightly bitter in flavor, slightly cold in nature and attributive to the heart, lung and stomach meridians.

【药性】 味甘、微苦,性微寒。归心、肺、胃经。

Actions Nourish yin and moisten the lung, benefit the stomach and regenerate the body fluids, clear away the heart-heat and relieve vexation.

【功效】 养阴润肺,益胃生津,清心除烦。

Application

【临床应用】

1. The medicinal herb is indicated for dry cough and sticky sputum due to lung-dryness and cough and hemoptysis due to asthenia of viscera. In treating pathogenic warm-dry invading the lung resulting in dry cough with less sputum that is difficult to be coughed out, dry nose and throat, it is usually combined with Sangye (*Folium Mori*), Xingren (*Semen Armeniacae Amarum*) and Shengshigao (*Gypsum Fibrosum*), such as Qingzhao Jiufei Tang (Decoction); in treating insufficiency of lung-yin manifested as cough and hemoptysis due to asthenia of viscera, usually combined with Tianmendong (*Radix Asparagi*), such as Erdong Gao (Soft extract).

1. 用于肺燥干咳,痰黏及劳嗽咯血。治温燥之邪犯肺干咳,痰少难咯,鼻咽干燥,常与桑叶、杏仁、生石膏同用,如清燥救肺汤;治肺阴亏损,劳嗽咯血,常与天门冬配伍,如二冬膏。

2. It is used for yin-syndromes of the stomach and intestine. For insufficiency of stomach-yin with dry tongue and thirst, it is usually combined with Shashen (*Radix Adenophorae*), Shengdihuang (*Radix Rehman-*

2. 用于胃肠阴虚证。胃阴不足,舌干口渴,常与沙参、生地黄、玉竹等同用,如益胃汤;治肠燥便秘,可与生地黄、

niae), Yuzhu (*Rhizoma Polygonati Odorati*), etc., such as Yiwei Tang (Decoction); for constipation due to dryness of the intestine, may be combined with Shengdihuang (*Radix Rehmannia*) and Xuanshen (*Radix Scrophulariae*) to compose a formula, that is Zengye Tang (Decoction).

玄参同用,即增液汤。

3. For vexation and palpitation caused by heat invading the heart, combined with Huanglian (*Rhizoma Coptidis*), Danshen (*Radix Salviae Miltiorrhizae*), and Zhuye (*Folium Phyllostachydis Henonis*), etc., such as Qingying Tang (Decoction); for that caused by yin-deficiency and interior heat, usually combined with Xuanshen (*Radix Scrophulariae*), Shengdihuang (*Radix Rehmanniae*), and Suanzaoren (*Semen Ziziphi Spinosae*), etc., such as Tianwang Buxin Dan (Bolus).

3. 用于心烦失眠。属热入心营而致者,配黄连、丹参、竹叶等,如清营汤;属阴虚内热所致者,常配玄参、生地黄、酸枣仁等,如天王补心丹。

Usage and Dosage 6 -12 g is used in decoction for oral use.

【用法用量】 水煎服,6~12克。

Notes It is not suitable for cough due to exogenous wind and cold, and obstruction of phlegm-dampness in the lung.

【使用注意】 外感风寒及痰湿阻肺的咳嗽,或脾胃虚寒泄泻者,均不宜服用。

Tianmendong *Radix Asparagi*

天门冬

The source is from the root tuber of *Asparagus cochinchinensis* (Lour.) Merr., family Liliaceae. The medicinal material is mainly produced in Sichuan, Guizhou, and Guangxi, etc., dug and collected in autumn and winter and cleaned, the fibrous roots being got rid of. Then it is boiled or steamed, after which the surface is removed, cleaned and dried. It is cut into thin slices and used crudely.

为百合科植物天门冬的块根。主产四川、贵州、广西等地。秋、冬两季采挖,洗净,除残茎及须根。煮或蒸透心,趁热除去外皮,洗净,干燥,切薄片。生用。

Medicinal Properties Sweet and bitter in flavor, cold in nature and attributive to the lung and kidney meridians.

【药性】 味甘、苦,性寒。归肺、肾经。

Actions Nourish yin and moisten the lung, clear away fire and regenerate the body fluids.

【功效】 养阴润肺,清火生津。

Application

1. It is indicated for dry cough due to yin-deficiency and lung-heat or cough and hemoptysis due to asthenia of viscera. In treating cough due to dryness-heat, it is usually combined with Maimendong (*Radix Ophiopogonis*), Shashen (*Radix Adenophorae*), and Chuanbeimu (*Bulbus Fritillariae Cirrhosae*), etc.; in treating cough and hemoptysis due to asthenia of viscera or dry cough and sticky sputum with blood, usually combined with Maimendong (*Radix Ophiopogonis*), Chuanbeimu (*Bulbus Fritillariae Cirrhosae*), Shengdihuang (*Radix Rehmanniae*), and Ejiao (*Colla Corii Asini*), etc..

2. It is used for insufficiency of kidney-yin and yin-deficiency causing hyperactivity of fire manifested as hectic fever, night sweat, nocturnal emission, diabetes due to interior heat, constipation due to dryness of the intestine. For yin-deficiency causing hyperactivity of fire marked by hectic fever, nocturnal emission, soreness and weakness of waist and knees, it is usually combined with Shudihuang (*Rhizoma Rehmanniae Praeparata*), Renshen (*Radix Ginseng*), etc., such as Sancai Fengsui Dan (Pellet); for internal heat with diabetes or febrile disease resulting in consumption of the body fluids manifested as thirst, usually combined with Maimendong (*Radix Ophiopogonis*), Tianhuafen (*Radix Trichosanthis*), and Zhimu (*Rhizoma Anemarrhenae*), etc., such as Erdong Tang (Decoction); for dryness of the intestine and constipation due to heat consuming the body fluids, may be combined with Shengdihuang (*Radix Rehmannia*), Danggui (*Radix Angelicae Sinensis*), etc..

Usage and Dosage 6 -12 g is used in decoction for oral use.

Huangjing *Rhizoma Polygonati*

The source is from the rhizome of *Polygonatum*

【临床应用】

1. 用于阴虚肺热燥咳或劳嗽咳血。治燥热咳嗽，常配麦门冬、沙参、川贝母等同用；治劳嗽咳血，或干咳痰黏，痰中带血，常配麦门冬、川贝母、生地黄、阿胶等同用。

2. 用于肾阴不足，阴虚火旺的潮热盗汗，遗精，内热消渴，肠燥便秘。治肾虚火旺，潮热遗精，腰膝酸软，常配熟地黄、人参等同用，如三才封髓丹；治内热消渴，或热病伤津口渴，常配麦门冬、天花粉、知母等同用，如二冬汤；治热伤津液的肠燥便秘，可与生地黄、当归等配伍。

【用法用量】 水煎服，6～12克。

黄　精

为百合科植物黄精、多花

sibiricum Red., *P. cyrtonema* Hua or the other species of the same genus, Family Liliaceae. The medicinal material is mainly produced in the areas of Hebei, Inner Mongolia, and Shaanxi, etc.. Duohuahuangjing in the areas of Guizhou, Hunan, and Yunnan, etc.. Zhenhuangjing in the areas of Yunnan, Guizhou and Guangxi. The rhizome is dug and collected in both spring and autumn, cleaned, scalded in boiling water or steamed thoroughly, and then dried in the sun. It is cut into thick slices and used crudely or prepared with wine for medication.

黄精及滇黄精的根茎。黄精主产于河北、内蒙古、陕西等，多花黄精主产于贵州、湖南、云南等，滇黄精主产于云南、贵州、广西。春、秋两季采挖，洗净，沸水中烫或蒸至透心。晒干，切厚片。生用或酒制用。

Medicinal Properties Sweet in flavor, mild in nature and attributive to the lung, spleen and kidney meridians.

【药性】 味甘，性平。归肺、脾、肾经。

Actions Moisten the lung and nourish the kidney, invigorate the kidney and benefit qi.

【功效】 润肺滋肾，补脾益气。

Application

【临床应用】

1. For dry cough with less sputum due to yin-deficiency and lung-dryness, it can be used alone and boiled into medicinal extract for oral use, or combined with Shashen (*Radix Adenophorae*), Chuanbeimu (*Bulbus Fritillariae Cirrhosae*), and Zhimu (*Rhizoma Anemarrhenae*), etc..

1. 用于阴虚肺燥，干咳少痰。可单用熬膏服，或配沙参、川贝母、知母等同用。

2. It can benefit spleen-qi as well as nourish spleen-yin, and used for deficiency of the spleen and stomach. For deficiency of spleen-qi and stomach-qi manifested as fatigue, poor appetite and feeble pulse, it can be combined with Dangshen (*Radix Codonopsis*), Baizhu (*Rhizoma Atractylodis Macrocephalae*), etc.; for deficiency of spleen-yin and stomach-yin causing dry mouth and poor appetite, red and uncoated tongue, can be combined with Shihu (*Herba Dendrobii*), Maimendong (*Radix Ophiopogonis*), and Shanyao (*Rhizoma Dioscoreae*), etc..

2. 用于脾胃虚弱。既补脾阴，又益脾气。脾胃气虚，倦怠乏力，食欲不振，脉虚者，可与党参、白术等同用；如脾胃阴虚而致口干食少，饮食无味，舌红无苔者，可与石斛、麦门冬、山药等同用。

3. For deficiency of the kidney and insufficiency of essence manifested as dizziness, weakness of the waist

3. 用于肾虚精亏的头晕，腰膝酸软，须发早白。常配枸

and knees and premature whitening of hair, it is usually combined with Gouqizi (*Fructus Lycii*) and others, such as Erjing Wan (Bolus).

杞子等同用,如二精丸。

In addition, it can also be used to treat diabetes, it is usually combined with Maimendong (*Radix Ophiopogonis*), Tianhuafen (*Radix Trichosanthis*), and Huangqi (*Radix Astragali*), etc..

此外还可用于消渴证,常配麦门冬、天花粉、黄芪等同用。

Usage and Dosage 10 -15 g is used in decoction for oral use.

【用法用量】 水煎服,10～15克。

Yuzhu *Rhizoma Polygonati Odorati*

玉 竹

The source is from the Rhizome of *Polygonatum odoratum* (Mill.) Druce, family Liliaceae. The medicinal material is mainly produced in the areas of Hebei, Jiangsu, etc.. The rhizome is dug and collected in autumn. After cleaned, it is exposed to the sun until it changes into softness and then rubbed, cooled and exposed to the sun until it has no hard mass, and meanwhile dried in the sun as well; or after steamed thoroughly, it is rubbed till it becomes translucent and then dried in the sun, cut into thick slices or segments for being used crudely or roasted for medication.

为百合科植物玉竹的根茎。主产河北、江苏等地。秋季采挖,洗净,晒至柔软后,揉搓,晾晒至无硬心,晒干;或蒸透后,揉至半透明,晒干,切厚片(段)。生用或炙用。

Medicinal Properties Sweet in flavor, slightly cold and attributive to the lung and stomach meridians.

【药性】 味甘,性微寒。归肺、胃经。

Actions Nourish yin and moisten the dryness, regenerate the body fluids to relieve thirst.

【功效】 养阴润燥,生津止渴。

Application

【临床应用】

1. For dry cough with less sputum due to yin-deficiency and lung-dryness, it is usually combined with Shashen (*Radix Adenophorae*), Maimendong (*Radix Ophiopogonis*), and Sangye (*Folium Mori*), etc., such as Shashen Maidong Tang (Decoction).

1. 用于阴虚肺燥的干咳少痰。常与沙参、麦门冬、桑叶等同用,如沙参麦冬汤。

2. For febrile disease with consumption of the body fluids manifested as fever accompanied with restlessness, it is usually combined with Shengdihuang (*Radix Reh-*

2. 用于热病伤津,烦热口渴及消渴。热病伤津的烦热口渴,常配生地黄、麦门冬等

manniae), Maimendong (*Radix Ophiopogonis*) and others, such as Yiwei Tang (Decoction); for diabetes due to internal heat, combined with Shengdihuang (*Radix Rehmanniae*), Tianhuafen (*Radix Trichosanthis*) and others.

同用,如益胃汤;内热消渴,可与生地黄、天花粉等同用。

In addition, it is tonic but not greasy, nourishes yin but does not make pathogenic factors linger, therefore, it can be used for exogenous wind and cold due to yin-deficiency, Jiajian Weirui Tang (Decoction) that is composed of Yuzhu (*Rhizoma Polygonati Odorati*) in combination with Bohe (*Herba Menthae*), Congbai (*Bulbus Allii Fistulosi*), Dandouchi (*Semen Sojae Praeparata*) and others.

此外,本品补而不腻,养阴而不恋邪。可治阴虚外感风热,加减葳蕤(玉竹)汤,即以此配伍薄荷、葱白、淡豆豉等同用。

Usage and Dosage 6 -12 g is used in decoction for oral use.

【用法用量】 水煎服,6～12克。

Shihu *Herba Dendrobii*

石　斛

The source is from the stem of the perennial herbage *Dendrobium nobil* Lindll., family Orchidaceae and other plants of the same genus. The medicinal material is mainly produced in the areas of Sichuan, Guizhou, and Yunnan, etc.. After it is collected, its fibrous roots and impurity are removed and then it is dried in the sun and cut into segments. The crude or fresh can be used for medication.

为兰科植物金钗石斛及同属多种植物的茎。主产于四川、贵州、云南等地。采后,除去须根和杂质,晒干,切段。生用,或鲜用。

Medicinal Properties Sweet in flavor, slightly cold in nature and attributive to the lung, stomach and kidney meridians.

【药性】 味甘,性微寒。归肺、胃、肾经。

Actions Nourish the stomach and regenerate the body fluids, and moisten yin and clear away heat.

【功效】 养胃生津,滋阴清热。

Application

【临床应用】

1. For dry mouth, excessive thirst, dry throat and dark red tongue due to consumption of the body fluids by febrile disease, it is usually combined with Shengdihuang (*Radix Rehmanniae*), Maimendong (*Radix Ophiopogonis*), etc.. For yin-deficiency causing insufficiency of the

1. 用于热病伤津,口燥烦渴,咽干,舌绛,多与生地黄、麦门冬等同用。如阴虚津亏,虚热不退,常与生地黄、白薇、麦门冬、玄参等同用。

body fluids and asthenic heat, it is usually combined with Shengdihuang (*Radix Rehmannia*), Baiwei (*Radix Cynanchi Atrati*), Maimendong (*Radix Ophiopogonis*), and Xuanshen (*Radix Scrophulariae*), etc..

2. For insufficiency of stomach-yin manifested as dull or burning pain in epigastric region, poor appetite, dry mouth, constipation, little coated tongue, it can be combined with Zhuru (*Caulis Bambusae in Taeniam*) Baishaoyao (*Radix Paeoniae Alba*), Lugen (*Rhizoma Phragmitis*), etc.; the fresh can also be used to treat diabetes and usually combined with Tianhuafen (*Radix Trichosanthis*), Huhuanglian (*Rhizoma Picrorhizae*), etc..

2. 用于胃阴不足，症见胃脘隐痛或灼痛，食欲减退，口干便秘，舌光少苔。可与竹茹、白芍药、芦根等同用；鲜品也用来治疗消渴证，多配天花粉、胡黄连等。

In addition, it has the action of improving visual acuity and strengthening the waist and knees, it is usually combined with Juhua (*Flos Chrysanthemi*), Gouqizi (*Fructus Lycii*) and others to treat vision decreasing; combined with Shudihuang (*Rhizoma Rehmanniae Praeparata*), Niuxi (*Radix Achyranthis Bidentatae*), etc., to treat weakness of waist and knees due to kidney-deficiency.

此外，本品还有一定的明目及强腰膝的作用，常配伍菊花、枸杞子等以治视力减退；配伍熟地黄、牛膝等以治肾虚腰膝软弱。

Usage and Dosage 6 -15 g is used in decoction for oral use, the fresh is 15 -30 g.

【用法用量】 水煎服，6～15克，鲜品 15～30 克。

Notes It is not suitable for early stage of seasonal febrile disease, and contraindicated for wet-warm or dampness-heat syndrome.

【使用注意】 温热病早期不宜用，湿温或湿热证忌用。

Gouqizi *Fructus Lycii*

枸杞子

The source is from the mature fruit of *Lycium barbarum* L., family Solanaceae. The medicinal material is mainly produced in the areas of Ningxia, Gansu, and Qinghai, etc.. After collected in summer and autumn, the fruits are exposed to the shade until the surface changes into rough, and then exposed to the sun until the peel becomes dry and hard and the sarcocarp soft. The raw can

为茄科植物宁夏枸杞的成熟果实。主产于宁夏、甘肃、青海等地。夏、秋季采摘后，先晾至皮皱，再曝晒至外皮干硬、果肉柔软。生用。

be used for medication.

Medicinal Properties Sweet in flavor, mild in nature and attributive to the liver, kidney and lung meridians.

【药性】味甘，性平。归肝、肾、肺经。

Actions Tonify the kidney and benefit essence, and nourish the liver and improve eyesight.

【功效】补肾益精，养肝明目。

Application

【临床应用】

1. For essence insufficiency of the liver and kidney manifested as sourness and weakness of waist and knees, and emission, it can be combined with Huangjing (*Rhizoma Polygonati*), Shudihuang (*Rhizoma Rehmanniae Praeparata*) and Shayuanzi (*Semen Astragali Complanati*).

1. 用于肝肾精亏，腰膝酸软，遗精。可与黄精、熟地黄、沙苑子同用。

2. For deficiency of liver-yin and kidney-yin manifested as dizziness and blurred vision, it is usually combined with Juhua (*Flos Chrysanthemi*), Shudihuang (*Rhizoma Rehmanniae Praeparata*), Shanzhuyu (*Fructus Corni*), and Shanyao (*Rhizoma Dioscoreae Hypogiaucae*), etc., such as Qi Ju Dihuang Wan (Bolus).

2. 用于肝肾阴虚、头晕目眩、视物模糊。常与菊花、熟地黄、山茱萸、山药等同用，如杞菊地黄丸。

3. For diabetes, it can be used alone, usually also combined with Shengdihuang (*Radix Rehmanniae*), Maimendong (*Radix Ophiopogonis*), and Tianhuafen (*Radix Trichosanthis*), etc..

3. 用于消渴。可单用本品，蒸熟嚼食，也常配生地黄、麦门冬、天花粉等同用。

In addition, it is also used for overstrain-cough due to asthenia of the lung.

此外，还可治肺阴虚劳嗽。

Usage and Dosage 6 -12 g is used in decoction for oral use.

【用法用量】 水煎服，6～12克。

Hanliancao *Herba Ecliptae*

旱莲草

The source is from the herb of *Eclipta prostrata* L., family Compositae. The medicinal material is mainly produced in all parts of China. The whole herb is pulled out in summer and autumn and cleaned. The fresh can be used or dried in the sun, and then cut into segments.

为菊科植物鳢肠的全草。主产于中国各地。夏、秋季拔取全草，洗净。鲜用，或晒干切段用。

Medicinal Properties Sweet and sour in flavor,

【药性】味甘、酸，性寒。

cold in nature and attributive to the liver and kidney meridians.

归肝、肾经。

Actions Nourish liver-yin and kidney-yin, cool the blood and arrest bleeding.

【功效】 补肝肾阴，凉血止血。

Application

【临床应用】

1. For deficiency of liver-yin and kidney-yin manifested as dizziness, premature whitening of hair, soreness and weakness of waist and knees, seminal emission and tinnitus, it is usually combined with Nüzhenzi (*Fructus Ligustri Lucidi*), such as Erzhi Wan (Pill).

1. 用于肝肾阴虚的头晕目眩，须发早白，腰膝酸软，遗精，耳鸣。常与女贞子相须配伍，如二至丸。

2. For yin deficiency and blood-heat manifested as hemoptysis, epistaxis, hemafecia, hematuria and metrorrhagia, it can be used alone or also usually combined with Shengdihuang (*Radix Rehmannia*), Ejiao (*Colla Corii Asini*), Puhuang (*Pollen Typhae*) and others that can moisten yin, cool the blood and arrest bleeding, so as to strengthen therapeutic effects. It is also used externally to treat bleeding due to wound.

2. 用于阴虚血热咯血，衄血，便血，尿血，崩漏。可单用，也常配生地黄、阿胶、蒲黄等滋阴凉血止血药，以增强疗效。外用可治创伤出血。

Usage and Dosage 10 –15 g is used in decoction for oral use, the fresh should be doubled in amount. Just right amount is used externally and pounded for application.

【用法用量】 水煎服，10～15克，鲜品用量加倍。外用，适量，捣敷。

Nüzhenzi *Fructus Ligustri Lucidi*

女贞子

The source is from the fruit of *Ligustrum lucidum* Ait., family Oleaceae. The herb is mainly produced in Shaanxi, Gansu and the south areas to the Yangtze River. The medicinal material is collected in winter when it is ripe, slightly steamed or scalded in boiling water, and then dried in the sun. It can be used crudely or prepared with wine for medication.

为木犀科植物女贞的成熟果实。主产于陕西、甘肃及长江以南地区。冬季果实成熟时采收，稍蒸或置沸水中略烫后，晒干。生用或酒制用。

Medicinal Properties Sweet and bitter in flavor, cool in nature and attributive to the liver and kidney meridians.

【药性】 味甘、苦，性凉。归肝、肾经。

Actions Moisten yin and clear away heat, and

【功效】 滋阴清热，乌须

blacken the hair and promote the eyesight.

明目。

Application

【临床应用】

1. For deficiency of liver-yin and kidney-yin manifested as blurred vision, eyesight being falling, whitening of hair, soreness of waist and tinnitus, it is usually combined with Hanliancao (*Herba Ecliptae*), or again with Shudihuang (*Rhizoma Rehmanniae Praeparata*), Tusizi (*Semen Cuscutae*), and Gouqizi (*Fructus Lycii*), etc.. For whitening of hair, it is usually combined with Heshouwu (*Radix Polygoni Multiflori*) and Gouqizi (*Fructus Lycii*).

1. 用于肝肾阴虚的目暗不明，视力减退，须发早白，腰酸耳鸣。常与旱莲草同用，或再配熟地黄、菟丝子、枸杞子等。治须发早白，多配何首乌、枸杞子。

2. It is also used for fever due to yin-deficiency, hectic fever and vexation. Its action of tonifying yin is not so effective as that of Hanliancao (*Herba Ecliptae*), but it has action of clearing away heat, so it can be often used in combination with Digupi (*Cortex Lycii*), Shengdihuang (*Radix Rehmanniae*), and Baiwei (*Radix Cynanchi Atrati*), etc..

2. 用于阴虚发热，潮热心烦。本品滋阴作用不及旱莲草，但有清虚热作用，常配地骨皮、生地黄、白薇等同用。

Usage and Dosage 10 - 15 g is used in decoction for oral use.

【用法用量】 水煎服，10～15克。

Guiban *Carapax et Plastrum Testudinis*

龟 版

The source is from the plastron of *Chinemys reevesii*, family Testudinidae. The medicinal material is mainly produced in the areas of Zhejiang, Hubei, Hunan, and Anhui, etc.. The animal can be caught all year round and after it is killed, the tendon and meat are removed, the plastron is remained and the plastron is cleaned and dried in the sun, which is called Xueban; after it is boiled in boiling water to death, the plastron is fetched out and dried in the sun, which is called Tangban. the crude one or the one roasted with vinegar can be used for medication after it is stir-baked with sand.

为龟科动物乌龟的背甲、腹甲。主产于浙江、湖北、湖南、安徽等地。全年均可捕捉，杀死，剔去筋肉，取其腹甲，洗净晒干者，称为“血版”；沸水煮死后取其腹甲，晒干者，称为“烫版”。生用，或沙炒后醋炙用。

Medicinal Properties Sweet and salty in flavor, cold in nature and attributive to the liver, kidney and heart meridians.

【药性】 味甘、咸，性寒。归肝、肾、心经。

Actions Nourish yin and suppress the hyperactive yang, benefit the kidney and strengthen the bone, enrich the blood and nourishing the heart, regulate menstruation and relieve bleeding.

【功效】 滋阴潜阳，益肾健骨，养血补心，固经止血。

Application

【临床应用】

1. It is used for deficiency of yin causing hyperactivity of yang with dizziness or yin-deficiency resulting in wind stirring manifested as convulsion of hands and feet. For the former, it is usually combined with Baishaoyao (*Radix Paeoniae Alba*), Niuxi (*Radix Achyranthis Bidentatae*), Longgu (*Os Draconis*), and Daizheshi (*Haematitum*), such as Zhengan Xifeng Tang (Decoction); for the latter, with Shengdihuang (*Radix Rehmannia*), Maimendong (*Radix Ophiopogonis*), Biejia (*Carapax Trionycis*), and Ejiao (*Colla Corii Asini*), etc., such as Da Dingfeng Zhu (Bolus).

1. 用于阴虚阳亢之头晕目眩或阴虚风动之手足抽搐。前者常配白芍药、牛膝、龙骨、代赭石等，如镇肝熄风汤；后者常配生地黄、麦门冬、鳖甲、阿胶等，如大定风珠。

2. For yin-deficiency with fire hyperactivity manifested as hectic fever, night sweat and nocturnal emission, it is usually combined with Shudihuang (*Rhizoma Rehmanniae Praeparata*), Zhimu (*Rhizoma Anemarrhenae*), and Huangbai (*Cortex Phellodendri*), etc., such as Da Buyin Wan (Pill).

2. 用于阴虚火旺，骨蒸潮热，盗汗遗精。常与熟地黄、知母、黄柏等配伍，如大补阴丸。

3. For insufficiency of the liver and kidney manifested as weakness of the tendons and bones, flaccidity of the neck and delayed closure of fontanel in infants, it is combined with Shudihuang (*Rhizoma Rehmanniae Praeparata*), Baishaoyao (*Radix Paeoniae Alba*), etc.

3. 用于肝肾不足，筋骨不健，颈项痿软及小儿囟门不合。配熟地黄、白芍药等同用。

4. For deficiency of the heart manifested as palpitation, insomnia and amnesia, it can be combined with Longgu (*Os Draconis*), Yuanzhi (*Radix Polygalae*), and Shichangpu (*Rhizoma Acori Graminei*), etc., such as Kongsheng Zhenzhong Dan (Bolus).

4. 用于心虚惊悸，失眠健忘。可与龙骨、远志、石菖蒲等同用，如孔圣枕中丹。

5. For yin-deficiency and blood-heat manifested as metrorrhagia and metrostaxis or menorrhagia, it is usually

5. 用于阴虚血热所致的崩漏或月经过多。常与白芍

combined with Baishaoyao (*Radix Paeoniae Alba*), Huangbai (*Cortex Phellodendri*), and Xiangfu (*Rhizoma Cyperi*), etc., such as Gujing Wan (Pill).

药、黄柏、香附等同用，如固经丸。

Usage and Dosage 10 - 30 g is used in decoction for oral use, which is broken and decocted first.

【用法用量】 水煎服，10～30克。打碎先煎。

Notes It is not suitable for deficiency of spleen-yang and stomach-yang.

【使用注意】 脾胃阳虚者不宜用。

Biejia *Carapax Trionycis*

鳖　甲

The source is from the shell of *Trionyx sinensis* Wiegmann, family Trionychidae. The medicinal material is mainly produced in the areas of Hebei, Hunan, and Anhui, etc.. The animal can be caught all year round. After it is caught and its head is removed, it is boiled in boiling water for one to two hours and then the shell is fetched out, the remaining meat in the shell being got rid of, and dried in the sun. The crude one or the one prepared with vinegar after stir-baked with sand can be used for medication.

为鳖科动物中华鳖或山瑞鳖的背甲。主产于河北、湖南、安徽等地。全年可捕捉，捕捉后去头，置沸水中煮1～2小时，取出背甲，去净残肉，晒干。生用或沙炒后醋淬用。

Medicinal Properties Salty in flavor, cold in nature and attributive to the liver and kidney meridians.

【药性】 味咸，性寒。归肝、肾经。

Actions Nourish yin and suppress the hyperactive yang, soften and disperse the lumps.

【功效】 滋阴潜阳，软坚散结。

Application

【临床应用】

1. It is used for febrile disease with consumption of yin, hyperactivity of liver-yang and deficiency-wind stirring inside. For deficiency of yin leading to hyperactivity of yang manifested as dizziness, it is combined with Shengdihuang (*Radix Rehmanniae*), Muli (*Concha Ostreae*) and Juhua (*Flos Chrysanthemi*); for the late stage of febrile disease and wind stirring inside due to yin-deficiency manifested as wriggling hands and feet, dry and dark red tongue, can be combined with Muli (*Concha Ostreae*), Ejiao (*Colla Corii Asini*), and Baishaoyao (*Radix Paeoniae Alba*), etc., such as Sanjia Fumai Tang

1. 用于热病伤阴，肝阳上亢，虚风内动。治阴虚阳亢，头晕目眩，配生地黄、牡蛎、菊花同用；治热病后期，阴虚风动、手足蠕动、舌干红绛等，可配与牡蛎、阿胶、白芍药等同用，如三甲复脉汤。

(Decoction).

2. For yin-deficiency with fever, hectic fever and night sweating, it is usually combined with Qinjiao (*Radix Gentianae Macrophyllae*), Digupi (*Cortex Lycii*), and Zhimu (*Rhizoma Anemarrhenae*), etc., such as Qinjiao Biejia San (Powder); for the late stage of febrile disease with consumption of yin fluid manifested as night fever that brings down in the morning, emaciation, rapid pulse, red tongue with little coating, also, usually combined with Qinghao (*Herba Artemisiae Annuae*), Mudanpi (*Cortex Moutan Radicis*), and Shengdihuang (*Radix Rehmanniae*), etc., such as Qinghao Biejia Tang (Decoction).

2. 用于阴虚发热，骨蒸盗汗。常与秦艽、地骨皮、知母等同用，如秦艽鳖甲散；若热病后期，阴液耗伤，症见夜热早凉、形瘦脉数、舌红少苔者，又常与青蒿、牡丹皮、生地黄等配伍，如青蒿鳖甲汤。

3. For abdominal mass and amenorrhea due to blood stasis, it is usually combined with Xiangfu (*Rhizoma Cyperi*), Qingpi (*Pericarpium Citri Reticulatae Viride*), Sanleng (*Rhizoma Sparganii*), and Ezhu (*Rhizoma Zedoariae*), etc., such as Biejiajian Wan (Pill).

3. 用于胁下癥块，腹中瘀块及血瘀经闭。常与香附、青皮、三棱、莪术等同用，如鳖甲煎丸。

Usage and Dosage 10 -30 g is used in decoction for oral use, broken and decocted first. The raw is suitable for nourishing yin and suppressing the hyperactive yang and the one roasted with vinegar for softening and dispersing the lumps.

【用法用量】 水煎服，10～30克，须打碎先煎。滋阴潜阳宜生用，软坚散结宜醋炙用。

15 Astringent Chinese Medicinal Herbs

第十五章 收敛固涩药

Chinese medicinal herbs with the main actions of inducing astringency and arresting discharge are called astringents.

This kind of Chinese medicinal herbs are mostly sour and astringent in flavor, respectively having the actions of stopping the excessive perspiration, relieving diarrhea, and nocturnal emission, reducing urination, stopping leucorrhea, bleeding, and cough, etc.. Therefore, they are indicated for abnormal leakage of body substances due to weakness and unconsolidation of healthy essence manifested as spontaneous sweating, night sweating, chronic diarrhea and dysentery, spermatorrhea, seminal emission, frequent micturition, chronic recurring cough and dyspnea, leucorrhea and others.

The purpose of using astringents is to induce astringency to prevent decline of anti-pathogenic factors and appearance of complications caused by involuntary discharge. But the principal cause of abnormal discharging of body substances is due to the deficiency of healthy qi, so astringents should be used in combination with appropriate tonics to treat both the principal and secondary aspects of diseases. For example, in treating spontaneous sweating due to deficiency of qi, or night sweating due to deficiency of yin, they should be used respectively in combination with qi invigorating tonics and yin nourishing tonics; in treating chronic diarrhea, dysentery and leucorrhea due to asthenia of the spleen and kidney, they should be used in combination with the spleen and kidney benefiting tonics;

凡以收敛固涩为主要作用的药物，称为收敛固涩药。又称固涩药、收涩药。

本类药物大多性味酸涩，分别具有敛汗、止泻、固精、缩尿、止带、止血、止嗽等作用，适用于体虚精气耗散所致的自汗、盗汗、久泻、久痢、遗精、滑精、遗尿、尿频，以及久咳虚喘、崩漏、带下不止等滑脱不禁证。

运用收敛固涩药，目的在于防止因滑脱不禁而导致正气衰竭，变生他证。但是滑脱证的根本原因是正气虚弱，治疗时必须与补益药配合应用，才能标本兼顾。如气虚自汗、阴虚盗汗，当分别与补气药、养阴药同用；脾肾虚弱所致的久泻、久痢及带下日久不愈，应与补益脾肾药同用；肾虚遗精、滑精、遗尿、尿频，当配伍补肾药；冲任不固、崩漏下血，当配伍固摄冲任药；肺肾虚损、久咳虚喘，应与补肺肾纳

in treating spermatorrhea, seminal emission, enuresis, frequent urination due to kidney deficiency, they should be used in combination with kidney tonifying medicinal herbs; in treating unconsolidation of thoroughfare and conception vessels, metrorrhagia, they should be used in combination with Chinese medicinal herbs that consolidate thoroughfare and conception vessels; in treating lung and kidney diseases due to asthenia of viscera, chronic cough with dyspnea resulting from asthenia, they should be used in combination with medicinal herbs that improve inspiration by invigorating lung and kidney qi.

气药同用。

Astringents have a "closing" effect on the body to prevent further discharge from the body, therefore, they are not suitable in the case with exogenous pathogenic factors that are not removed or interior stagnation of any dampness and domination of sthenia pathogenic factors.

收涩药有恋邪之弊，所以表邪未解、内有湿滞，以及实邪盛者，均不宜用。

Mahuanggen *Radix Ephedrae*

麻黄根

The source is from the root of *Ephedra sinica* stapf., *E. Intermedia* Schrenk et C. A. Mey., and *E. Equisetina* Bunge, family Ephedraceae. The medicinal material is collected in autumn, the fibrous roots being removed, then cut into thick slices and dried in the sun. The raw is used.

为麻黄科植物草麻黄、木贼麻黄或中麻黄的根。秋天采挖。剪去须根，切段，晒干。生用。

Medicinal Properties Sweet in flavor, mild in nature and attributive to the lung meridian.

【药性】 味甘，性平。归肺经。

Actions Arrest sweating.

【功效】 止汗。

Application

【临床应用】

The medicinal herb is indicated for spontaneous perspiration and night sweat. For spontaneous perspiration, it can be used in combination with Danggui (*Radix Angelicae Sinensis*) and Huangqi (*Radix Astragali*), such as Mahuanggen San (Powder) and also with Muli (*Concha Ostreae*) prepared as powder for external use, for night sweat due to yin deficiency, it is usually used together

用于自汗、盗汗。治自汗不止，可配伍当归、黄芪，如麻黄根散；也可以配伍牡蛎，研细末外扑；治阴虚盗汗，常与熟地黄、山茱萸、龙骨、牡蛎等同用。

with Shudihuang (*Radix Rehmanniae Praeparata*), Shanzhuyu (*Fructus Corni*), Longgu (*Os Draconis*) and Muli (*Concha Ostreae*), etc..

Usage and Dosage　3 -10 g is used in decoction for oral use. For external use, the amount should be appropriate.

【用法用量】　水煎服，3～10克。外用，适量。

Notes　It is contraindicated in those affected by exogenous pathogenic factors.

【使用注意】　有表邪者忌用。

Fuxiaomai　*Fructus Tritici Levis*

浮小麦

The source is from the blighted caryopsis of *Triticum aestivum* L., family Gramineae. The medicinal material is produced all over China. The wheat is washed, the floated one is picked out, and then dried in the sun. The raw or stir-baked one is used for medication.

为禾本科植物小麦未成熟的颖果。中国各地均产。以水淘小麦，取浮起者，晒干。生用或炒用。

Medicinal Properties　Sweet in flavor, cool in nature, and attributive to the heart meridian.

【药性】　味甘，性凉。归心经。

Actions　Replenish qi, clear away heat and arrest sweating.

【功效】　益气，除热，止汗。

Application

【临床应用】

1. It is used for spontaneous perspiration and night sweat. It can be used alone to treat night sweat and persistent deficient sweating. For persistent spontaneous perspiration due to weakness of the body, it is usually used together with Muli (*Concha Ostreae*), Mahuanggen (*Radix Ephedrae*) and Huangqi (*Radix Astragali*) to compose a formula, that is, Muli San (Powder).

1. 用于自汗、盗汗。治盗汗及虚汗不止，可单用本品；治体虚自汗不止，常与牡蛎、麻黄根、黄芪同用，即牡蛎散。

2. In treating hectic fever and overstrain-fever, it is often used together with the medicinal herbs that nourish yin and clear asthenia-heat such as Shengdihuang (*Radix Rehmanniae*, unprepared), Maimendong (*Radix Ophiopogonis*), and Digupi (*Cortex Lycii*).

2. 用于骨蒸劳热。多与生地黄、麦门冬、地骨皮等养阴清虚热药同用。

Usage and Dosage　15 -30 g is used in decoction, or stir-fried until burnt and then ground into powder for oral use.

【用法用量】　水煎服，15～30克。或炒焦研末服。

Wuweizi *Fructus Schisandrae*

The source is from the ripe fruit of *Schisandra chinensis* (Tuecz.) Bail. And *S. Sphenanthera* Rehd. Et Wils., family Magnoliaceae. The former is called Beiwuweizi, mainly produced in the Northeast, Hebei and Shanxi provinces of China. The latter is called Nanwuweizi, mainly produced in the Southwest China and the south areas to the Yangtze River. The medicinal material is collected in autumn when the fruits are ripe and dried in the sun. The raw form can be used, or used after the fruit steamed with vinegar and honey and dried in the sun for medication.

Medicinal Properties Sour in flavor, warm in nature, and attributive to the lung, heart and kidney meridians.

Actions Astringe the lung to treat cough and asthma and nourish the kidney, promote the production of body fluid and constrain perspiration, astringe the essence and stop diarrhea, nourish the heart and calm the mind.

Application

1. It is used for chronic cough and dyspnea resulting from asthenia. In treating chronic cough due to deficiency of the lung, it is used in combination with Wumei (*Fructus Mume*) and Yingsuke (*Pericarpium Papaveris*), such as Wuweizi Wan (Pill). For syndrome of kidney deficiency manifested as dyspnea and shortness of breath, it can be used in Liuwei Dihuang Wan (Pill). It can also be used in Duqi Wan (Pill) which can invigorate the kidney for improving inspiration and astringe the lung to treat cough and asthma. In treating cough and dyspnea caused by lung cold, it should be used together with pungent-warm Chinese medicinal herbs such as Xixin (*Herba Asari*) and Ganjiang (*Rhizoma Zingiberis*) functioning in dispersing, such as in Xiao Qinglong Tang (Decoction).

五味子

为木兰科植物五味子和华中五味子的成熟果实。前者称北五味子,主产于东北、河北、山西等地;后者称南五味子,主产于西南及长江以南地区。秋季果实成熟时采收,晒干。生用或经醋、蜜拌蒸,晒干用。

【药性】 味酸,性温。归肺、肾、心经。

【功效】 敛肺滋肾,生津敛汗,涩精止泻,宁心安神。

【临床应用】

1. 用于久咳,虚喘。治肺虚久咳,配乌梅、罂粟壳同用,如五味子丸;肾虚喘促短气,可用之配六味地黄丸,补肾敛肺纳气,如都气丸。治肺寒咳喘,则需配辛温宣散之细辛、干姜,如小青龙汤。

2. It is used for thirst due to consumption of the body fluids, spontaneous perspiration and night sweat. In treating damage of qi and yin due to excessive heat manifested as palpitation, feeble pulse, thirst and hyperhidrosis, it is often used in combination with Renshen (*Radix Ginseng*) and Maimendong (*Radix Ophiopogonis*), such as in Shengmai San (Powder), it can also be used together with Huangqi (*Radix Astragali*), Shengdihuang (*Radix Rehmanniae*), Maimendong (*Radix Ophiopogonis*), and Tianhuafen (*Radix Trichosanthis*), etc. for diabetes with frequent drink and polyuria, such as Huangqi Tang (Decoction). In treating incessant sweating due to deficienfy, it is often used in combination with Baiziren (*Semen Biotae*), Renshen (*Radix Ginseng*), Mahuanggen (*Radix Ephedrae*), and Muli (*Concha Ostreae*), etc., such as Baiziren Wan (Pill).

2. 用于津伤口渴,自汗盗汗。治热盛气阴两伤,心悸、脉虚、口渴多汗,多与人参、麦门冬相配,如生脉散;消渴病多饮、多尿,可与黄芪、生地黄、麦门冬、天花粉等同用,如黄芪汤;治虚汗不止,常与柏子仁、人参、麻黄根、牡蛎等同用,如柏子仁丸。

3. The medicinal herb is indicated for emission, spermatorrhea and chronic diarrhea. It can be used alone to treat emission and spermatorrhea due to kidney-deficency, or combined with Sangpiaoxiao (*Ootheca Mantidis*) and Longgu (*Os Draconis*). In treating deficiency and cold of the spleen and kidney with diarrhea at dawn, it is often used together with Buguzhi (*Fructus Psoraleae*), Wuzhuyu (*Fructus Evodiae*), Roudoukou (*Semen Myristicae*), such as Sishen Wan (Pill).

3. 用于遗精,滑精,久泻不止。治肾虚遗精、滑精,单用本品即效,亦可以配伍桑螵蛸、龙骨等;治脾肾虚寒,黎明泄泻,常配补骨脂、吴茱萸、肉豆蔻等,如四神丸。

4. For insufficiency of heart-blood and kidney-yin manifested as vexation, palpitation, insomnia and frequent dreaminess, it can be used in combination with Shengdihuang (*Radix Rehmanniae*), Maimendong (*Radix Ophiopogonis*), Danshen (*Radix Salviae Miltiorrhizae*), Suanzaoren (*Semen Ziziphi Spinosae*), such as Tianwang Buxin Dan (Bolus).

4. 用于心血虚、肾阴亏损所致的虚烦心悸,失眠多梦。可配伍生地黄、麦门冬、丹参、酸枣仁等,如天王补心丹。

In addition, its powder preparation is used for chronic hepatitis with elevation of serum transaminase.

此外,本品研末内服,还可用于慢性肝炎转氨酶升高者。

Usage and Dosage 2 -6 g is used in decoction for oral use or 1 -3 g of its powder is taken orally.

【用法用量】 水煎服，2～6克。或研末服，1～3 克。

Note It is contraindicated in those with exopathogenic factors which have not been eliminated, sthenic heat in the interior, cough and measles at the initial stage.

【使用注意】 表邪未解，内有实热，咳嗽初起，麻疹初起患者均不宜用。

Wumei *Fructus Mume*

乌 梅

The source is from smoked unripe fruit of Prunus mume (*Sieb*) Sieb. Et Zucc., family Rosaceae. The medicinal material is mainly produced in Zhejiang, Fujian, and Yunnan provinces. The medicinal material is collected in the early summer, baked at a low temperature until the pulp is yellowish-brown with the peel wrinkled, and then braised until it turns black. The crude or carbonized is used for medication after the pit is removed.

为蔷薇科植物梅未成熟果实的加工熏制品。主产于浙江、福建、云南等地，初夏采收，低温焙至果肉呈黄褐色，呈皱皮，再焖至黑色。去核生用或炒炭用。

Medicinal Properties Sour in flavor, mild in nature and attributive to the liver, lung and large intestine meridians.

【药性】 味酸，性平。归肝、脾、肺、大肠经。

Actions Astringe the lung to relieve cough, astringe the intestine to arrest diarrhea, promote production of the body fluids to quench thirst, relieve ascaris colic and alleviate pain.

【功效】 敛肺止咳，涩肠止泻，生津止渴，安蛔止痛。

Application

【临床应用】

1. In treating prolonged cough with little sputum due to deficiency of the lung, or dry cough without sputum, it is often used together with Xingren (*Semen Armeniacae Amarum*), Banxia (*Rhizoma Pinelliae*), and Ejiao (*Collo Corii Asini*), etc., to strengthen the effect of astringing the lung to relieve cough.

1. 用于肺虚久咳少痰，或干咳无痰。常与杏仁、半夏、阿胶等配伍，加强敛肺止咳之效。

2. In treating prolonged diarrhea or dysentery, it can be used in combination with Roudoukou (*Semen Myristicae*), Hezi (*Fructus Chebulae*), such as in Guchang Wan (Pill).

2. 用于久泻久痢。可配肉豆蔻、诃子等同用，如固肠丸。

3. Its single form is effective in treating diabetes due to heat of deficiency type, or used together with

3. 用于虚热消渴。单用煎服有效，或与天花粉、麦门

Tianhuafen (*Radix Trichosanthis*), Maimendong (*Radix Ophiopogonis*), Gegen (*Radix Puerariae*), and Renshen (*Radix Ginseng*), such as Yuquang Wan (Pill).

冬、葛根、人参等同用,如玉泉丸。

4. In treating abdominal pain and vomiting caused by intestinal ascariasis, it is often used in combination with Xixin (*Herba Asari*), Ganjiang (*Rhizoma Zingiberis*), and Huanglian (*Rhizoma Coptidis*), etc., such as Wumei Wan (Pill).

4. 用于蛔虫引起的腹痛,呕吐。常配细辛、干姜、黄连等,如乌梅丸。

In addition, it has the action of arresting bleeding, such as hemafecia, hematuria, metrorrhagia and metrostaxis. Dermatopathy and hemorrhoids can be treated by the application.

此外,本品还有止血作用,可治便血、尿血、崩漏下血等;外敷能消疮毒,并治痔疮。

Usage and Dosage It is usually decocted for oral use. The usual dosage is 6 -12 g and large dosage may be up to 30 g. Proper amount can be used in external treatment. To arrest bleeding and diarrhea, the carbonized is used, and to promote production of the body fluids and relieve the ascaris colic, the crude is used.

【用法用量】 水煎服,6～12克,大剂量可用至30克。外用,适量。止血、止泻宜炒炭用,生津、安蛔宜生用。

Notes In oral use, it is contraindicated in those with exogenous factors or those with stagnation of sthenic heat.

【使用注意】 有表邪或内有实热积滞者均不宜内服。

Roudoukou *Semen Myristicae*

肉豆蔻

The source is from the ripe seed of the arbor *Myristica fragrans* Houtt., family Myristicacene. The medicinal material is mainly produced in Malaysia and Indonesia. In China it is cultivated in Guangdong and other places. The ripe fruit is collected in winter and spring. The shell being removed, the seeds are dried, and then roasted to get rid of the oil for medication.

为肉豆蔻科植物肉豆蔻树的成熟种仁。主产马来西亚、印度尼西亚。中国广东等地有栽培。冬、春季采收成熟果实,除去皮壳后干燥。煨制去油用。

Medicinal Properties Pungent in flavor, warm in nature and attributive to the spleen, stomach and large intestine meridians.

【药性】 味辛,性温。归脾、胃、大肠经。

Actions Astringe the intestine to arrest diarrhea and warm the middle energizer to promote flow of qi.

【功效】 涩肠止泻,温中行气。

Application

1. It is indicated for chronic diarrhea. For that due to asthenia and cold of the spleen and stomach, it can be used in combination with Dangshen (*Radix Codonopsis*), Baizhu (*Rhizoma Atractylodis Macrocephalae*), Rougui (*Cortex Cinnamomi*), etc., such as Yangzang Tang (Decoction); for that with diarrhea at dawn due to yang-deficiency of the spleen and kidney, it can be used in combination with Buguzhi (*Fructus Psoraleae*), Wuzhuyu (*Fructus Evodiae*) and Wuweizi (*Fructus Schisandrae*), such as Sishen Wan (Pill).

2. In treating stomach-cold with stagnation of qi manifested as abdominal pain, poor appetite and vomiting, it is often used in combination with Muxiang (*Radix Aucklandiae*), Ganjiang (*Rhizoma Zingiberis*) and Banxia (*Rhizoma Pinelliae*), etc..

Usage and Dosage 3 -10 g is used in decoction and 1.5 -3 g is used in pill or powder.

Notes It is contraindicated in those with dysentery due to damp and heat.

【临床应用】

1. 用于久泻不止。脾胃虚寒者，与党参、白术、肉桂等同用，如养脏汤；若脾肾阳虚，黎明泄泻，可与补骨脂、吴茱萸、五味子等同用，如四神丸。

2. 用于胃寒气滞，脘腹胀痛，食少呕吐。常与木香、干姜、半夏同用。

【用法用量】 水煎服，3～10 克。入丸、散，1.5～3 克。

【使用注意】 湿热泻痢者忌用。

Chishizhi *Halloysitum Rubrum*

The source is from a mineral of silicate salt of polyhydrate kaolinate group, containing mainly hydrated Aluminum silicate. The medicinal material is mainly produced in Fujian, Shandong, and Henan provinces, and collected all year around. The impurity being removed from it, it is ground into powder with water or calcined and then ground into powder with water for medication.

Medicinal Properties Sweet, sour and astringent in flavor, warm in nature and attributive to the large intestine and stomach meridians.

Actions Astringe the intestine to arrest diarrhea and bleeding, and promote tissue regeneration and healing

赤石脂

为硅酸盐类矿物多水高岭石族多水高岭石。主要成分为含水硅酸铝。主产于福建、山东、河南等地。全年均可采挖，去杂质。研粉水飞或火煅水飞用。

【药性】 味甘、酸、涩，性温。归大肠、胃经。

【功效】 涩肠止泻，收敛止血，敛疮生肌。

of wounds.

Application

1. It can be applied for hypofunction of the lower energizer manifested as uncontrollable diarrhea, hemafecia, prolapse of the rectum. In treating prolonged and uncontrollable lingering diarrhea, it is usually used together with Yuyuliang (*Limonitum*), such as Chishizhi Yuyuliang Tang (Decoction); in treating dysentery caused by cold and deficiency, endless pus and blood in the stool, it is often combined with Ganjiang (*Rhizoma Zingiberis*), Jingmi (*Semen Oryzae Sativae*), such as Taohua Tang (Decoction).

2. For metrostaxis that lingers for a long time, it can be used in combination with Cebaiye (*Cacumen Biotae*) and Wuzeigu (*Os Sepiellae seu Sepiae*), which are calcined and ground into powder for oral administration, such as Chishizhi San (Powder). It can also be used to treat leukorrhagia with bloody discharge together with Baishaoyao (*Radix Paeoniae Alba*) and Ganjiang (*Rhizoma Zingiberis*) in decoction for oral use.

3. For unhealed chronic ulcer with rupture, it can be used together with Longgu (*Os Praconis*), Luganshi (*Calamina*), Xuejie (*Resina Draconis*), and Ruxiang (*Olibanum*), etc., which are ground into powder for applying on the ulcer.

In addition, it can also be applied externally for skin pyogenic infection and traumatic bleeding because of its action of eliminating dampness and arresting bleeding.

Usage and Dosage 10 -20 g is used in decoction, pill or powder, and just right amount for external use.

Notes It is contraindicated in those with stagnantion of dampness and heat and should be used with great caution in pregnant women. It is incompatible with Rougui

【临床应用】

1. 用于下焦不固,泻痢不止,便血脱肛。治泻痢日久,滑泄不禁,多与禹余粮相须同用,如赤石脂禹余粮汤;治虚寒下痢,便脓血不止,配干姜、粳米同用,如桃花汤。

2. 用于妇人漏下,日久不愈。以本品配侧柏叶、乌贼骨,煅为末服,如赤石脂散;治赤白带下,还可配白芍药、干姜水煎服。

3. 用于溃疡久溃不敛。可与龙骨、炉甘石、血竭、乳香等,共研细末,掺于疮口。

此外,外用也可治湿疮流水、外伤出血,可以收湿,止血。

【用法用量】 水煎服,10～20克,或入丸、散服。外用,适量。

【使用注意】 有湿热积滞者忌服。孕妇慎用。畏肉桂。

(*Cortex Cinnamomi*).

Shanzhuyu *Fructus Corni*

The source is from the ripe sarcocarp of the deciduous arbor *Cornus officinalis* Sieb. et Zucc., family Cornaceae. The medicinal material is mainly produced in Zhejiang, Anhui, and Henan provinces. The fruit is collected in autumn when it is ripe, baked over a soft fire or treated with boiling water for a moment, the kern being removed, and then dried in the sun or baked for medicinal use.

Medicinal Properties Sour in flavor, slightly warm in nature, and attributive to the liver and kidney meridians.

Actions Invigorate the liver and kidney, astringe and preserve the essence.

Application

1. It can be used for deficiency of the liver and kidney manifested as dizziness, soreness of the waist and knees, impotence, emission, spermatorrhoea, enuresis. For those with deficiency of the liver-yin and kidney-yin, it is often used together with Shudihuang (*Radix Rehmanniae Praeparata*), Shanyao (*Rhizoma Dioscoreae*), and Zexie (*Rhizoma Alismatis*), etc., such as Liuwei Dihuang Wan (Pill). For those with insufficiency of kidney-yang, it is often used in combination with Buguzhi (*Fructus Psoraleae*), Danggui (*Radix Angelicae Sinensis*), and Shexiang (*Moschus Artifactus*), etc., such as Caohuan Dan (Bolus). It is often combined with Sangpiaoxiao (*Ootheca Mantidis*), Yizhiren (*Fructus Alpiniae Oxphyllae*), Shayuanzi (*Semen Astragali Complanati*) to treat incontinence.

2. It is used for excessive sweat due to deficiency. In treating debility after illness, hypofunction of connective tissue, profuse perspiration, it can be used together with

山茱萸

为山茱萸科植物山茱萸的成熟果肉。主产于浙江、安徽、河南等地。秋季果实成熟时采摘，烘或沸水中略烫后，挤除果核，晒干或烘干备用。

【药性】 味酸，性微温。归肝、肾经。

【功效】 补益肝肾，收敛固涩。

【临床应用】

1. 用于肝肾虚损，头晕目眩，腰膝酸软，阳痿，遗精，滑精，小便不禁。属肝肾阴虚者，多配伍熟地黄、山药、泽泻等，如六味地黄丸；属肾阳不足者，多配补骨脂、当归、麝香等同用，如草还丹。治小便不禁，还常配桑螵蛸、益智仁、沙苑子等同用。

2. 用于虚汗不止。病后体虚，腠理不固，遍身汗出，可与人参、黄芪、白芍药等同用；

Renshen (*Radix Ginseng*), Huangqi (*Radix Astragali*), and Baishaoyao (*Radix Paeoniae Alba*), etc.; for profuse cold sweat and collapse due to weakness of the body, its large dosage together with Renshen (*Radix Ginseng*) should be decocted for oral use immediately, or Fuzi (*Radix Aconiti Lateralis Praeparata*), Longgu (*Os Draconis*), and Muli (*Concha Ostreae*) are added again to those to astringe and preserve the essence.

若冷汗不止,体虚欲脱,可急用大剂量本品与人参煎服,或再加附子、龙骨、牡蛎等,以收敛固脱。

In addition, it can be used to arrest bleeding due to its astringing property. For metrorrhagia and metrostaxis and menorrhagia, it is often used together with Haipiaoxiao (*Os Sepiellae seu Sepiae*), Qiancaotan (*Radix Rubiae*, Carbonized), such as Guchong Tang (Decoction).

此外,本品收敛之性还可用于止血。治妇女崩漏及月经过多,常配海螵蛸、茜草炭等,如固冲汤。

Usage and Dosage 5 -10 g is used in decoction for oral use, the large dosage may be up to 30 g, and 1 -3 g is used in pill or powder.

【用法用量】 水煎服,5~10克,大剂量可用至30克。入丸散,1~3克。

Notes It should be used with caution in those with excessive fire from the gate of life (due to deficiency of kidney-yin), or damp-heat or dysuria.

【使用注意】 命门火炽,素有湿热及小便不利者慎用。

Lianzi *Semen Nelumbinis*

莲 子

The source is from the ripe seed of the *Nelumbo nucifera* Gaertn, family Nymphaeaceae. The medicinal material is mainly produced in Hunan, Fujian, Jiangsu, and Zhejiang provinces. It is collected in August and September, the seeds being taken out from the seed pod and the pericarp being removed, and then dried in the sun. The crude is broken into pieces for medicinal use.

为睡莲科植物莲的成熟种仁。主产于湖南、福建、江苏、浙江等地,8~9月采收成熟莲房,取出果实,除去果皮,晒干。打碎生用。

Medicinal Properties Sweet and astringent in flavor, mild in nature, and attributive to the spleen, kidney and heart meridians.

【药性】 味甘、涩,性平。归脾、肾、心经。

Actions Benefit the kidney to preserve the essence, invigorate the spleen and relieve diarrhea, nourish the heart and tranquilize the mind.

【功效】 益肾固精,补脾止泻,养心安神。

Application

1. For poor nocturnal emission and spermatorrhea due to kidney-deficiency, it is often used in combination with Shayuanzi (*Semen Astragali Complanati*), Longgu (*Os Draconis*), Muli (*Concha Osteae*), and Lianxu (*Stamen Nelumbinis*), etc., such as Jinsuo Gujing Wan (Pill).

2. For poor appetite and chronic diarrhea due to deficiency of the spleen, it is usually used together with Renshen (*Radix Ginseng*), Baizhu (*Rhizoma Atractylodis Macrocephalae*), Fuling (*Poria*), Shanyao (*Rhizma Dioscoreae*), etc., such as Shen Ling Baizhu San (Powder).

3. For asthenia-dysphoria, palpitation and insomnia, it can be used in combination with Suanzaoren (*Semen Ziziphi Spinosae*), Maimendong (*Radix Ophiopogonis*), and Yuanzhi (*Radix Polygalae*), etc..

In addition, it can also be used to treat metrorrhagia and metrostaxis and excessive leukorrhea, etc..

Usage and Dosage 6 -15 g is used in decoction for oral use.

Notes Lianxu (*Stamen Nelumbinis*) is also a medicinal part. It is sweet and astringent in flavor, mild in nature and it has the actions of strengthening the kidney to stop seminal emission. It is indicated for seminal emission, spermatorrhea, leukorrhea, and frequent micturition, etc..

Jinyingzi *Fructus Rosae Laevigatae*

The source is from the ripe fruit of *Rosa laevigata* Michx, family Rosaceae. The medicinal material is mainly produced in Guangdong, Sichuan, Yunnan, and Guizhou provinces and collected in September, October and November when the fruit is ripe. After the kernel is removed from the fruit, it is dried in the sun. The crude one is

【临床应用】

1. 用于肾虚遗精，滑精。常配沙苑子、龙骨、牡蛎、莲须等同用，如金锁固精丸。

2. 用于脾虚食少，久泻。多与人参、白术、茯苓、山药等同用，如参苓白术散。

3. 用于虚烦、心悸、失眠。可配酸枣仁、麦门冬、远志等同用。

此外，还可用于妇女崩漏、白带过多等证。

【用法用量】 水煎服，6～15克。

【说明】 莲花中的雄蕊亦作药用，名莲须。味甘、涩，性平。功能固肾涩精。主治遗精，滑精，带下，尿频等。

金樱子

为蔷薇科植物金樱子的成熟果实。主产于广东、四川、云南、贵州等地。9～11月果实成熟时采收，去核，晒干。生用。

used.

Medicinal Properties Sour and astringent in flavor, mild in nature, and attributive to the kidney, bladder and large intestine meridians.

【药性】 味酸、涩，性平。归肾、膀胱、大肠经。

Actions Relieve nocturnal emission and reduce the frequency of urination, astringe the intestine to relieve diarrhea.

【功效】 固精缩尿，涩肠止泻。

Application

【临床应用】

1. For kidney-deficiency manifested as nocturnal emission, sperma torrhoea, enuresis, frequent micturition and excessive leukorrhea, it can be decocted singly into soft extract for oral use, that is, Jinyingzi Gao (Soft extract) or used together with Qianshi (*Semen Euryales*), such as Shuilu Erxian Dan (Bolus).

1. 用于肾虚精气不固的遗精滑精，遗尿尿频，白带过多。单用熬膏服有效，如金樱子膏；亦可与芡实为丸服，如水陆二仙丹。

2. For chronic diarrhea and lingering dysentery, it can be decocted alone or used together with such Chinese medicinal herbs for benefiting qi and tonifying the spleen as Dangshen (*Radix Codonopsis*), Baizhu (*Rhizoma Atractylodis Macrocephalae*), and Shanyao (*Rhizoma Dioscoreae*).

2. 用于久泻久痢。可单味煎服，也可配益气健脾药党参、白术、山药等同用。

In addition, it can also be applied for prolapse of the rectum, uterine prolapse, and metrorrhagia and metrostaxis because of its astringing property.

此外，还可用于脱肛、子宫下垂、崩漏等证，皆取其收涩作用。

Usage and Dosage 6 -12 g is used in decoction for oral use. It can also be made into pills or soft extract for oral use.

【用法用量】 水煎服，6～12克。或熬膏、为丸服。

Notes It is not suitable for those with sthenic fire and/or sthenic pathogenic factors.

【使用注意】 有实火、实邪者不宜用。

Haipiaoxiao　*Os Sepiellae seu Sepiae*

海螵蛸

The source is from the internal shell of the mollusc *sepiella maindroni* de Rochebrune., or *Sepia esculenta* Hoyle, family Sepidae. The medicinal material is mainly produced in such coastal provinces as Liaoning, Jiangsu, and Zhejiang and collected from April to August. The in-

为乌贼科动物无针乌贼或金乌贼等多种乌贼的贝壳。主产于辽宁、江苏、浙江等沿海地区。4～8月捕捞，取其内壳洗净，日晒夜露至无腥味，

ternal shell is taken out, cleaned, dried in the open air until the smell of seafood disappears. The crude is used.

生用。

Medicinal Properties Salty and astringent in flavor, slightly warm in nature, and attributive to the liver and kidney meridians.

【药性】 味咸、涩,性微温。归肝、肾经。

Actions Astringe to stop bleeding, stop emission and leukorrhea, control acid regurgitation to arrest pain, eliminate dampness and promote sore healing.

【功效】 收敛止血,固精止带,制酸止痛,收湿敛疮。

Application

【临床应用】

1. It is used for metrorrhagia and metrostaxis and bleeding from the lung or stomach, and that due to trauma. In treating metrorrhagia and metrostaxis, it is often used in combination with Qiancaogen (*Radix Rubiae*), Zonglütan (*Petioulus Trachycarpi Carbonisatus*), and Wubeizi (*Galla Chinensis*), etc., such as Guchong Tang (Decoction). In treating bleeding from the lung or stomach, the powder is used together with same amount of the powder of Baiji (*Rhizoma Bletillae*), that is, Wu Ji San (Powder). In treating traumatic bleeding, the powder can be applied to the local area.

1. 用于崩漏下血,肺、胃出血及外伤出血。治妇女崩漏下血,多配茜草根、棕榈炭、五倍子等同用,如固冲汤;治肺胃出血,可与白及等分为末服,即乌(海螵蛸)及散;单用研末外敷,可止外伤出血。

2. It is used for emission and leukorrhea. In treating emission, it is used together with such Chinese medicinal herbs for benefiting the kidney to stop nocturnal emission as Shanzhuyu (*Fructus Corni*), Tusizi (*Semen Cuscutae*), and Shayuanzi (*Semen Astragali Complanati*). In treating abnormal leukorrhea with bloody discharge, it can be used in combination with Baizhi (*Radix Angelicae Dahuricae*) and Xueyutan (*Crinis Carbonisatus*), such as Baizhi San (Powder).

2. 用于遗精,带下。治遗精,配山茱萸、菟丝子、沙苑子等益肾固精药同用;治妇女赤白带下,可配白芷、血余炭同用,如白芷散。

3. For stomachache with acid regurgitation, it can be used together with Beimu (*Bulbus Fritillariae*), such as Wu Bei San (Powder).

3. 用于胃痛泛酸。多与贝母同用,即乌(海螵蛸)贝散。

4. It is used for skin pyogenic infection, eczema, ulcer with profuse pus. In treating skin pyogenic infection

4. 用于湿疮、湿疹及溃疡多脓。治湿疮、湿疹,多与黄

and eczema, it is used together with Huangbai (*Cortex Phellodendri*) and Qingdai (*Indigo Naturalis*), which can be ground into powder and applied to the local area. In treating ulcer with profuse pus, it can be ground into powder and applied to the local area, or used together with Duanshigao (*Gypsum Fibrosum Usta*) and Duanlonggu (*Os Draconis Usta*), Baizhi (*Radix Angelicae Dahuricae*), and Bingpian (*Borneolum*), etc. which are ground into fine powder for applying to the wound areas.

柏、青黛研末外敷；治疮疡多脓，可单用研末外敷，也可配煅石膏、煅龙骨、白芷、冰片等，共研细末，撒敷患处。

Usage and Dosage　6 -12 g is used in decoction for oral use and 1. 5 -3 g in powder. Just right amount is used for external use.

【用法用量】　水煎服，6～12克；研末服，1. 5～3 克。外用，适量。

Notes　It is not suitable for those with heat of yin-deficiency type.

【使用注意】　阴虚有热者不宜服。

16 Chinese Medicinal Herbs for External Application

第十六章 外用药

Most of the kind of Chinese medicinal herbs are for external use. They respectively have such actions as removing toxin, subduing swelling, draining the pus, and promoting tissue regeneration. Therefore, they can be used respectively to treat various carbuncle, furuncle, scabies, trauma, snake or insect bite and diseases of five sensory organs.

本类药物大多以外用为主，分别具有解毒消肿、化腐排脓、生肌敛疮等功效，适用于痈疽疮疖、疥癣、外伤、蛇虫咬伤以及五官科疾患。

Liuhuang *Sulphur*

硫 黄

The source is from the refined product of the natural ore Sulphur. The medicinal material is mainly produced in Shanxi, Shandong and Henan provinces. For oral use, the clean sulfur is boiled with bean curd until the bean curd shows a blackish-green color, then remove the bean curd and dry it in the shade. It is used in powder form.

为天然硫黄矿的提炼加工品。主产于山西、山东、河南等省。供内服的硫黄须与豆腐同煮至豆腐呈墨绿色为度，然后除去豆腐，阴干。研末用。

Medicinal Properties Sour in flavor, warm in nature, toxic and attributive to the kidney and large intestine meridians.

【药性】 味酸，性温。有毒。归肾、大肠经。

Actions Clear away toxic materials, kill parasites when externally used; strengthen yang to relax bowel when used orally.

【功效】 外用解毒杀虫；内服壮阳通便。

Application

【临床应用】

1. It can be used to treat scabies, eczema and alleviate itching. In treating scabies, mixed with sesame oil, its powder can be applied alone to the local area, or its extract is used externally. Together with Qiandan (*Plumbum Preparatium*), it is pounded into powder for all tineas of dry or damp type. In treating pruritus vulvae

1. 用于疥癣，湿疹，皮肤瘙痒。治疥疮，可单用研末，麻油调涂，也可以制成膏剂外用；用硫黄配铅丹等研末调涂，能治一切干湿癣证；配蛇床子、明矾煎水洗，又可治阴

caused by dampness, it can be used together with Shechuangzi (*Fructus Cnidii*) and Mingfan (*Alumen*), which are decocted for washing.

部湿痒。

2. It is used for syndromes caused by insufficiency of kidney-yang and deficiency and cold of the lower energizer. For cold dyspnea due to kidney-deficienty failing to receive qi, it is often used together with Fuzi (*Radix Aconiti Lateralis Praeparata*), and Rougui (*Cortex Cinnamomi*), such as Heixi Dan (Pill). It is often used in combination with Lurong (*Cornu Cervi Pantotrichum*), Buguzhi (*Fructus Psoraleae*) for impotence, frequent micturition, and pain of the loin and knees, etc..

2. 用于肾阳不足,下焦虚冷诸证。治肾虚不能纳气的寒喘,多与附子、肉桂配伍,如黑锡丹;治阳痿,小便频数、腰膝冷痛,常与鹿茸、补骨脂等同用。

3. It is often used together with Banxia (*Rhizoma Pinelliae*), such as in Banliu Wan (Pill), to treat the elder's constipation due to deficiency and cold.

3. 用于老人虚寒便秘。多与半夏同用,如半硫丸。

Usage and Dosage For external application, its powder can be applied to the local area or mixed with oil, and the amount should be proper. For oral administration, 1-3 g is taken after made into pills or powder.

【用法用量】 外用,适量,研末撒,或油调涂。内服,入丸、散,1～3 克。

Notes It is contraindicated in those with deficiency of yin and hyperactivity of fire, or pregnant women.

【使用注意】 阴虚火旺者及孕妇忌服。

Shengyao *Hydrargyri Oxydum*

升 药

The source is from the compound prepared from equal amount of mercury, nitre and alum through sublimation. The medicine may be red or yellow in color, the red one is called Hongsheng; the yellow one Huangsheng. It is mainly produced in Hebei, Hunan, and Jiangsu provinces. It is ground into powder for medicinal use and more effective if stored over a long time.

为粗制氧化汞,由水银、火硝、明矾各等分混合升华而成。红色者称红升,黄色者称黄升。主产于河北、湖南、江苏等地。研细末入药,陈久者良。

Medicinal Properties Pungent in flavor and hot in nature, toxic and attributive to the lung and spleen meridians.

【药性】 味辛、热。有大毒。归肺、脾经。

Actions Remove toxin and necrotic tissue to regenerate tissues.

【功效】 搜脓拔毒,化腐生肌。

Application

In treating ulceration from carbuncle or phlegmon failing to evacuate pus smoothly and necrotic tissue, it is often used in combination with Duanshigao (*Gypsum Fibrosum Usta*), which is ground into powder for external use. The ratio of Duanshigao (*Gypsum Fibrosum Usta*) and Hongsheng is 9 : 1, which is called Jiuyi Dan (Pill) with weak action of removing toxin. When the ratio of the two is 1 : 1, the composition is called Wuwu Dan (Pill) with strong action of removing toxin. When the ratio is 1 : 9, the composition is called Jiuzhuan Dan (Pill), its action of removing toxin being strongest. These can be selected according to disease conditions. They can be applied to the local area, or stuck to a paper spill and inserted into the vomica.

【临床应用】

用于痈疽破溃后，流脓不畅，或腐肉不去，新肉难生。临床多配伍煅石膏研细末外用。煅石膏与红升的比例为9∶1者称九一丹，拔毒力较轻；1∶1者称五五丹，拔毒力较强；1∶9者称九转丹，拔毒力更强。根据病情需要选用，掺于患处，也可将药粘附于纸捻上插入脓腔中。

Usage and Dosage Proper amount is for external use. It is usually used in combination with other Chinese herbs and is not used singly.

【用法用量】 外用，适量，多配伍使用，不用纯品。

Notes It has strong toxicity, is only for external use but not for oral use. It is not suitable for pyocutaneous dosease without necrotic tissues or pus.

【使用注意】 本品毒性强，只可外用，不可内服。疮疡腐肉已去或脓水已净者，不宜用。

Luganshi *Calamina*

炉甘石

The source is from smithsonite of carbonate of calcite group, mainly containing zinc carbonate. The medicine is mainly produced in Guangxi, Hunan, and Sichuan. Impurity is removed from the material after being collected. It is calcined, or quenched with vinegar or with Sanhuang Tang (Decoction), containing Huanglian (*Rhizoma Coptidis*), Huangbai (*Cortex Phellodendri*) and Dahuang (*Radix et Rhizoma Rhei*)) and then dried in the sun and ground into fine powder with water for use.

为碳酸类矿物方解石族菱锌矿，主要成分为碳酸锌。主产于广西、湖南、四川等地。采后除杂石，火煅、醋淬及三黄汤（黄连、黄柏、大黄）淬制后，晒干研末，水飞后用。

Medicinal Properties Sweet in flavor, mild in nature, and attributive to the liver and stomach meridians.

【药性】 味甘，平。归肝、胃经。

Actions Remove nebula to improve eyesight, eliminate dampness and promote tissue regeneration.

【功效】 明目去翳,收湿生肌。

Application

【临床应用】

1. It can be used to treat eye diseases. For conjunctivitis, equal amount of the Chinese medicinal herbs such as Fenghuaxiao (*Natrii Sulfas*, weathering) and Mangxiao (*Natrii Sulfas*) can be elutriated and used as eye drops. For nebula, it is used in combination with Mangxiao (*Natrii Sulfas*) to wash the local area, and also with Haipiaoxiao (*Os Sepiellae seu Sepiae*) and Pengsha (*Borax*) as eye drops.

1. 用于目疾。治目暴赤肿,以之与风化硝(芒硝)等分,化水点眼;治目生翳膜,配芒硝等,外洗,还可以配海螵蛸、硼砂研末,点眼。

2. For ulceration that does not heal and purulent skin lesion, together with Hai'ercha (*Catechu*) it is ground into powder after mixed with sesame oil and applied to the local area. For yin ulcer and damp itching due to yin perspiration, it is alone ground into powder and applied to the local area.

2. 用于溃疡不敛,皮肤湿疮。多配伍孩儿茶,研末麻油调敷;治阴疮和阴汗湿痒,多单味研末调敷。

Usage and Dosage Proper amount is used for external application. It can be elutriated and used as an eye drops. The powder can be applied externally or mixed with water for application.

【用法用量】 外用,适量,水飞点眼,研末撒或调敷。

Mingfan *Alumen*

明 矾

The source is from the refined product of the mineral Alunite of sulphate, mainly containing potassium aluminium sulfate. The medicinal material is mainly produced in Hubei, Anhui, Zhejiang, and Fujian provinces. The crude or calcined one (the latter called kufan in Chinese) is used for medication.

为硫酸盐类矿物明矾石的提炼品。主要成分含水硫酸铝钾。主产于湖北、安徽、浙江、福建等地。生用或煅用,煅用名枯矾。

Medicinal Properties Sour in flavor, cold in nature and attributive to the lung, liver, spleen, stomach and large intestine meridians.

【药性】 味酸,性寒。归肺、肝、脾、胃、大肠经。

Actions Remove toxin and kill parasites, eliminate dampness and relieve itching, stop bleeding and diarrhea, clear away heat and eliminate phlegm.

【功效】 解毒杀虫,燥湿止痒,止血止泻,清热消痰。

Application

1. For pyocutaneous disease, scabies and tinea, eczema with itching. In treating malignant sore, equal amount of Mingfan (*Alumen*) and Huangdan (*Minium*) can be ground into powder for application, such as Erxian San (Powder). In treating pustulosis bullous, equal amount of the calcined one, Shusongxiang (*Colophonium Praeparata*) and Huangdan (*Minium*) is ground into powder that is mixed with sesame oil and applied to the local area. In treating scabies and tinea, and eczema with itching, it is often used together with Liuhuang (*Sulphur*) and Xionghuang (*Realgar*). When taken orally, it is effective in subduing swelling and removing toxin. The drug together with Huangla (yellow wax) is taken orally with liquor to treat all syndroms of carbuncle, phlegmon, and malignant boil, such as La Fan Wan (Pill).

2. For haematemesis and bleeding due to trauma, epistaxis, prolonged diarrhea. In treating haematemesis and epistaxis, it is ground together with Hai'ercha (*Catuchu*) into powder for external or oral use. In treating the old man's prolonged diarrhea, the calcined one with Weihezi (*Fructus Chebulae*, roasted) is ground into powder for oral use.

3. It is used for epilepsy. In treating epilepsy due to wind and phlegm, it is used in combination with Xicha (Fine tea), such as Huatan Wan (Pill). In treating accumulation of phlegm-heat in the interior manifested as insanity, it is prepared with Yujin (*Radix Curcumae*) into pill for oral use, such as in Baijin Wan (Pill).

Usage and Dosage For external application, its powder can be applied to the local area or mixed with water for application. The amount should be proper. 0.6 – 1.5 g is used in pills or powder for oral administration.

Notes It is contraindicated in those with debility

【临床应用】

1. 用于疮疡疥癣，湿疹瘙痒。治恶疮，以白矾、黄丹各等分研末外敷，如二仙散；治黄水疮，以枯矾、熟松香、黄丹等分研末，麻油调涂患处。治疥癣，湿疮瘙痒，常配伍硫黄、雄黄等。本品内服，亦有消疮解毒之效，可治一切痈肿恶疮，如蜡矾丸，由白矾、黄蜡组成，酒送服。

2. 用于吐衄下血，泻痢不止。治吐衄下血及外伤出血，以之配孩儿茶，研末内服或外用；治老人久泻不止，以枯矾配煨诃子，研末内服。

3. 用于癫痫发狂。治风痰癫痫，配白矾、细茶，如化痰丸；治痰热内郁，发为癫狂，以白矾、郁金两药为丸服，如白金丸。

【用法用量】 外用，适量，研末撒或调敷。内服，入丸散，0.6～1.5 克。

【使用注意】 体虚胃弱

of the stomach or those without damp-heat and phlegm-fire.

及无湿热痰火者忌服。

Pengsha *Borax*

硼砂

The source is from the crystals prepared from the ore *Borax*. The medicinal material is mainly produced in the areas of Tibet and Qinghai of China. The crude or calcined one is used for medication.

为硼砂矿石提炼出的结晶体。主产于西藏、青海等地。生用或火煅用。

Medicinal Properties Sweet and salty in flavor, cool in nature, and attributive to the lung and stomach meridians.

【药性】 味甘、咸，性凉。归肺、胃经。

Actions Clear away heat and toxin (external use); clear away lung heat and eliminate phlegm (oral use).

【功效】 外用清热解毒；内服清肺化痰。

Application

【临床应用】

1. It is used for aphthae, sore throat, conjunctivitis and nebula. In treating thrush, it is used together with Xionghuang (*Realgar*), Bingpian (*Borneolum*) and Gancao (*Radix Glycyrrhizae*), such as Sibao Dan (Bolus). In treating sore throat, it is often used in combination with Bingpian (*Borneolum*), Xuanmingfen (*Natrii Sulfas Exsiccatus*), Zhusha (*Cinnabar*), such as Bing Peng San (Powder). In treating conjunctivitis and nebula, it is prepared to be a water solution as eyewash, or used together with Luganshi (*Calamina*), Bingpian (*Borneolum*), and Xuanmingfen (*Natrii Sulfas Exsiccatus*), such as Bailong Dan (Bolus).

1. 用于口舌生疮，咽喉肿痛，目赤翳障。治鹅口疮，配硼砂、雄黄、冰片、甘草，蜜水调涂或干掺，即四宝丹；治咽喉肿痛，以之配冰片、玄明粉、朱砂，如冰硼散；治目赤肿痛或生翳膜，可用本品水溶液洗眼，也可与炉甘石、冰片、玄明粉等配用，如白龙丹。

2. For cough due to phlegm-heat with yellow, sticky and thick sputum that is not easy to expectorate out, it is often used in combination with Sangbaipi (*Cortex Mori Radicis*), Beimu (*Bulbus Fritillariae*), and Gualou (*Fructus Trichosanthis*), etc..

2. 用于痰热咳嗽，痰黄黏稠，咯吐不利。多配桑白皮、贝母、瓜蒌等同用。

Usage and Dosage For external use, the fine powder can be applied to the local area or used with water. The amount should be proper. 0.6-1.5 g is taken as a dose in pill or powder for oral use.

【用法用量】 外用，适量，研细末撒或调敷。内服，入丸、散，0.6～1.5 克。

Notes It is usually used externally but should be taken with caution for oral use.

【使用注意】多作外用，内服宜慎。

Fengfang *Nidus Vespae*

蜂房

The source is from the honeycomb of *Polistes olivaceous* Degeer, *Polistes japonicus* Saussure or *Parapolybia varia* Fabricius, family Vespidae. The medicinal material is produced all over China, and the yield of it in the South is much larger. The honeycomb can be collected at any time; dried in the sun, or steamed briefly, dead pupae and wapes being removed, it is cut into small pieces. The crude or stir-baked one is used.

为胡蜂科昆虫果马蜂、日本长脚胡蜂或异腹胡蜂的巢。中国各地均有，南方地区尤多。随时可采。晒干或略蒸过，取出死蛹、死蜂，剪成小块。生用或炒用。

Medicinal Properties Sweet in flavor, mild in nature, toxic and attributive to the stomach meridian.

【药性】味甘，性平。有毒。归胃经。

Actions Remove toxin, destroy parasites and dispel wind.

【功效】攻毒，杀虫，祛风。

Application

【临床应用】

1. It can be used for carbuncle, scrofula, toothache and tinea. In treating acute mastitis at the early stage, it can be alone baked till it turns brown and ground into powder for oral use. In treating ulcerate carbuncle, the decoction is used to wash the local area. In treating scrofula with pus, it is made together with Xuanshen (*Radix Scrophulariae*) and Huangqi (*Radix Astragali*) into soft extract for external application, such as Fengfang Gao (Soft extract). In treating toothache due to wind and parasites, its decoction can be used to rinse the mouth. In treating head tinea, it can be used externally together with Wugong (*Scolopendra*) and Mingfan (*Alumen*).

1. 用于痈疽、瘰疬、牙痛、癣疮。治乳痈初起，可单用本品焙黄研末服；痈疽溃烂，可用水煎液冲洗；瘰疬脓水不干，配伍玄参、黄芪等熬膏外贴，即蜂房膏；治风虫牙痛，可煎水漱牙；治头癣，以之配蜈蚣、明矾外用。

2. For itching caused by urticaria, it is used together with Chantui (*Periostracum Cicadae*).

2. 用于瘾疹瘙痒。可配蝉蜕内服。

In addition, it is often used in combination with Quanxie (*Scorpio*), Baijiangcan (*Bombyx Batryticatus*), and Shancigu (*Bulbus Talipae*) to treat various cancers.

此外，还可用于多种癌肿，常与全蝎、白僵蚕、山慈姑等药同用。

Usage and Dosage For external application, its powder or decoction can be applied to or used to wash the local area. For oral administration, 3 -5 g is used in decoction, or 1.5 -3 g in powder.

【用法用量】 外用，适量，研末调敷或煎水冲洗。水煎内服，3～5 克；研末服，1～1.5 克。

Notes It is not suitable for those with deficiency of qi and blood.

【使用注意】 气血虚弱者不宜服。

Maqianzi *Semen Strychni*

马钱子

The source is from the dried ripe seed of *Strychnos nuxvomica* L. or *Strychnos pierriana* A. W. Hill, family Loganiaceae. The medicinal material is mainly prouded in India, Vietnam, Thailand, and the *Strychnos pierriana* A. W. is mainly produced in Yunnan and Guangdong provinces of China. It is collected in summer and autumn, the pulp being removed and the seed being taken out and then dried in the sun. It is processed before being used.

为马钱科植物马钱或云南马钱的成熟种子。马钱主产于印度、越南、泰国；云南马钱主产于云南、广东等地。夏、秋季摘取成熟果实，去除果肉，取出种子，晒干。经炮制后入药。

Medicinal Properties Bitter in flavor, cold in nature, toxic and attributive to the liver and spleen meridians.

【药性】 味苦，性寒。有毒。归肝、脾经。

Actions Remove obstruction in the channels, relieve pain and subdue swelling.

【功效】 通络散结，消肿定痛。

Application

【临床应用】

1. It can be used in combination with Baijiangcan (*Bombyx Batryticatus*) to treat carbuncle or fracture with stasis of the blood, swelling and pain, such as Qinglong Wan (Pill). For laryngalgia, it is used in combination with equal amount of Shandougen (*Radix Sophorae Subprostratae*) and Qingmuxiang (*Radix Aristolochiae*), which is ground into powder and insufflated into the local area.

1. 用于痈疽或跌打损伤肿痛。可配白僵蚕等，如青龙丸；也治喉痹作痛，以之配山豆根、青木香等分研末吹喉。

2. In treating Bi-syndrome with pain of wind and dampness type or spasm and numbness, it can be used in combination with Mahuang (*Herba Ephedrae*), Ruxiang (*Olibanum*), Moyao (*Myrrhae*), etc..

2. 用于风湿痹痛或拘挛麻木。配麻黄、乳香、没药等同用。

Usage and Dosage For external use, proper

【用法用量】 外用，适

amount is ground into powder, which is insufflated into the local area or applied to the local area with water. 0.3-0.6 g is processed into pill or powder for oral use.

量,研末吹喉或调涂。内服,炮制入丸散服,0.3～0.6克。

Notes It is toxic and therefore it should not be taken over a long time and the dosage should be strictly controlled. It is contraindicated in pregnant women. Overdosage may lead to such symptoms as tremor of the limbs, infantile convulsion, dyspnea and even coma.

【使用注意】 本品有毒,不可久服多服;孕妇忌用。服用过量,可引起肢体颤动,惊厥,呼吸困难,甚至昏迷等中毒症状。

Shechuangzi *Fructus Cnidii*

蛇床子

The source is from the dried ripe fruit of *Cnidium onnierii* (L.) cusson, family Umbelliferae. The medicinal material is produced all over China, collected in summer and autumn when the fruit is ripe, the stems of the plant being cut down, dried in the sun, threshed to get the fruits and then sieved. The crude is used for medication.

为伞形科植物蛇床的成熟果实。中国各地均产。夏、秋季果实成熟时,割取全株,晒干,打下果实,筛净。生用。

Medicinal Properties Pungent and bitter in flavor, mild in nature, slightly toxic and attributive to the kidney meridian.

【药性】 味辛、苦,性温。有小毒。归肾经。

Actions Eliminate dampness and destroy parasites, warm the kidney and strengthen yang.

【功效】 燥湿杀虫,温肾壮阳。

Application

【临床应用】

1. It can be used for pudendum itching caused by dampness, eczema, exudative ulcer and tinea. In treating pudendum itching, eczema of scrotum, it is alone decocted to wash the local area, or together with Mingfan (*Alumen*), Kushen (*Radix Sophorae Flavescentis*), and Huangbai (*Cortex Phellodendri*). In treating tinea, it can be ground into powder and applied to the local area with oil.

1. 用于阴部湿痒,湿疹,湿疮,疥癣。治妇女阴痒,男子阴囊湿疹,可单用本品煎汤外洗,也可配明矾、苦参、黄柏同用;治疥癣,可研末用油脂调敷。

2. For leukorrhea of cold-damp type, lumbago caused by damp-Bi-syndrome. In treating leukorrhea of cold-damp type, it can be used in combination with Shanzhuyu (*Fructus Corni*), Cheqianzi (*Semen Plantaginis*), and Xiangfu (*Rhizoma Cyperi*), etc.. In trea-

2. 用于寒湿带下,湿痹腰痛。治寒湿带下,配山茱萸、车前子、香附等同用;治湿痹腰痛,配桑寄生、杜仲、秦艽等同用。

ting lumbago caused by damp-Bi-syndrome, it is used in combination with Sangjisheng (*Ramulus Taxilli*), Duzhong (*Cortex Eucommiae*), and Qinjiao (*Radix Gentianae Macrophyllae*), etc..

3. For deficiency of kidney-yang, deficiency-cold of the lower energizer manifested as impotence and sterility, it can be used together with Wuweizi (*Fructus Schisandrae*) and Tusizi (*Semen Cuscutae*), which are ground together into powder and made into pill with honey for oral use.

3. 用于肾阳虚衰、下焦寒湿诸证。如治男子阳痿,女子不孕,可配五味子、菟丝子,研末作蜜丸服。

Usage and Dosage For oral use, 3 -10 g is used in decoction, or in pill or powder. For external use, it is decocted to wash the local area, or ground into powder and applied to the local area. The amount should be proper.

【用法用量】 水煎服,3～10克,或入丸、散。外用,适量,水煎洗或研末敷。

Notes It is not suitable for those with hyperactivity of fire due to yin deficiency or those with dampness and heat in the lower energizer.

【使用注意】 阴虚火旺或下焦有湿热者不宜内服。

Index : Herbs by Latin Names

附录：拉丁名索引

A

Agkistrodon Acutus	Qishe	蕲蛇	145
Aloe	Luhui	芦荟	129
Alumen	Mingfan	明矾	362

B

Bombyx Batryticatus	Baijiangcan	白僵蚕	282
Borax	Pengsha	硼砂	364
Borneolum Syntheticum	Bingpian	冰片	286
Bulus Allii Macrostemi	Xiebai	薤白	185
Bulus Fritillariae	Beimu	贝母	246

C

Cacumen Biotae	Cebaiye	侧柏叶	203
Calamina	Luganshi	炉甘石	361
Calculus Bovis	Niuhuang	牛黄	271
Calyx Kaki	Shidi	柿蒂	192
Carapax et Plastrum Testudinis	Guiban	龟版	340
Carapax Trionycis	Biejia	鳖甲	342
Caulis Akebiae	Mutong	木通	161
Caulis Sargentodoxae	Hongteng	红藤	114
Caulis Spatholobi	Jixieteng	鸡血藤	231
Cinnabaris	Zhusha	朱砂	258
Colla Corii Asini	Ejiao	阿胶	327
Concha Haliotidis	Shijueming	石决明	269
Concha Ostreae	Muli	牡蛎	270
Cordyceps	Dongchongxiacao	冬虫夏草	315
Cornu Bubali	Shuiniujiao	水牛角	100

Cornu Cervi Pantotrichum	Lurong	鹿茸	307
Cornu Saigae Tataricae	Lingyangjiao	羚羊角	274
Cortex Acanthopanacis Radicis	Wujiapi	五加皮	147
Cortex Albiziae	Hehuanpi	合欢皮	266
Cortex Cinnamomi	Rougui	肉桂	171
Cortex Eucommiae	Duzhong	杜仲	316
Cortex Lycii Radicis	Digupi	地骨皮	118
Cortex Magnoliae Officinalis	Houpo	厚朴	153
Cortex Moutan Radicis	Mudanpi	牡丹皮	97
Cortex Phellodendri	Huangbai	黄柏	88
	E		
Endothelium Corneum Gigeriae Galli	Jineijin	鸡内金	197
	F		
Flos Carthami	Honghua	红花	227
Flos Caryophylli	Dingxiang	丁香	190
Flos Chrysanthemi	Juhua	菊花	58
Flos Genkwa	Yuanhua	芫花	135
Flos Inulae	Xuanfuhua	旋覆花	252
Flos Lonicerae	Jinyinhua	金银花	101
Flos Magnoliae	Xinyi	辛夷	56
Flos Sophorae	Huaihua	槐花	203
Folium Artemisiae Argyi	Aiye	艾叶	211
Folium Eriobotryae	Pipaye	枇杷叶	254
Folium Mori	Sangye	桑叶	62
Folium Sennae	Fanxieye	番泻叶	130
Folium Perillae	Zisuye	紫苏叶	45
Fructus Alpiniae Oxyphyllae	Yizhiren	益智仁	311
Fructus Amomi	Sharen	砂仁	154
Fructus Arctii	Niubangzi	牛蒡子	61
Fructus Aurantii Immaturus	Zhishi	枳实	183
Fructus Cnidii	Shechuangzi	蛇床子	367
Fructus Corni	Shanzhuyu	山茱萸	353
Fructus Crataegi	Shanzha	山楂	194

Fructus Evodiae	Wuzhuyu	吴茱萸	174
Fructus Foeniculi	Xiaohuixiang	小茴香	175
Fructus Forsythiae	Lianqiao	连翘	103
Fructus Gardeniae	Zhizi	栀子	75
Fructus Hordei Germinatus	Maiya	麦芽	196
Fructus Kochiae	Difuzi	地肤子	163
Fructus Ligustri Lucidi	Nüzhenzi	女贞子	339
Fructus Lycii	Gouqizi	枸杞子	337
Fructus Meliae Toosendan	Chuanlianzi	川楝子	189
Fructus Mume	Wumei	乌梅	349
Fructus Perillae	Zisuzi	紫苏子	250
Fructus Psoraleae	Buguzhi	补骨脂	313
Fructus Rosae Laevigatae	Jinyingzi	金樱子	355
Fructus Schisandrae	Wuweizi	五味子	347
Fructus Trichosanthis	Gualou	瓜蒌	244
Fructus Tritici Levis	Fuxiaomai	浮小麦	346
Fructus Xanthii	Cang'erzi	苍耳子	55

G

Gypsum Fibrosum	Shigao	石膏	72

H

Haematitum	Daizheshi	代赭石	273
Halloysitum Rubrum	Chishizhi	赤石脂	351
Herba Agastaches	Huoxiang	藿香	149
Herba Agrimoniae	Xianhecao	仙鹤草	207
Herba Andrographitis	Chuanxinlian	穿心莲	108
Herba Artemisiae Annuae	Qinghao	青蒿	117
Herba Artemisiae Scopariae	Yinchenhao	茵陈蒿	166
Herba Asari	Xixin	细辛	53
Herba Cephalanoploris	Xiaoji	小蓟	201
Herba Cistanches	Roucongrong	肉苁蓉	310
Herba Dendrobii	Shihu	石斛	336
Herba Ecliptae	Hanliancao	旱莲草	338
Herba Ephedrae	Mahuang	麻黄	42

Herba Elsholtziae	Xiangru	香薷	47
Herba Epimedii	Yinyanghuo	淫羊藿	309
Herba Eupatorii	Peilan	佩兰	151
Herba Lobeliae Chinensis	Banbianlian	半边莲	109
Herba Leonuri	Yimucao	益母草	228
Herba Lophatheri	Danzhuye	淡竹叶	80
Herba Lysimachiae	Jinqiancao	金钱草	165
Herba Houttuyniae	Yuxingcao	鱼腥草	112
Herba Menthae	Bohe	薄荷	57
Herba Patriniae	Baijiangcao	败酱草	115
Herba Schizonepetae	Jingjie	荆芥	48
Herba Violae	Zihuadiding	紫花地丁	104
Hirudo	Shuizhi	水蛭	234
Hydragyri Oxydum	Shengyao	升药	360
	I		
Indigo Naturalis	Qingdai	青黛	106
	L		
Lignum Aquilariae Resinatum	Chenxiang	沉香	191
Lumbricus	Dilong	地龙	280
	M		
Magnetitum	Cishi	磁石	259
Massa Medicata Fermentata	Shenqu	神曲	196
Mel	Fengmi	蜂蜜	305
Moschus	Shexiang	麝香	285
Myrrha	Moyao	没药	224
	N		
Natrii Sulfas	Mangxiao	芒硝	127
Nidus Vespae	Fengfang	蜂房	365
	O		
Olibanum	Ruxiang	乳香	223

Os Draconis	Longgu	龙骨	260
Os Sepiellae seu Sepiae	Haipiaoxiao	海螵蛸	356

P

Pericarpium Citri Reticulatae Viride	Qingpi	青皮	180
Pericarpium Citri Tangerinae	Jupi	橘皮	179
Pericarpium Zanthoxyli	Huajiao	花椒	176
Periostracum Cicadae	Chantui	蝉蜕	60
Pollen Typhae	Puhuang	蒲黄	210
Polyporus	Zhuling	猪苓	157
Poria	Fuling	茯苓	156

R

Radix Achyranthis Bidenatatae	Niuxi	牛膝	229
Radix Aconiti	Chuanwu	川乌	142
Radix Aconiti Lateralis Praeparata	Fuzi	附子	169
Radix Angelicae Pubescentis	Duhuo	独活	139
Radix Angelicae Sinensis	Danggui	当归	319
Radix Asparagi	Tianmendong	天门冬	332
Radix Astragali	Huangqi	黄芪	296
Radix Aucklandiae	Muxiang	木香	182
Radix Bupleuri	Chaihu	柴胡	63
Radix Cirsii Japonici	Daji	大蓟	200
Radix Clematidis	Weilingxian	威灵仙	141
Radix Codonopsis	Dangshen	党参	293
Radix Curcumae	Yujin	郁金	220
Radix Cynanchi Atrati	Baiwei	白薇	119
Radix Ephedrae	Mahuanggen	麻黄根	345
Radix Euphorbiae Kansui	Gansui	甘遂	133
Radix Euphorbiae Pekinensis	Daji	大戟	134
Radix Gentianae	Longdan	龙胆	90
Radix Gentianae Macrophyllae	Qinjiao	秦艽	144
Radix Ginseng	Renshen	人参	290
Radix Glehniae	Beishashen	北沙参	329
Radix Glycyrrhizae	Gancao	甘草	303

Radix Isatidis	Banlangen	板蓝根	105
Radix Linderae	Wuyao	乌药	186
Radix Morindae Officinalis	Bajitian	巴戟天	308
Radix Notoginseng	Sanqi	三七	208
Radix Ophiopogonis	Maimendong	麦门冬	331
Radix Paeoniae Rubra	Chishaoyao	赤芍药	98
Radix Panacis Quinquefolii	Xiyangshen	西洋参	295
Radix Peucedani	Qianhu	前胡	243
Radix Platycodi	Jiegeng	桔梗	249
Radix Polygalae	Yuanzhi	远志	265
Radix Polygoni Multiflori	Heshouwu	何首乌	323
Radix Puerariae	Gegen	葛根	65
Radix Pulsatillae	Baitouweng	白头翁	111
Radix Rehmanniae	Shengdihuang	生地黄	93
Radix Rehmanniae Praeparata	Shudihuang	熟地黄	322
Radix Rubiae	Qiancaogen	茜草根	209
Radix Salviae Miltiorrhizae	Danshen	丹参	215
Radix Sanguisorbae	Diyu	地榆	201
Radix Saposhnikoviae	Fangfeng	防风	50
Radix Sanguisorbae	Digupi	地骨皮	118
Radix Scrophulariae	Xuanshen	玄参	95
Radix Scutellariae	Huangqin	黄芩	83
Radix Sophorae Flavescentis	Kushen	苦参	91
Radix Stellariae	Yinchaihu	银柴胡	122
Radix Stemonae	Baibu	百部	254
Radix Stephaniae Tetrandrae	Fangji	防己	143
Radix Trichosanthis	Tianhuafen	天花粉	79
Ramulus Cinnamomi	Guizhi	桂枝	43
Ramulus Taxilli	Sangjiseng	桑寄生	146
Ramulus Uncariae cum Uncis	Gouteng	钩藤	275
Rhizoma Acori Graminei	Shichangpu	石菖蒲	287
Rhizoma Alismatis	Zexie	泽泻	158
Rhizoma Anemarrhenae	Zhimu	知母	74
Rhizoma Arisaematis	Tiannanxing	天南星	241
Rhizoma Atractylodis	Cangzhu	苍术	151

Rhizoma Atractylodis Macrocephalae	Baizhu	白术	298
Rhizoma Bletillae	Baiji	白及	205
Rhizoma Chuanxiong	Chuangxiong	川芎	217
Rhizoma Cimicifugae	Shengma	升麻	67
Rhizoma Coptidis	Huanglian	黄连	85
Rhizoma Corydalis	Yanhusuo	延胡索	219
Rhizoma Curcumae	Ezhu	莪术	233
Rhizoma Curcumae Longae	Jianghuang	姜黄	222
Rhizoma Cynanchi Stautonii	Baiqian	白前	243
Rhizoma Cyperi	Xiangfu	香附	181
Rhizoma Dioscoreae	Shanyao	山药	301
Rhizoma Dioscoreae Hypoglaucae	Bixie	萆薢	164
Rhizoma Dryopteris Crassirhizomae	Guanzhong	贯众	110
Rhizoma et Radix Notopterygii	Qianghuo	羌活	52
Rhizoma Fagopyri Cymosi	Jinqiaomai	金荞麦	113
Rhizoma Gastrodiae	Tianma	天麻	276
Rhizoma Imperatae	Baimaogen	白茅根	204
Rhizoma Phragmitis	Lugen	芦根	77
Rhizoma Picrorrhizae	Huhuanglian	胡黄连	120
Rhizoma Pinelliae	Banxia	半夏	238
Rhizam Polygonati	Huangjing	黄精	333
Rhizoma Polygonati Odorati	Yuzhu	玉竹	335
Rhizoma Sparganii	Sanleng	三棱	232
Rhizoma Zingiberis	Ganjiang	干姜	173
Rhizoma Zingiberis Praeparata	Paojiang	炮姜	213

S

Scolopendra	Wugong	蜈蚣	279
Scorpio	Quanxie	全蝎	278
Semen Arecae	Binglang	槟榔	187
Semen Armeniacae Amarum	Xingren	杏仁	248
Semen Biotae	Baiziren	柏子仁	264
Semen Cannabis	Huomaren	火麻仁	131
Semen Cassiae	Juemingzi	决明子	81
Semen Coicis	Yiyiren	薏苡仁	158

Semen Cuscutae	Tusizi	菟丝子	314
Semen Lepidii seu Descurainiae	Tinglizi	葶苈子	251
Semen Myristicae	Roudoukou	肉豆蔻	350
Semen Nelumbinis	Lianzi	莲子	354
Semen Persicae	Taoren	桃仁	225
Semen Pharbitidis	Qianniuzi	牵牛子	136
Semen Plantaginis	Cheqianzi	车前子	160
Semen Pruni	Yuliren	郁李仁	132
Semen Astragali Complanati	Shayuanzi	沙苑子	318
Semen Strychni	Maqianzi	马钱子	366
Semen Ziziphi Spinosae	Suanzaoren	酸枣仁	263
Spica Prunellae	Xiakucao	夏枯草	76
Spora Lygodii	Haijinsha	海金沙	163
Succinum	Hupo	琥珀	261
Sulfur	Liuhuang	硫黄	359

T

Tabanus	Mengchong	虻虫	235

Postscript

The compilation of *A Newly Compiled Practical English-Chinese Library of TCM* was started in 2000 and published in 2002. In order to demonstrate the academic theory and clinical practice of TCM and to meet the requirements of compilation, the compilers and translators have made great efforts to revise and polish the Chinese manuscript and English translation so as to make it systematic, accurate, scientific, standard and easy to understand. Shanghai University of TCM is in charge of the translation. Many scholars and universities have participated in the compilation and translation of the Library, i.e. Professor Shao Xundao from Xi'an Medical University (former Dean of English Department and Training Center of the Health Ministry), Professor Ou Ming from Guangzhou University of TCM (celebrated translator and chief professor), Henan College of TCM, Guangzhou University of TCM, Nanjing University of TCM, Shaanxi College of TCM, Liaoning College of TCM and Shandong University of TCM.

The compilation of this Library is also supported by the State Administrative Bureau and experts from other universities and colleges of TCM. The experts on the Compilation Committee and Approval Committee have directed the compilation and translation. Professor She

后　记

《(英汉对照)新编实用中医文库》(以下简称《文库》)从2000年中文稿的动笔，到2002年全书的付梓，完成了世纪的跨越。为了使本套《文库》尽可能展示传统中医学术理论和临床实践的精华，达到全面、系统、准确、科学、规范、通俗的编写要求，全体编译人员耗费了大量的心血，付出了艰辛的劳动。特别是上海中医药大学承担了英语翻译的主持工作，得到了著名医学英语翻译家、原西安医科大学英语系主任和卫生部外语培训中心主任邵循道教授，著名中医英语翻译家、广州中医药大学欧明首席教授的热心指导，河南中医学院、广州中医药大学、南京中医药大学、陕西中医学院、辽宁中医学院、山东中医药大学等中医院校英语专家的全力参与，确保了本套《文库》具有较高的英译水平。

在《文库》的编撰过程中，我们始终得到国家主管部门领导和各中医院校专家们的关心和帮助。编纂委员会的国内外学者及审定委员会的

Jing, Head of the State Administrative Bureau and Vice-Minister of the Health Ministry, has showed much concern for the Library. Professor Zhu Bangxian, head of the Publishing House of Shanghai University of TCM, Zhou Dunhua, former head of the Publishing House of Shanghai University of TCM, and Pan Zhaoxi, former editor-in-chief of the Publishing House of Shanghai University of TCM, have given full support to the compilation and translation of the Library.

专家对编写工作提出了指导性的意见和建议。尤其是卫生部副部长、国家中医药管理局局长佘靖教授对本书的编写给予了极大的关注,多次垂询编撰过程,并及时进行指导。上海中医药大学出版社社长兼总编辑朱邦贤教授,以及原社长周敦华先生、原总编辑潘朝曦先生及全体编辑对本书的编辑出版工作给予了全面的支持,使《文库》得以顺利面世。在此,一并致以诚挚的谢意。

With the coming of the new century, we have presented this Library to the readers all over the world, sincerely hoping to receive suggestions and criticism from the readers so as to make it perfect in the following revision.

在新世纪之初,我们将这套《文库》奉献给国内外中医界及广大中医爱好者,恳切希望有识之士对《文库》存在的不足之处给予批评、指教,以便在修订时更臻完善。

Zuo Yanfu
Pingju Village, Nanjing
Spring 2002

左言富
于金陵萍聚村
2002年初春

A Newly Compiled Practical English-Chinese Library of Traditional Chinese Medicine

(英汉对照)新编实用中医文库

Basic Theory of Traditional Chinese Medicine	中医基础理论
Diagnostics of Traditional Chinese Medicine	中医诊断学
Science of Chinese Materia Medica	中药学
Science of Prescriptions	方剂学
Internal Medicine of Traditional Chinese Medicine	中医内科学
Surgery of Traditional Chinese Medicine	中医外科学
Gynecology of Traditional Chinese Medicine	中医妇科学
Pediatrics of Traditional Chinese Medicine	中医儿科学
Traumatology and Orthopedics of Traditional Chinese Medicine	中医骨伤科学
Ophthalmology of Traditional Chinese Medicine	中医眼科学
Otorhinolaryngology of Traditional Chinese Medicine	中医耳鼻喉科学
Chinese Acupuncture and Moxibustion	中国针灸
Chinese Tuina (Massage)	中国推拿
Life Cultivation and Rehabilitation of Traditional Chinese Medicine	中医养生康复学